MULTICULTURAL ISSUES IN REHABILITATION AND ALLIED HEALTH

Edited by

Paul Leung
University of North Texas

Carl R. Flowers
Southern Illinois University Carbondale

William B. Talley
University of Maryland-Eastern Shore

Priscilla Sanderson
University of Arizona

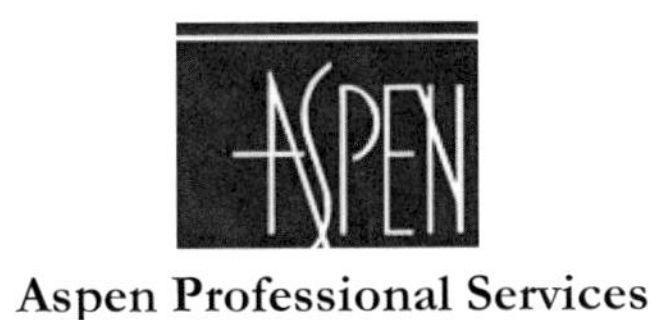

Aspen Professional Services

PUBLISHED BY
Aspen Professional Services
63 Duffers Drive
Linn Creek, MO 65052

Includes bibliographical references and subject index
ISBN 0-9721642-2-7

The cover: Many fabrics represent the range of cultures in the global village we all live in. It is the hand of understanding we all lend; to help heal the global issues we face everyday.

Cover design by: Vincent E. Gardner

Production Editor: Jason D. Andrew, Ph.D., CRC/R, NCC

To secure additional copies, contact:

**Aspen Professional Services
63 Duffers Drive
Linn Creek, MO 65052
jandrew@socket.net
573.317.0907
573.286.0418 (Cellular)**

Acknowledgements

The editors wish to acknowledge the work of the chapter authors. Their contributions have required time and energy that could have been devoted to their own projects, their families and loved ones. All were open to the suggestions from the editors not only in framing their chapters, but also in their presentations. This book would not have been possible without their cooperation.

Special recognition goes to our publisher who has been committed to the project from the beginning and who has spent countless hours behind the scenes.

We want to dedicate this book to those who paved the way and whose lives provided the guidance and inspiration to recognize and include all people regardless of creed, religion, and color.

Table of Contents

Acknowledgements iii

The Editors vi

The Contributors viii

Preface xii

Chapter 1   **Multicultural Rehabilitation: An Historical Perspective** 1
Paul Leung and Bobbie Atkins

Chapter 2   **Legislative Aspects of Rehabilitation** 17
Madan M. Kundu and Chrisann Schiro-Geist

Chapter 3   **Ethical Issues in Diversity** 44
Jeanne B. Patterson and Janet Spry

Chapter 4   **Preparing Culturally Competent Practitioners For Rehabilitation and Allied Health** 68
William Talley and Chandra Donnell

Chapter 5   **Case Management and Vocational Rehabilitation Counseling** 108
Keith B. Wilson, Tyra N. Turner Whittaker, And Virginia Black

Chapter 6   **Diversity Issues in Psychological Assessment** 128
Chow S. Lam, Debra B. Homa, and Amy Buser

Chapter 7   **Psychosocial Adjustment to Disability: A multi-ethnic approach** 155
Alo Dutta and Madan M. Kundu

Chapter 8   **Addressing the Independent Living Needs Of Ethnic-Racial Minority Groups** 176
Joan Looby

Chapter 9   **Human Resources Development and Issues in Rehabilitation** 201
Michelle P. Pointer

Chapter 10   **Rehabilitation Technology:
More than assistive technology for
multicultural consumers**.................................224
*Yolanda V. Edwards, Dothel W. Edwards, Jr.,
and Dion F. Porter*

Chapter 11   **Rehabilitation Research from a
Multicultural Perspective**...............................240
*Paul Leung, Catherine Marshall,
and Keith Wilson*

Chapter 12   **The Spiritual Realm of Rehabilitation
Counseling**...266
Joseph Keferl and Marti Riemer-Reiss

Chapter 13   **Partnering With Families for Successful
Career Outcomes**..281
Stacie L. Robertson and Carl R. Flowers

INDEX 302

The Editors

Paul Leung, Ph.D., CRC

Dr. Leung is professor and Chair of the Department of Rehabilitation, Social Work, and Addictions at the University of North Texas. His interests include disability and rehabilitation related to persons with diverse backgrounds in both his teaching and research. He is a Fellow of the American Psychological Association.

Dr. Leung has held teaching and administrative appointments at the University of Arizona, the University of North Carolina at Chapel Hill, the University of Illinois/Champaign-Urbana, and Deakin University, Melbourne, Australia.

Dr. Leung has been a practicing counselor and psychologist, a principal as well as co-investigator of numerous grants, and has published extensively. He was Editor of the Journal of Rehabilitation from 1987 to 1996. He was President of the National Council on Rehabilitation Education, Division 22 (Rehabilitation Psychology) of the American Psychological Association and the National Association of Multicultural Rehabilitation Concerns. Dr. Leung received his doctorate in Psychology at Arizona State University.

Carl R. Flowers, Ph.D., CRC, CLPC

Dr. Flowers is an Associate Professor in the Rehabilitation Institute at Southern Illinois University Carbondale where he teaches classes in the Rehabilitation Administration and Rehabilitation Counseling Programs.

Dr. Flowers has published and presented widely on issues associated with diversity, ethics, and leadership and serves on the editorial boards of several journals. He has consulted with organizations and governmental agencies in the United States and abroad, including Korea and Russia.

Dr. Flowers is former president of the National Association of Multicultural Rehabilitation Concerns (NAMRC) and President Elect of the National Rehabilitation Association (NRA). He is a NRA Switzer Scholar (2001), member of Phi Delta Kappa and a number of other education and social issue focused organizations.

William B. Talley, Rh.D.

Dr. Talley is Chair of the Department of Rehabilitation Services and an Associate Professor at the University of Maryland Eastern Shore. He previously served as Chair of the Department of Rehabilitation and Director of the Institute for Social and Rehabilitation Services at Assumption College. He spent more than twenty-five years working first as a practitioner and, more recently, as an educator and administrator in the field of rehabilitation.

He received his doctorate in Rehabilitation from Southern Illinois University at Carbondale, IL and the M.A. in Rehabilitation from South Carolina State University, Orangeburg, SC.

Priscilla R. Sanderson, Ph.D., CRC

Dr. Sanderson is a Navajo. Her clan is Táchii'nii (Red-Running-Into-The Water Clan), born for kinyaa'ánii (Towering House Clan), maternal grandparents clan are Naakaii Dine'é (Mexican Clan) and paternal grandparents clan are Bit'ahnii (Leaf Clan). Dr. Sanderson is a Postdoctoral Fellow with the Arizona Cancer Center, Cancer Prevention and Control, University of Arizona.

She is a co-founder of the Consortia of Administrators for Native American Rehabilitation and served as a consulting editor for the *Journal of Rehabilitation Administration*. She received her B.A. in Psychology from Southwestern College, M.S. in Rehabilitation Counseling from Oklahoma State University, and her doctorate in Rehabilitation Education from the University of Arizona.

The Contributors

Bobbie J. Atkins, Ph.D., is Professor Emeritus, Department of Administration, Rehabilitation and Postsecondary Education, San Diego State University. She has over 30 years of experience in teaching, research, publications, and service in rehabilitation counseling. Atkins currently serves as Project Director for several grants for training, technical assistance, and teaching.

Virginia H. Black, B.A. in Psychology from Hendrix College. She was a Peace Corps volunteer in Poland for two years.

Amy Buser, received her Ph.D. in Clinical Psychology from Illinois Institute of Technology, specializing in Rehabilitation Psychology. She is currently a postdoctoral student at the Center for Neurovisceral Sciences and Women's Health at University of California Los Angeles.

Chow S. Lam, Ph.D., CRC, is Distinguished Professor of Psychology and Director of the Rehabilitation Psychology of the Institute of Psychology at Illinois Institute of Technology. He is Fellow of the American Psychological Association (APA and Distinguished Research Fellow of the National Institute on Disabilities and Rehabilitation Research (NIDRR). He holds several visiting and honorary professorships at the universities in Hong Kong and China.

Chandra M. Donnell, Ph.D., CRC, LLPC, is an Assistant Professor of rehabilitation counseling in the Department of Counseling, Educational Psychology, and Special Education at Michigan State University. She is an editorial board member for the Journal of Multicultural counseling and Development and president-elect for the National Association of Multicultural Rehabilitation Concerns.

Alo Dutta, Ph.D., CRC, is an Assistant Professor in the Department of Rehabilitation and Disability Studies at Southern University, Baton, Rouge, LA. She received an MA in Rehabilitation Counseling from SU and a Ph.D. in Community Health with a specialization in rehabilitation from the University of Illinois at

Urbana-Champaign. She is the principal investigator of a NIDRR funded project.

Dothel W. Edwards, Jr., Rh.D., is Coordinator and Assistant Professor in the Rehabilitation Counseling and Case Management program at Fort Valley State University. He received an M.A. degree in Rehabilitation Counseling from South Carolina State University and the Doctor of Rehabilitation from Southern Illinois University at Carbondale.

Yolanda V. Edwards, Ph.D., is Assistant Professor with the Department of Neuropsychiatry and Behavioral Science in the Rehabilitation Counseling Program at the University of South Carolina in Columbia, SC. She earned her M.A. in rehabilitation counseling from South Carolina State University and the Ph.D. in Rehabilitation Counseling from the University of Iowa.

Debra B. Homa, Ph.D., CRC, CVE, is an Assistant Professor in the Department of Rehabilitation and Counseling at the University of Wisconsin-Stout. She has over 20 years of experience in rehabilitation counseling and assessment.

Joseph E. Keferl, Rh.D., CRC, is Assistant Professor and Advisor of the Graduate Rehabilitation Counseling, Chemical Dependency Program at Wright State University. He holds two Masters Degrees in Rehabilitation Counseling in the areas of severe disabilities and chemical dependency. Dr. Keferl received his doctorate in Rehabilitation from Southern Illinois University at Carbondale.

Madan M. Kundu, Ph.D., CRC, NCC, LRC, FNRCA, is a Professor and Chair of the Department of Rehabilitation and Disability Studies at Southern University, Baton Rouge, LA. Dr. Kundu was a Fulbright Scholar and has over 40 years in national and international rehabilitation. He is the Project director of a NIDRR funded project entitled the Rehabilitation Research Institute for Underrepresented Populations. He is the North American Chair for the Work and Employment Commission of Rehabilitation International and Board Member of the U.S. International Council on Disability.

E. Joan Looby, Ph.D., LPC, NCC, is a Professor of Counselor Education and former Assistant Dean of the College of Education, Mississippi State University. Dr. Looby has over 20 years of clinical experience working with individuals across the developmental spectrum (children, adolescents, adults) providing individual, group, and family counseling for a wide range of personal, social, and developmental issues.

Catherine A. Marshall, Ph.D., is a Research Professor in the Department of Educational Psychology at Northern Arizona University and Adjunct Professor in the Centre for Work, Leisure, and Community Research at Griffith University near Brisbane, Australia. She is the founder and President of a non-profit organization, the Women's International Leadership Institute that benefits low-income women seeking to improve their educational and economic status.

Jeanne Boland Patterson, Ed.D., CRC, is Professor and Director of the Rehabilitation Counseling Program at the University of North Florida. She is Past President of the National Council on Rehabilitation Education and President of the National Rehabilitation Counseling Association. Dr. Patterson has over 30 years experience in rehabilitation counseling.

Michelle Phillips Pointer, Ed.D., CRC, NCC, LCPC, is an Associate Professor at Coppin State University, Baltimore, MD and Project Director for two Rehabilitation Services Long-Term Training Grants.

Dion F. Porter, Rh.D., is an Assistant Professor in the Department of School, Community, and Rehabilitation Counseling at Jackson State University in Jackson, MS. He teaches in the rehabilitation counseling program as well as the counseling education program. He received the Masters degree from Jackson State University in Rehabilitation Counseling and his Rh.D. from the University of Southern Illinois at Carbondale.

Marti Riemer-Reiss, Ph.D., CRC, is a faculty member of the Human Services and Rehabilitation Program at Western Washington University. Her doctorate is in Human Rehabilitation from the University of Northern Colorado and her Master's degree is from San Diego State University.

Stacie L. Robertson, Ph.D., CRC, is an Assistant Professor in the Rehabilitation Institute at Southern Illinois University at Carbondale. She teaches courses in Rehabilitation Counselor Training and provides consultation to the Center for Autism and Spectrum Disorders (CASD). Dr. Robertson received her doctorate from The Pennsylvania State University. She serves on the Board of Directors for the National Association of Multicultural Rehabilitation Concerns (NAMRC) and is President of the Illinois Association of Multicultural Rehabilitation Concerns.

Chrisann Schiro-Geist, Ph.D., is Vice Provost for Academic Affairs at the University of Memphis and a Professor in the Department of Counseling, Educational Psychology and Research. She received her Ph.D. in Counseling Psychology from Northwestern University.

Janet D. Spry, Ed.D., CRC, LCPC, CVE, is an Associate Professor and Director of the Masters Rehabilitation Counseling Program at Coppin State University. Dr. Spry received her Doctorate and Ed.S. from The George Washington University and her M.Ed. from Coppin State College in Rehabilitation Counseling.

Tyra Turner Whittaker, Rh.D., CRC, is an Associate Professor of Counseling and the Rehabilitation Counseling Program Coordinator in the Department of Human Development and Services at North Carolina Agricultural and Technical State University.

Keith B. Wilson, Ph.D., CRC, NCC, LPC, ABDA, is an Associate Professor and Program Chair of Rehabilitation Programs in the Department of Counselor Education, Counseling Psychology, and Rehabilitation Services at The Pennsylvania State University.

PREFACE

$\mathcal{A}$merica's population has been changing. Not only are we growing in numbers, but we are also getting chronologically older; and, at the same time, we are also becoming more and more culturally diverse. Regardless, the bottom line is that we are having a difficult time dealing with the myriad of changes. Witness the debate occurring at all levels of American society regarding immigration, English only, and whether we have anything in common with one another.

Rehabilitation has been a bit behind the eight-ball with regard to exploring how multiculturalism impacts rehabilitation and other allied health professions. Psychology, mental health, and counseling have forged ahead with opinions and research on multiculturalism that is a rich source of ideas and practical applications, while rehabilitation is only at the starting gate. There is very little opinion or research in the field of rehabilitation that is specific to culture and ethnicity.

This textbook is arguably the first attempt to synthesize and integrate the meaning of living in a multicultural society as it relates to rehabilitation practitioners and educators. It is a book written by persons from diverse backgrounds and experiences. The emphasis has been on the traditional "ethnic minority" populations with no intent to diminish other aspects of diversity such as age, sexual orientation, or disability itself. We have chosen to review more traditional rehabilitation topics from the perspective of "persons of color." We know that as members of minority populations, we have not always paid enough attention to disability and what disability (and, therefore, rehabilitation) means in our groups. Our attitudes and behavior, unfortunately, mirror those of the larger American society. Persons with disabilities have had to fight their way into our organizations and culture. It is the belief of the Editors that each of our many ethnic groups has much to offer to the larger society as America looks for ways to better and more effectively serve all of its citizens. That is our starting point, and we hope that this book will provoke you to think and to act to better the lives of persons with disabilities, regardless of their race or ethnicity.

We have not covered all that could be explored. We see this book as the first of many that will enhance the available literature from perspectives that have often been left out. To paraphrase a cliché, as history is often written from the eyes of the victor so too has disability and rehabilitation been recorded only from the narrow perspective of the predominant culture.

The Editors are hopeful that this book is a beginning to diversity being fully integrated into the rehabilitation literature and research.

THIS PAGE IS INTENTIONALLY LEFT BLANK

CHAPTER 1

MULTICULTURAL REHABILITATION: AN HISTORICAL PERSPECTIVE

PAUL LEUNG
BOBBIE ATKINS

Chapter Highlights

- Multicultural counseling

- Rehabilitation

- The mental health multicultural movement

- Access to rehabilitation

- Legislative mandates

- Future

While some professionals in rehabilitation still believe a multicultural approach (we will use diversity and multicultural as interchangeable terms) to be debatable (Middleton, et al., 2002; Thomas & Weinrach, 2002), multiculturalism in rehabilitation and human services is almost taken for granted today as a natural part of the fabric of all human service interactions. Yet, much remains to be done to ensure that diversity is accepted as a natural part of the rehabilitation process and practice. Business and industry have adopted diversity as a benchmark of good business practice (http://www.diversityinc. com/).

Multiculturalism and diversity have become accepted within the context of an America that is drastically different (Leung, 1993) than that found in the past, but that reality may still be difficult to accept when actual practices must change. The population estimates from the U.S. Census Bureau (2001) for the near future are that no one group will make up a majority. We have become a nation of many rich, diverse backgrounds and experiences. This chapter is an attempt to chronicle the impact of this change within the rehabilitation arena.

The history of anything is not always easy to describe. Quite often, what is written is the perspective of those who have prevailed and who remain on top, leaving out those who were left behind. Feminists have long suggested that history has not been "her" story. Moreover, we know that contributions of ethnic and racial groups have not been well documented in mainstream history. A comprehensive look at the history of multicultural activity within an area such as rehabilitation requires far more resources than what we had available for this chapter. As a result, we consider this an incomplete account in anticipation of a time when a more complete story can be told.

How far along rehabilitation is on this road of multiculturalism is open to question. Part of it depends on the same dynamics that govern the greater society. Perspectives differ dependent upon personal experience and on the color of one's skin. The struggle that has brought rehabilitation to where it is now in terms of diversity is illuminating, interesting, and perhaps an indictment of our profession. As suggested by the word struggle, the road to diversity in rehabilitation is still being paved. Multiculturalism in rehabilitation, not unlike multiculturalism in other areas, came about because of the vision of a courageous few who were willing to step forward to take a stand. These individuals came from the ranks of consumers, practitioners, and educators as well as researchers. This chapter is an attempt to tell that story. As suggested earlier, it will not be the complete story and is certainly limited by the memories of the authors and the availability of sources.

The movement toward full inclusion is not only of ethnicity and culture, but of disability as well. The multicultural movement in rehabilitation has been intertwined with the broader social changes that have occurred in American society. Those of us in rehabilitation and disability must acknowledge the debt owed to the broader civil rights movement as well as the disability movement. At the same time, the focus of the civil rights and disability movements has not always been inclusive of the interests of persons of color with disabilities or of the field of rehabilitation.

Ethnic/racial civil rights groups have not always included disability as part of their overall agenda, and even now, many persons with disabilities from diverse groups do not feel included or welcome among many mainstream civil rights organizations. In like manner, the disability movement has often been led by white, middle class persons whose perspective did not often include persons with disabilities from ethnic/racial backgrounds (NCD, 1997). Just as the impetus for the civil rights and disability movement came about because of inequities and injustice, so is the current desire that there be a place for persons with disabilities who are members of diverse ethnic/racial populations.

Rehabilitation, and rehabilitation counseling as an area or field of study, are related to many other disciplines. These disciplines include medicine and allied health professions; other helping professions such as counseling and psychology; and the broader area of mental health. Rehabilitation's multicultural history is, in part, the history of these movements, and some summary is included here in order to provide further context.

MULTICULTURAL COUNSELING

Morris Jackson (1995) captured the history of the multicultural counseling movement in a chapter written for *The Handbook of Multicultural Counseling*. Jackson suggested that the roots of the guidance and counseling movement are based on the premise of choosing a vocation. Because African Americans and other minorities faced extreme discrimination and prejudice, African Americans had limited choice in selecting a vocation. Some counseling professionals excluded minority clients or only matched clients with employment where it was felt by the counselor that the clients were most likely to be hired (Jackson, 1995). This type of career counseling, clearly, was not in the best interest of consumers who have disabilities, let alone persons of color.

Jackson (1995) also suggested that counseling during this era emphasized the assimilation of immigrant and minority populations into the "mainstream" of American society, and that assimilation counseling "proved to be ineffective for a large segment of the American population, as counselors worked with theories and techniques that were at odds with the cultural backgrounds of their clients" (p. 6). Jackson's review of the counseling literature found little information on the role of culture or race in counseling prior to the 1960's. Much of the emphasis in those years was not on counseling, but rather on the significance of culture for the administration of standardized tests. This limitation in the literature provides a background for understanding some of the current challenges related to multicultural counseling in rehabilitation and related counseling areas.

The decade of the 1960's was a particularly prescient time for the multicultural counseling movement. The Civil Rights Act of 1964 certainly paved the way for an exploration and discussion of race. Within the counseling profession, special legislation was passed by the 1966 American Personnel and Guidance Association (APGA) that called for the inclusion of "guidance and counseling of persons who were 'culturally disadvantaged' (Jackson, 1995). The use of the term "culturally disadvantaged" is interesting as the term suggested that cultures of people of color were somehow lacking. Atkinson, Morten, and Sue (1998) articulated this when they wrote, "The term culturally disadvantaged suggests the person to whom it is applied is at a disadvantage because he/she lacks the cultural background formed by the controlling social structure….we seriously object, however, to any inference that racial/ethnic groups have less culture" (p. 10).

Jackson (1995) saw this as an "indictment of previous counseling practice," and as recognition that a new paradigm would have to emerge. Jackson (1995) related other events within the counseling profession including the call for establishing an Office of Non-White Concerns at the 1969 APGA conference. The petition calling for the office was the beginning of the Association's first Black caucus (Jackson, 1995). The office soon led to the Association for Non-White Concerns (ANWC) in 1972 and to the Association for Multicultural Counseling and Development in 1985.

REHABILITATION

Within the field of rehabilitation, parallel events occurred though again only after long continuing neglect by the primary rehabilitation professional association. In 1969, nine members of the National Rehabilitation Association (NRA), 46 years after the founding of the NRA, presented a document entitled "Non-White Caucus Demands" to the NRA Board of Directors (McConnell, Keener, & Farish, 1995). These nine included some early multicultural pioneers including Thomas Washington, George Ayers, Vernon Hawkins, Beth

Anderson, and Jose Rodriguez. The document listed issues long ignored by the NRA related to the need for expanding the Non-White voting membership, employing Non-Whites in NRA, increasing Non-White involvement in the NRA legislative agenda, and expanding NRA support related to directing public resources to Non-White rehabilitation and community organizations. The NRA Board accepted the document and agreed on a resolution to be voted on at the NRA Delegate Assembly that year. The passage of Resolution 14 became the first formal recognition by NRA that race and ethnicity were issues (McConnell et al, 1995) in the organization, and more broadly in rehabilitation. This recognition eventually evolved into the current NRA division known as the National Association of Multicultural Rehabilitation Concerns.

The struggle to bring a multicultural perspective to rehabilitation also includes stories of many individuals with and without disabilities who were pioneers in the effort. We reiterate that this chapter can only partially cover this history. It is important to acknowledge the authors' gratitude as well as apology to the many who may have been omitted.

It is essential, as rehabilitation professionals, that we appreciate what brought us to where we are today, as it demonstrates our interdependence on each other along with knowing that we are not alone in the struggle. As many pioneers age and gray, it becomes ever more critical that this legacy not be lost, especially to those who are now entering rehabilitation and are emerging to become rehabilitation's new pioneers. One movement that has had influence repeatedly on rehabilitation is mental health.

THE MENTAL HEALTH MULTICULTURAL MOVEMENT

The multicultural movement within the mental health community also brought recognition that the needs and requirements of ethnic/racial minority groups were not equivalent to the issues and needs that the majority society presented. Researchers such as Stanley Sue (1970) found an underutilization of mental health services by different ethnic/racial groups, as well as different help seeking behaviors that affected how various populations accessed, or did not access, mental health services. Atkinson (2004) further elaborated that when "sociodemographic data have been controlled, mental illness is not related to ethnicity per se…." (p.75). People of color, however, are often differentiated from their white peers in terms of mental health access, utilization, quality, and research. These disparities provided continuing motivation for exploring and expanding a multicultural emphasis in rehabilitation counseling and related professions.

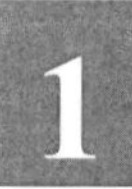

The United States Department of Health and Human Services funded several centers with the mission of addressing through research the requirements of different racial and ethnic groups. These centers also provided an impetus to look beyond the traditional mental health services, and the one size fits all approach. Each center has made substantial contributions to our understanding that cultural variables are critical and must be addressed in any service delivery system.

- National Center for American Indian and Alaska Native Mental Health Research has explored some of the specific requirements of American Indians and Alaska natives, the populations indigenous to the United States, but often left out of the loop with regard to appropriate and relevant mental health services. The rates of post-traumatic stress disorder in American Indian and Alaska Native veterans have always been high, but mental health services were not available for the population, according to a study conducted by the National Center for American Indian and Alaska Native Mental Health Research. The findings of this study revealed that current services for American Indian veterans rank low in availability, accessibility, and acceptability. The Center is located at the University of Colorado Health Sciences Center in Denver.

- The National Research Center on Asian American Mental Health, also funded by the National Institute for Mental Health (NIMH), conducts research on various Asian groups, including Koreans, Filipinos, and Southeast Asians. The center has looked at mental health problems among Asians including the rates of mental disturbance and factors that affect utilization of health services. Researchers there conducted a study looking at whether it is better for therapists and clients to be of the same race and ethnicity. "We found that Asian clients who had Asian therapists stayed in treatment longer and were more likely to have better treatment outcomes," said Stanley Sue, PhD, director of the center located at the University of California, Davis, Department of Psychology.

- The African American Mental Health Research Center is part of the Program for Research on Black Americans established by an interdisciplinary team of social scientists. The NIMH started the research center with the goal of studying African American mental health, and evaluating the way African Americans seek help for mental illness. In 1993, the grant was expanded to study issues surrounding the mental health of children and adolescents, including the plight of the chronically mental ill in urban areas. The Program for Research on Black Americans is located at the University of Michigan, Institute for Social Research, in Ann Arbor.

- The Center for Hispanic Mental Health Research was established through a grant from the NIMH with a charge to explore mental health research and the fast growing Hispanic population. The Mission of the Center is to conduct innovative applied mental health research on Hispanic populations with a goal of generating new knowledge in order to provide improved services. The Center's objectives include conducting epidemiological research identifying mental health needs of Hispanic populations; studying how standard assessment, treatment interventions, and prevention approaches can be modified to enhance outcomes for Hispanics; conducting psychotherapeutic intervention studies testing new culturally competent psychosocial services; and disseminating research findings through scholarly publications, a Center newsletter, colloquia, and conferences. The center is located at Fordham University, New York.

The issues that led to the formation of these research centers have not diminished and a recent release by the Surgeon General of the U.S. suggests that there is much work yet to be done. The supplemental report (2001) of the Surgeon General pointed out that disparities affecting mental health care of racial and ethnic minorities, compared with whites, continue to exist. The conclusions included the following:

- Minorities have less access to, and availability of, mental health services.
- Minorities are less likely to receive needed mental health services.
- Minorities in treatment often receive a poorer quality of mental health care.
- Minorities are underrepresented in mental health research.

These disparities correspond to those cited by Atkinson (2004) specific to the mental health needs of ethnic minority populations. Mental illness continues to affect racial and ethnic populations disproportionately creating disabling conditions that affect their ability to participate fully in society and to be employed. The Supplemental report found that racial and ethnic minorities

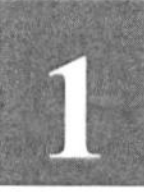

collectively experience a greater disability burden from mental illness than do whites. This higher level of burden stems from minorities receiving less care and poorer quality of care. This is in distinct contrast to the notion that mental illnesses are inherently more severe or prevalent in minority communities. Awareness of these issues is essential for rehabilitation providers, educators, and researchers if there is to be truly equitable programs and services based or grounded on an "asset orientation" (Atkins, 1988) rather than a deficit approach that undermines what consumers of color have to offer. This perspective is akin to the unacceptable use of "disadvantaged" (Atkinson et al., 1998) and brings about a negative bias in understanding and relating to various ethnic populations.

ACCESS TO REHABILITATION

One of the earliest publications regarding vocational rehabilitation and Blacks appeared in 1938 in the *Journal of Negro Education* (Wilkerson & Penn, 1938) regarding "The Participation of Negroes in the Federally-aided Program of Civilian Vocational Rehabilitation." Based on data obtained in 1935-36, Wilkerson and Penn (1938) explored the "relative extent to which Negro and white persons participate in the rehabilitation services of the 15 Southern states and District of Columbia." Wilkerson and Penn (1938), in an attempt to make sense of the data, speculated "One wonders if the predominating practice of rehabilitation agencies is to fit a Negro client with a cork arm or leg, or a pair of spectacles, find him a job, and close his case, without having afforded him the opportunity for vocational training which a similarly handicapped white client would normally enjoy" (p. 325). Recommendations offered by Wilkerson and Penn (1938) included the need for Federal laws to "be amended to require a 'just and equitable' distribution of funds and services to minority racial groups" and that annual reports be published "showing the extent to which Negroes and other minority racial groups share in the funds and services." Inequities and disparities obviously existed during these years and continued to be carried over into the 1980's.

A second watershed event in multicultural rehabilitation occurred in 1980, further accentuating the need for attention to minority populations and specifically African Americans. An article based on the doctoral dissertation of Bobbie J. Atkins (Atkins & Wright, 1980) was published in the *Journal of Rehabilitation.* The Atkins & Wright article had major impact on rehabilitation, and specifically the state federal public vocational rehabilitation program, as Atkins drew attention to inequalities that existed. For example, Atkins and

Wright (1980) found that "Blacks entered and exited the public VR programs in a proportionately more disadvantaged status than Whites (p. 45). Atkins and Wright (1980) further suggested, "fewer VR resources were employed to help improve the overall status of disabled Blacks" (p. 45). Their conclusion was that "while it is clear from this study that Blacks are proportionately in greater need of compensatory VR services, the actual amount of such assistance was generally less for Blacks than Whites" (p. 45). Atkins and Wright (1980) are significant not only for their findings and subsequent publication, but as the authors of the first of a number of studies and related publications that explored the relationship between service provision and race or ethnicity (Bowe, 1983, 1985; Asbury et al, 1994).

Dr. Bobbie Atkins, being the first contemporary to draw attention to the treatment of racial minorities in rehabilitation, also encountered obstacles that future researchers were less likely to face. Because Atkins (1980) suggested what many perceived to be a negative reflection on the state federal vocational rehabilitation program, scrutiny at a level seldom seen before or since was placed on publication of her data. The article was not published after acceptance for the reader to draw their own conclusions about the validity of the data and their implications, as is generally the case. The *Journal of Rehabilitation* editors sought out two additional reactions or responses. In what was perhaps an unprecedented act, commentary from the RSA Commissioner and Deputy Commissioner, along with invited comments from two other researchers were obtained. Given the implied criticism of the public rehabilitation program by Atkins & Wright (1980), this certainly seemed a somewhat transparent and defensive way to lessen the impact.

The RSA Commissioner's and Deputy RSA Commissioner's (1980) response was that the conclusions of Atkins & Wright (1980) were possible, but the analysis did not clearly indicate where the problem was. The response from the two researchers (Bolton and Cooper, 1980) suggested that statistical differences could be interpreted in a different way than Atkins & Wright (1980). Bolton & Cooper (1980) took the position that the percentage of Blacks accepted into the public VR program exceeded the proportion of Blacks in the U.S. and, at the same time, acknowledging that Blacks have higher rates of disability. Bolton and Cooper (1980) went on to suggest that clients who lack education be thoroughly assessed to determine who would benefit from "vocational adjustment and/or intensive job placement." In the end, even the responses could not lessen the impact of a study that confirmed what many in the African American community felt to be true.

It was also during this time period that a Rehabilitation Research and Training Center (R & T) was funded through the National Institute on

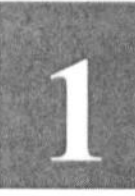

Disability and Rehabilitation Research that was perhaps the only Center that maintained an agenda related to underserved populations. Based in Howard University and directed by Dr. Sylvia Walker, the Center for Access to Rehabilitation and Economic Opportunity was the only federally funded R & T Center with the expressed mission to study underserved and underrepresented populations, such as African Americans.

Two other R & T Centers were established to explore rehabilitation and the American Indian, and were located at the University of Arizona in Tucson (UA) and at Northern Arizona University (NAU). The NAU and UA were both called the Native American Research and Training Center (NARTC). Historically, UA focused on the health and well-being of Native Americans while NAU focused on vocational rehabilitation and independent living of American Indians. Since 1983, the NARTCs have conducted research and training to improve rehabilitation services for American Indians with disabilities. The centers serve as a national resource for Native American communities and for persons working with Native American populations, especially those with chronic diseases or disabilities.

In the early part of 1987, a subproject was funded to NAU and UA to conduct a national study at the request of Congress. Dr. Joanne O'Connell, NAU Research Director was the lead researcher and editor for the subproject and worked with the primary researcher, Dr. Jim Morgan

In the 1988 grant application, the NAU center changed its name from Native American Research and Training Center to American Indian Rehabilitation Research, primarily for the sake of brevity (NIDRR Competitive Grant Application, December 15, 1988, p.4)

The research center on the campus of Howard University, founded by Dr. Sylvia Walker, focused on populations that were not well served by rehabilitation programs. Based on the inclusive vision of Dr. Walker, the R&T Center for Access to Rehabilitation took upon itself to collaborate with not only the African American community, but also the Hispanic American and Asian American communities in its research and training agenda. A number of significant documents resulted from the research done during those early years. The study titled "Disability Prevalence and Demographic Association Among Race/Ethnic Minority Populations in the United States: Implications for the 21st Century" (Asbury, Walker, Maholmes, Rackley, & White1991) was perhaps the first major documentation of disability prevalence within diverse communities. In addition, The Research and Training Center at Howard University hosted numerous workshops, training opportunities, and seminars focusing on multicultural issues and concerns. It is especially noteworthy because many of these conferences and meeting were held without widespread

10

support from those who were not people of color. The Howard Center also collaborated with the President's Committee on Employment of People with Disabilities and coordinated numerous sessions in conjunction with the President's Committee annual meeting.

Several rehabilitation educators also sensed a need for an academic base to address issues related to a multicultural approach to rehabilitation counseling. A special issue of the *Journal of Applied Rehabilitation Counseling* appeared in 1988 devoted to the multicultural aspects of rehabilitation counseling (Leal, Leung, Martin, & Harrison, 1988). Not long after, Tennyson Wright and William Emener (1989) published the first annotated bibliography consisting of 526 entries between 1952-1988 related to ethnic minority populations, disability, and rehabilitation.

At about the same time, the National Council on Disability (NCD), an independent federal agency charged with oversight related to disability and the federal government, identified needs in diverse populations that were not met. With an African American woman, Ethel Briggs (formerly with the District Vocational Rehabilitation Program under Vernon Hawkins), as their Executive Director, inroads were made toward examining needs of minority persons with disabilities. This focus by NCD led to a national conference in Jackson, Mississippi in 1992 targeting the unique needs of minorities with disabilities. One hundred eighty-six persons participated, including a majority from minority communities, and produced 11 major findings along with recommendations for policy for the National Council. In October 1992, the NCD held a daylong meeting in San Francisco as a follow-up to the national conference.

LEGISLATIVE MANDATES

Two pieces of legislation were instrumental in moving the multicultural rehabilitation agenda forward. The first was Section 610(j) of the Individuals with Disabilities Education Act (IDEA), and its mirror in Section 21 of the Rehabilitation Act Amendments of 1992. Both of these pieces of legislation grew from Congressman Major Owens of New York, who was Chair of the Subcommittee on Select Education (Zawaiza, 2002). Changes mandated by these two pieces of legislation involved funds specifically set aside to ensure outreach and capacity building for institutions such as historically black colleges and universities and other high minority enrollment institutions. The additional emphasis was brought by legislative mandate; suggesting perhaps that the state federal program did not make the needed effort to outreach to

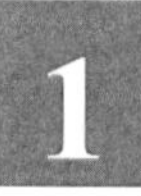

those populations that are in particular need of rehabilitation. In addition, it was a strategy that helped keep multicultural issues in the forefront of rehabilitation public policy.

The initial phase for implementing Section 21 by the Rehabilitation Services Administration was through development of the Rehabilitation Cultural Diversity Initiative (RCDI). Housed within San Diego State University and led by Dr. Bobbie Atkins, the RCDI vision was for rehabilitation to reflect the cultural diversity of American society with the mission to promote opportunities to enhance equal access and quality services for individuals who are culturally diverse. The RSA designated the Regional Rehabilitation Continuing Education Programs (RRCEPs) as the avenue for implementation, with each of the ten RRCEPs funded to perform outreach services to minority institutions of higher learning.

Most RRCEPs designated or hired a staff member to serve in the outreach effort. RSA has also established a National Rehabilitation Cultural Diversity Initiative (RCDI) Committee composed of individuals from around the country to provide input into policies established by RSA and to provide recommendations for systemic change.

Some of the values driving the RCDI were the empowerment of persons with disabilities; diversity is perceived as an asset; partnership and collaboration; awareness that all people have talents and values; realization that all people deserve respect and equal opportunity; and maximizing human resources in rehabilitation organizations. RCDIs' operating principles were articulated to promote diversity in all aspects of rehabilitation; model diversity inclusion in all interaction with other organizations; work in partnership with its constituency to ensure empowerment and use of talents; practice and promote the highest standard of human behaviors, products, and interactions; and develop and implement policy changes as needed.

The RCDI utilized a lead specialist (experts in diversity issues) approach in each region to obtain baseline data, to establish research agendas, and to develop programmatic strategies. RCDI proposed to extend beyond the quantitative measures of numbers and statistics to attitudinal and systemic changes. The RCDI, in the words of Dr. Atkins, was not about the Noah's Ark Syndrome (two by two), but rather about system and paradigm shifts and change. (Atkins, 1994)

An outgrowth of the RCDI was the establishment of the Consortia of Administrators for Native American Rehabilitation (CANAR) in 1993 by Dr. Ken Galea'I, who was then the RCEP VIII director. CANAR functioned as a national platform for drawing attention to the need for effective rehabilitation service delivery for American Indians and Alaska Natives with disabilities.

12

CANAR continues to serve as the official voice of Native American rehabilitation programs, which provide VR services to American Indians and Alaska Natives with disabilities who reside on or near Federal or State reservations, Alaska Native villages, rancheros, and pueblos. Under the leadership of Ms. Treva Roanhorse, CANAR has established itself as a viable political voice using a collaborative and cooperative partnership approach. Membership in CANAR includes Indian Country leaders able to work with a wide variety of constituencies. Due in part to CANAR, rehabilitation programs serving American Indians and Alaska natives have grown. After approximately three years, RSA abandoned the RCDI approach involving the RCEP's and followed a system involving a call for proposals to build capacity. These capacity-building projects are doing much to expand rehabilitation services and education through Indian Tribes and minority institutions of higher education, including minority serving institutions, historically black colleges, and universities and American Indian Tribal colleges. Much of the initial effort was directed toward conducting training sessions on how to access and write grants to support rehabilitation efforts. These sessions, along with related technical assistance, continue at this time.

More recently, the Rehabilitation Services Administration, perhaps sensing a need to focus more directly on underserved populations, completed three technical assistance centers. These centers were to assist vocational rehabilitation programs and partners to better respond to the cultural requirements that hve been documented as barriers for vocational rehabilitation service delivery. The American Indian Disability Technical Assistance Center was located in Montana. Projecto Vision was housed within the World Institute on Disability in California. The National Technical Assistance Center – Asian Americans and Pacific Islanders was established in Hawaii. With a three-year time frame, the RSA ceased competitions to extend these centers.

FUTURE

This chapter only scratches the surface regarding the rich and diverse history of multicultural rehabilitation. It is, in many ways, only the reflections of the two authors, based on their own experiences.

What are the lessons of history and rehabilitation? Nothing happens without commitment and struggle for what one believes to be important. A place at the table for persons of color resulted in greater emphasis on the importance of values, family, religion, and other cultural attributes more often found in communities of color. This chapter focused on what has occurred, but we would be remiss not to think about what our legacy means for the future.

We need to always be "asset oriented" (Atkins, 1988) and focus on the strengths that are brought to the table by so many diverse groups. Education and research must be inclusive of all, but in particular, those who have been so long ignored. Rehabilitation is not "nice" or even "interesting," but must be meaningful so that there is an improvement in the quality of life for all persons with disabilities. There will be a continuing need to dispel myths about not only disability, but also race and ethnicity.

Finally, there is need to enlist partners who may have interest in other issues of civil rights, race, and ethnicity to include disability as part of their agenda. Many organizations continue to leave out disability as part of the consideration of diversity. A major challenge for emerging leaders is not to abandon the struggle for equality. There is a tremendous need for all the talents of persons committed to ensuring that disability is embraced as a natural part of the human experience that includes people of color.

REFERENCES

Asbury, C. A., Walker. S. Maholmes, V., Rackley, R., & White, S. (1991). *Disability prevalence and demographic association among race/ethnic minority populations in the United States: Implications for the 21st century.* Washington, DC: Howard University Research and Training Center.

Asbury, C. A. Walker, S. Belgrave, FZ. Maholmes, V. Green, L. (1994). Psychosocial, Cultural, and Accessibility Factors Associated With Participation of African-Americans in Rehabilitation. *Rehabilitation Psychology, 39*(2), 113-121.

Atkins, B. J. & Wright, G.N. (1980). The vocational rehabilitation of blacks, *Journal of Rehabilitation, 42*(2), 40-46.

Atkins, B. J. (1988). An asset-oriented approach to cross cultural issues: blacks in rehabilitation. *Journal of Applied Rehabilitation Counseling, 19*(4) 45-49

Atkins, B. J. (1995). Diversity: A Continuing Rehabilitation Challenge and Opportunity. In *Disability and Diversity: New Leadership for a New Era.* President's Committee on Employment of People with Disabilities. Washington, D.C.

Atkinson, D.R. (2004). *Counseling American Minorities*. Boston:McGraw Hill.

Bolton, B., & Cooper, P. G. (1980). Three views: Vocational rehabilitation of Blacks: The comment. *Journal of Rehabilitation, 46*(41) 41-49.

Bowe, F. (1983). *Demography and disability: A chartbook for rehabilitation*. Little Rock, AR: Arkansas Rehabitation and Training Center, University of Arkansas.

Bowe, F. (1995). *Black Adults with disabilities: A statistical report from Census Bureau Data*. Little Rock, AR: Arkansas Rehabilitation and Research Training Center, University of Arkansas.

Doxey A. Wilkerson & Lemuel A. Penn (July, 1938). The Participation of Negroes in the Federally-Aided Program of Civilian Vocational Rehabilitation. *The Journal of Negro Education, Vol. 7(*3) 319-330.

Jackson, M. L. (1995). Multicultural Counseling: Historical Perspectives In J.G. Ponterotto, J.M. Casas, L.A. Suzuki, C.M. Alexander (Eds.) *Handbook of Multicultural Counseling*, Thousand Oaks, CA: Sage

Leal, A., Leung, P., Martin, W.E., & Harrison, D.K. (1988). Multicultural aspects of rehabilitation counseling: Issues and challenges. *Journal of Applied Rehabilitation Counseling, 19*(4) 3.

Leung, P. (1993). A changing demography and its challenge to vocational rehabilitation. *Journal of Vocational Rehabilitation 3*(1) 3-11.

McConnell, L. R., J. M. Keener, J. Farish (1995). National Association of Multicultural Rehabilitation Concerns - Special Anniversary Issue 1925-1995. *Journal of Rehabilitation 61*(3) 58-60.

Mental health: Culture, race, and ethnicity (2001). Retrieved July 8, 2003, from the U.S. Dept. of Health and Human Services, Office of the Surgeon General at http://www.surgeongeneral.gov/library/mentalhealth/cre/.

Middleton, R.A., Rollins, C.W., Sanderson, P.L., Leung, P., Harley, D.A., Ebener, D., et al. (2000). Endorsement of professional multicultural rehabilitation competencies and standards: A call to action. In *Rehabilitation Counseling Bulletin, 4*(4), 219-240.

National Council on Disability (1997). *Outreach to minorities with disabilities and people with disabilities in rural communities: roundtable report of findings*. Washington, D.C.

O'Connell, J. C. (Ed.) (1987). *A study of the special problems and needs of American Indians with handicaps both on and off the reservations*. Flagstaff, AZ: Northern Arizona University, and Tucson, AZ: University of Arizona, Native American Research and Training Center.

Sue, S. (2002). Asian American mental health: What we know and what we don't know. In W. J. Lonner, D. L. Dinnel, S. A. Hayes, & D. N. Sattler (Eds.), *Online Readings in Psychology and Culture* (Unit 3, Chapter 4) Retrieved April 10, 2006 at http://www.wwu.edu/~culture, Center for Cross-Cultural Research, Western Washington University, Bellingham, Washington USA.

Thomas, K. R. and Weinrach, S. G. (2002). Multiculturalism, Cultural Diversity and Affirmative Action Goals: A Reconsideration, *Rehabilitation Education,* (12), 65-75.

U.S. Census Bureau (2001). http://www.census.gov/, retrieved March 31, 2006.

Wright, T. J., & Emener, W. G. (Eds.) (1989). *Ethnic Minorities with Disabilities: An Annotated Bibliography of Rehabilitation Literature.* Tampa, FL: University of South Florida.

Zawaiza, T., Walker, S., & Ball, S. (2002, May). *Diversity matters: Infusing issues of people with disabilities from underserved communities into a trans-disciplinary research agenda in the behavioral and social sciences.* Washington, DC: Howard University, Center for Disability and Socioeconomic Policy Studies.

CHAPTER 2

LEGISLATIVE ASPECTS OF REHABILITATION

MADAN M. KUNDU

CHRISANN SCHIRO-GEIST

Chapter Highlights

➡ The depression and pre-World War II years: 1920-1939

➡ Accelerated growth era: 1940-1959

➡ The legislative era: 1960-1979

➡ The 1980s and beyond

➡ The Americans with Disabilities Act

➡ Implications

2

*T*his chapter provides a historical overview of legislation in rehabilitation. The early legislation, designed to establish a foundation for rehabilitation, is summarized briefly, and the later legislative mandates are discussed in detail. Prevailing social attitudes and language describing people with disabilities are kept intact, so that the reader has an opportunity to comprehend the socio-political dynamics that moved the field of rehabilitation. The concept of multiculturalism and issues affecting rehabilitation outcomes of people with disabilities of diverse backgrounds, are also discussed.

The legislation discussed in this chapter is the basis of both the process of vocational rehabilitation and the cornerstone of professionalism in the field. Legislation can only reflect the spirit of the legislators and their constituents at the time. Many of the acts cited in this chapter are mute on issues related to persons of diverse backgrounds. They say nothing about the cultural context of the United States at the time the legislation was passed. The legislation often accurately reflects the spirit of the time. Diversity was not a focus. Multiculturalism was not perceived to be an issue and, therefore, the legislation is barren of language from this perspective. However, that does not mean that there were not multicultural issues underlying the need for rehabilitation legislation during the legislative history. This chapter will look at some of the most critical pieces of legislation that relate to the field of vocational rehabilitation and some of the culturally relevant issues of the time.

The legislative history of vocational rehabilitation begins around 1916, focusing on World War I and the issues of veterans with disabilities who were returning to civilian life in the United States. This early period only occasionally highlights cultural issues, which reflects the country's lack of focus and even denial of diversity during that period. The sections of the chapter beginning in about 1992 to the present reflect a much more culturally rich, diversity-focused legislative period, reflective of the cultural changes taking place in the United States that also reflect the spirit of the times from a cultural perspective.

The **National Defense Act of 1916** provided educational and vocational instruction for soldiers in active military service to increase their military efficiency and return to civil life with better occupational skills.

The **Smith-Hughes Act of 1917** (Public Law 64-347) created the Federal Board for Vocational Education to administer federal monies on a matching basis to the states for vocational education programs. The Act provided for the physical restoration and vocational retraining of disabled veterans of World War I and dislocated industrial workers.

The **Soldier's Rehabilitation Act of 1918** (Public Law 65-178, **The Smith-Sears Act**) expanded the Federal Board of Vocational Education to offer programs of vocational rehabilitation exclusively to disabled veterans. The disabled veteran had to be vocationally handicapped in a gainful occupation to qualify for services.

It is quite obvious that the early legislative focus was on veterans, and especially those whose contributions to our country's war efforts had caused them serious impairment. Job placement was the obvious goal, with soldiers given an alternative to being on welfare rolls after their war-related disability. Due to industrial and farm mechanization, many could not, with their disabilities, return to their former work.

Cost was an issue and return for the tax dollar has always been the goal. Bitter (1979) notes that between 108% and 133% of the tax dollars spent on vocational rehabilitation are returned to the United States coffers from the income taxes of the rehabilitants. This was seen not as a welfare program, but a jobs program. Obviously, no money can be returned to government without successful job placement.

THE DEPRESSION AND PRE-WORLD WAR II YEARS:
1920-1939

The **Smith-Fess Act of 1920** (Public Law 66-236) established the First Civilian Vocational Rehabilitation Act that provided vocational rehabilitation services to those "physically disabled" due to industrial accidents, or other injuries not related to war injury. It established the state-federal program on a 50-50 matching basis to provide vocational guidance, vocational education, training, occupational adjustment, prostheses, and placement services. The act emphasized services for civilians with physical disabilities and was definitely vocational in nature. Other relevant legislation during this time period included the **Social Security Act of 1935** (Public Law 74-271), the **Randolph-- Sheppard Act of 1936** (Public Law 74-732) that authorized the states to license qualified vending machine operators who were blind, in federal buildings, and the **Wagner-O'Day Act of 1938** (Public Law 75-739), later amended by Public Law 92-28 of 1971, that mandated the federal government to purchase items produced in workshops by persons who are blind or visually impaired.

The Great Depression of the 1930s had a severe impact on placement. Even the best placement counseling could not help procure jobs if there were none. Consequently, this was where learning job-seeking skills to sell oneself to the employer became most relevant. "Mr. Employer, you need me because..."

helped keep many off the bread lines. Wilkerson and Penn (1938) found that, in the years leading up to the World War, disabled African Americans received vocational rehabilitation significantly less than White Americans, although as a group, African Americans had a greater need.

ACCELERATED GROWTH ERA: 1940-1959

As a result of the GI Bill, established by the federal government after World War II to financially assist veterans in their educational endeavors, colleges and universities experienced an increase in enrollment. Retraining and skill development were crucial in this period's unstable job market. In addition to training, the transition from wartime production to peacetime growth increased demand on the educational system. A liberal arts education was now deemed important. An individual needed to possess a basic education to become a "well-rounded" individual. It was believed that this preparation would best serve a peacetime economy. The transition toward long-range goals and individual planning now became reality.

Veterans Administration (VA) physicians made assessments of Black ex-GI's based on racialized concepts of normality, i.e. by assuming that a disability was merely typical of a "normal" African American. In 1948, for example, chief medical officers told black veterans at a VA hospital in Virginia, "there is nothing wrong with your nose, that's your natural look; nature made all Negroes to look that way." (Jefferson, 2003, pp. 1104-1105)

Officials at VA hospitals and rehabilitation centers in states such as Mississippi, South Carolina, Georgia, Virginia, Missouri, and Alabama enforced racial segregation and often provided blacks with less than adequate health care, personal adjustment counseling, and physical rehabilitation (Jefferson, 2003, p. 1110). African American veterans often found themselves barred from access to the special vocational compensation and rehabilitation allotted to them under Public Law 16 and the GI Bill of Rights (Jefferson, 2003, p. 1119). In addition to the persistence of the racism against which they fought, activist black veterans were hampered by the advent of the Cold War and subsequent anticommunist hysteria that forced the protest politics developed by wounded black World War II servicemen, underground (Jefferson, 2003, p. 1124).

J. C. Lee wrote to NAACP Executive Secretary Walter White, "Is this the Democracy that I've spent nearly three years defending in the Pacific? I am a disabled veteran, but the deplorable conditions that exist here in this country makes me wonder if I'm going to survive as a Negro" (Lee, 1948). White physician Harold Blackwell commented to NAACP Secretary of Veterans Affairs in 1945 about black disabled veterans "The time that Negro disabled GIs spent in the service does not qualify them for royalties from this man's Army. The only legitimate patients in this hospital are free, white and twenty-one" (Blackwell, 1945).

The **Vocational Rehabilitation Act Amendments of 1943** (Public Law 78-113, **Barden-LaFollette Act**) superseded the original 1920 Act, and brought many significant changes. The new law deleted the word "physical" from the earlier definition and, for the first time, made eligible persons with mental retardation and mental illness. In addition, for the first time, separate state agencies for persons who are blind and visually impaired were established. The concept of rehabilitation was widened by broadening the scope of services to include any services necessary for persons with disabilities to engage in remunerative occupations. These services include medical, surgical, and physical restoration; hospitalization; corrective surgery or therapeutic treatment; prosthetic devices to obtain or retain employment; transportation; occupational licenses; occupational tools and equipment; maintenance; and books and training materials (McGowan & Porter, 1967; Oberman, 1965).

The **Vocational Rehabilitation Act Amendments of 1954** (Public Law 83-565, **Hill-Burton Act**) provided training grants to colleges and universities to develop master's degree programs for rehabilitation counselors; in-service grants for staff development of state vocational rehabilitation agencies; and short-term grants for seminars, workshops, specialized institutes, and rehabilitation research fellowships. It expanded resources for restoring persons with disabilities to productive employment. Funds were available to expand community based rehabilitation facilities and workshops as opposed to traditional institutional settings; for research and demonstration grants to state rehabilitation agencies, rehabilitation facilities, universities, and institutions to harness new knowledge for better rehabilitation and information dissemination throughout the country. The act also strengthened the provisions of the Randolph-Sheppard Act with Vending Stand Programs for persons who are blind or visually impaired; expanded services for persons who are mentally ill; provided greater financial support to the states, and established a working relationship between public (state-federal) and private (rehabilitation facilities) agencies for rehabilitation to attain goals for persons with disabilities.

THE LEGISLATIVE ERA: 1960-1979

The 1960s through the 1970s were a time of great social consciousness in the United States. The Great Society of Lyndon B. Johnson and a tremendous amount of social legislation, from civil rights and women's rights issues to environmental concerns, were approved by Congress.

As the United States became more socially conscious during this period, the legislative activity and the acts began to include themes addressing culturally relevant issues. This was particularly true following the assassination of Dr. Martin Luther King in 1968. Rehabilitation legislation finally began to include language about social disadvantages and eventually became honest and bold enough to enumerate the needs of specific populations that had been largely ignored.

The **Vocational Rehabilitation Act Amendments of 1965** (Public Law 89-333) eliminated economic need as a prerequisite for vocational rehabilitation services. Services were expanded to include the socially disadvantage and behavior disorders such as juvenile offenders, adult public offenders, alcoholics, and drug abusers. Six-month evaluation and 18-month extended evaluation services to determine employment potential were established for persons with mental retardation and severe disability. Reader services for the blind and visually impaired and interpreter services for the deaf and hard of hearing were provided. Funds were provided to construct new centers, workshops, and residential accommodations for the mentally retarded; improve existing workshops and facilities to provide better job training, state-wide planning, and project development; and expand working relationships between public and voluntary agencies for vocational rehabilitation services and return to gainful employment for handicapped citizens. Professional training assistance in vocational rehabilitation was extended from 2 to 4 years. Finally, the Act created the National Commission on Architectural Barriers to enhance employment opportunities (McGowan & Porter, 1967).

Other legislation during this period included the **Social Security Amendments of 1965** (of the original Social Security Act of 1935) that targeted state vocational rehabilitation (VR) agencies to assure that insurance beneficiaries who are disabled receive vocational rehabilitation services. The **Vocational Rehabilitation Act Amendments of 1968** (Public Law 90-391) broadened eligibility criteria to include persons who are "socially disadvantaged" due to environmental deprivation, and provided for vocational evaluation and work adjustment programs.

The **Rehabilitation Act of 1973** (Public Law 93-112), which was a major overhaul of the original Vocational Rehabilitation Act of 1920 and its subsequent amendments, emphasized priority services to persons with severe disabilities, client's rights, the individualized written rehabilitation program (IWRP), annual reviews, accountability, post-employment services, the promotion of consumer involvement, and support for research and the advancement of civil rights for person with disabilities (Rehabilitation Act Amendments of 1986, p. 181011).

One of the landmark accomplishments of the 1973 Rehabilitation Act were the title V provisions to advance the *civil rights* of persons with disabilities. Persons with severe disabilities had been barred from *mainstreaming* into society mainly due to discrimination, and inaccessible housing and work sites. Sections 501, 502, 503, and 504 of the title enforced affirmative action, non-discrimination in employment, and accessibility in place of residence and work.

SECTION 501: Non-discrimination in hiring practices in the Federal government. It requires each Federal department and agency in the executive branch to submit an Affirmative Action Program plan to the U.S. Civil Service Commission for the hiring, placement, and advancement of workers with disabilities in Federal employment. Such public agency plans should act as a model for other private agencies, businesses, and industries to emulate. An Interagency Committee on Handicapped Employees was established to oversee the effective implementation of affirmative action plans, make reviews and updates annually, and provide sufficient assurances and commitment to the intent of section 501. The committee included the chairman of the Civil Service Commission, the Administrator of Veterans' Affairs, the Secretary of Labor, and the Secretary of Health, Education, and Welfare (now, the Department of Health and Human Resources and the Department of Education).

SECTION 502: Accessibility established the Architectural and Transportation Barriers Compliance Board (ATBCB) that modified the provisions of the Architectural Barriers Act of 1968 (Public Law 90-480), and its subsequent amendment of 1970 (Public Law 91-205). The major functions of the Board were to investigate alternative approaches to the architectural, transportation, and attitudinal barriers confronting the handicapped; determine measures to be taken by federal, state, and local governments and other public or non-profit agencies to eliminate transportation barriers or subsidize travel expenses for those unable to use mass transit to work; and determine the housing needs, availability, and accessibility to handicapped individuals. The Board was empowered to hold public hearings and conduct investigations of those not in compliance with the provisions of the Act, and to report the results and make administrative and legislative recommendations to Congress and to the President to eliminate barriers (Public Law 93-112, p. 36-37).

SECTION 503: Affirmative Action requires any contractor or subcontractor for a federal department or agency receiving in excess of $2,500 to take affirmative action to employ and advance the employment of qualified handicapped individuals. In addition, any contractor or subcontractor for the federal government receiving in excess of $50,000 or employing 50 or more people must develop a written affirmative action plan and submit it to the Employment Standards Administration of the Department of Labor. "Affirmative action under this program requires that qualified handicapped individuals be actively recruited, considered, and employed, and that all qualified handicapped employees not be discriminated against for promotions, training, transfers, and other job opportunities" (Thoben, 1975, p. 243-244). Persons with disabilities may not be discriminated against in employment on the basis of physical or mental handicaps, and may file complaints with the Department of Labor concerning contractors or subcontractors failing or refusing to comply with the provisions of their contracts.

SECTION 504: Nondiscrimination in programs or institutions receiving federal grants prohibits discrimination on the basis of physical or mental handicap, against otherwise qualified persons with disabilities, from participation in programs or institutions receiving federal financial assistance. Not only employers, but also educational and social services programs (such as vocational schools, training centers, rehabilitation facilities, work-study centers, work-activity centers, day care centers, hospitals, nursing homes, housing programs, transportation programs, school districts, and colleges and universities that receive grants or financial assistance from the federal government are expected to make "reasonable accommodation." Examples of such accommodations are, but are not limited to, the provision of reader services, Braille reading materials, talking books, talking calculators for the blind; large print material for the partially sighted; interpreter services for the deaf and hearing impaired; alternative test-taking procedures for persons with specific learning disabilities; accessibility to buildings, classrooms, and restrooms; designated parking facilities close to buildings; prevention of architectural barriers in new building construction and renovation of inaccessible buildings and facilities.

Employers' hiring criteria should be based on the actual skills required to perform the job, and refrain from artificial or superfluous requirements unrelated to job performance, designed to discriminate against persons with disabilities. Pre-employment tests unrelated to job tasks are forbidden. The implementation of alternative testing procedures is required for persons with specific learning disabilities, dyslexia, visual impairment, or other conditions that interfere with reading, writing, and taking tests. Physical and medical examinations will be allowed only if they are related to job performance and are required of other non-disabled individuals. Employers are required to make reasonable accommodations to create a receptive work environment by modifying work schedules; revising job descriptions; restructuring jobs; modifying equipment, devices, and the environment; and removing attitudinal barriers. Employers must make reasonable accommodations for employees with physical or mental limitations, unless employers demonstrate that making such accommodations would cause "undue hardship" in conducting the business. In cases where employment is denied due to disability and the employer failed to make reasonable accommodations, affected persons can file complaints with the nearest office of the employment Standards Administration of the Department of Labor (Department of Labor, 1975).

In summary, Sections 501 though 504 provided civil rights and employment rights for people who have disabilities. The major thrusts of these provisions are integration, mainstreaming, and holistic participation at all levels in society. These sections of the Rehabilitation Act of 1973 provide four major tools for rehabilitation counselors and placement specialists to use in enhancing client employment potential and the education of persons with respect to their civil rights.

A major amendment to the Rehabilitation Act of 1973 was the **Rehabilitation Comprehensive Services and Developmental Disabilities Amendments of 1978** (Public Law 95-602) that strengthened the existing provisions and expanded new services for persons with severe disabilities. *Section 130* of Title I and Part D of the act extended *vocational rehabilitation services to include members of American Indian tribes who are disabled and residing on or around reservations and trust lands*. It authorized the Rehabilitation Services Administration (RSA) to offer competitive grants to the governing bodies of federal and state recognized American Indian tribes for the establishment of vocational rehabilitation programs. These programs were designed to act as a supplement to the state-federal vocational rehabilitation agencies so that American Indian consumers can receive culturally appropriate services (e.g., ceremonial healing) on the reservation. The Navajo Vocational Rehabilitation Program was the first one to be funded (Guy, 1991).

The act also established the National Institute of Handicapped Research (now, the *National Institute on Disability and Rehabilitation Research*) to promote and coordinate research activities that enhance the quality of life for persons with disabilities. It established an *Integrating Committee on Handicapped Research* to avoid duplications and promote coordination and cooperation in Federal departments and agencies conducting rehabilitation research, and established the National Council on the Handicapped (now, *National Council on Disability*) to increase consumer involvement in the rehabilitation movement. Consumer involvement was further strengthened by reconstituting and expanding the Architectural and Transportation Barriers Act.

Persons with disabilities have received attention from the federal government in over 200 pieces of legislation. Past legislation, however, tended to be of intent only and provided for minimal services, often in highly segregated settings. The 1970s, however, saw renewed attention focused on the rights of adults and children with disabilities. The principle that all persons, even if unequal in abilities, should be granted equal opportunities found implementation in another important piece of legislation, the **Education for All Handicapped Children Act** of 1975 (renamed **Individuals with Disabilities Education Act in** Public Law 94-142). This act, together with the Rehabilitation Act of 1973, provided the mechanism to assure that children and adults with disabilities are given a chance to be integrated into American society in the least restrictive manner possible. The right to a free and appropriate public education was mandated by this act (Jenkins, 1980).

In 1979, for effective management, the Carter administration reorganized the U. S. Department of Health, Education, and Welfare (DHEW) into the Department of Health and Human Resources (DHHR) and the Department of Education (DOE). An **Office of Special Education and Rehabilitative Services** (OSERS) was created under the U. S. Department of Education. The **Rehabilitation Services Administration** (RSA) administers the Rehabilitation Acts, and the **Office of Special Education Programs** (OSEP) administers grants for special services and education for children with disability. Both agencies are now administered by an Assistant Secretary of OSERS, resulting in programs for persons with disabilities becoming more closely linked.

THE 1980s AND BEYOND

The 1980s began with inflation and recession. While the fully functional worker had more than enough to do to keep up with double-digit inflation and was lucky to keep a job in those times of recession, the person with a disability was at a tremendous disadvantage when trying to work and make a decent living. Many rehabilitationists were concerned about the political conservatism that swept the United States, beginning with California's "Proposition 13," through the presidencies of Ronald Reagan and George H. W. Bush. At this time, Bowe (1985) found disability to be more common in black adults than it is among whites and Hispanics; blacks must confront discrimination on the basis of race as well as disability; and black adults with work disabilities are much less likely to be employed as professional or managerial workers than are other disabled individuals.

The **Rehabilitation Amendments of 1984** (Public Law 98-221) reauthorized the earlier provisions through 1986, reemphasizing the activities of the National Institute of Handicapped Research (NIHR) and the National Council on the Handicapped (NCOH). The NIHR was authorized to establish a program of pediatric rehabilitation research; a research and training center in the Pacific Basin; and demonstration projects for persons with spinal cord injuries. NIHR was also authorized to conduct projects to provide job training, on-the-job training, job search assistance, job development, work site modification using the latest technology, and follow-up services for youth having disabilities entering the labor force.

The National Council on the Handicapped became an independent agency, and no longer an agency of the Department of Education. The Council was given added responsibility to promote full integration of individuals with disabilities in all walks of life and to study the process of eliminating disincentives in federal programs and increasing incentives, thus allowing persons with disabilities to become more productive members of society.

The 1984 amendment assured that consumers with disabilities would receive rehabilitation services from qualified rehabilitation professionals. The National Council on Rehabilitation Education defines the qualified rehabilitation professional as (Graves, Coffey, Habeck, & Stude, 1987):

> an individual who has received an academic degree from an accredited education program accepted by the rehabilitation profession as denoting professional status; is certified and/or licensed to practice in accordance with the rehabilitation profession's national certification board or commission and/or the state's licensing board; maintains her or his certification and/or licensure by completing continuing education units approved by the certification/licensure boards for renewal of certification/licensure; and has completed the amount of time on the job specified by the profession as denoting achievement of journeyman status.

p.5-6

The Rehabilitation Act Amendments of 1986 (Public Law 99-506) extended and improved the Rehabilitation Act of 1973 and authorized appropriations for 1986-1991. The amendment used gender-neutral terminology, changing the language to convey a positive attitude and the functional aspects of disability. For example, the phrase "handicapped individual" was replaced with "individual with handicaps," and "a handicapped individual" with "an individual with handicaps." The "National Institute of Handicapped Research" became the **National Institute on Disability and Rehabilitation Research** (NIDRR). In 1988, the "National Council on the Handicapped" was renamed The **National Council on Disability** (NCD), and the "President's Committee on the Employment of the Handicapped" became the **President's Committee on the Employment of People with Disabilities** (PCPED). It is imperative that words reflect positive attitudes, convey functional aspects of the person, and create an image of ability and independence, which helps placement counselors facilitate placement of their clients.

New provisions were added in the development of IWRP to include statements of determination of employability; long-range rehabilitation goals and intermediate objectives, based on an evaluation of rehabilitation potential; rehabilitation engineering services, when appropriate, to achieve rehabilitation goals and objectives; an evaluation procedure and schedule to determine whether such goals and objectives are met; an assessment of the need for post-employment services prior to case closure; annual review and revision as needed; and description of the availability of Client Assistance Programs.

The same Act added a number of responsibilities to NIDRR, including disseminating information to Indian tribes and conducting studies of the rehabilitation needs of Indians. Other responsibilities included establishing a center for research and training concerning the delivery of rehabilitation services to rural areas; reporting to Congress on the development and distribution of cost-effective technological devices for persons with disabilities; studying health insurance practices and policies affecting persons with disabilities; authorizing grants for studies and analyses related to supported employment; demonstrating and disseminating innovative models for the delivery of cost-effective rehabilitation engineering services to assist in meeting the employment and independent living needs of individuals with severe handicaps in rural and urban areas; establishing two rehabilitation engineering centers, one in Connecticut and one in South Carolina, to demonstrate and disseminate innovative models to assist in meeting the needs of, and addressing the barriers confronted by, individuals with handicaps; and conducting research relating to children with disabilities and individuals 60 and over (55 for Indians) with disabilities. Finally, to carry out joint projects, the National Institute of Mental Health was added to the list of agencies.

The purpose statement of the National Council on Disability was amended to include "promot[ing] the full integration, independence, and productivity of handicapped individuals in the community, schools, the work place and all other aspects of American life" (p. 1828). The duties of the Council were expanded to include review and evaluation of all statutes pertaining to Federal programs that assist individuals with disabilities and to assess the extent to which these policies, programs, and activities provide incentives or disincentives to the establishment of community-based services for individuals with disabilities promoting integration and independence in the community, in schools, and in the work place.

SERVICES FOR INDEPENDENT LIVING

The act requires each state to establish an Independent Living Council to provide guidance in developing and expanding independent living programs, including recreational services (Jones, 1986), on a statewide basis through state agencies and local entities. Members of the Council are appointed by the state agency director and include representatives of state and local agencies, groups, persons with disabilities, parents, and guardians of individuals with disabilities, directors of independent living centers, private businesses, and other appropriate individuals or organizations. The majority of each Council membership tends to be individuals with disabilities, including parents and guardians of persons with disabilities. Recreational services were added to the list of possible services that may be provided by the Centers for Independent Living (Jones, 1986).

In summary, the changes in the Rehabilitation Act Amendments of 1986 have had significant impact on the delivery of services and outcomes in the rehabilitation of persons with severe handicaps. Previously, the functional aspects of severe handicapping conditions had been overemphasized in language and in the provision of services made for supported employment. Transitional employment and part-time employment are now considered viable outcomes of rehabilitation services.

THE AMERICANS WITH DISABILITIES ACT

The landmark legislation, the **Americans With Disabilities Act** (ADA), Public Law 101-336 signed by President George H. W. Bush on July 26, 1990, ushered in "another Independence Day" and "a bright new era of equality, independence, and freedom" for 43 million Americans (17% of the U. S. population) with disabilities. The ADA is patterned after Section 504 of the 1973 Rehabilitation Act and the Civil Rights Act of 1964. The ADA is one of the most comprehensive civil rights laws ever enacted and has made sweeping changes in every sphere of life for persons both with and without disabilities.

The Act may be viewed as central to achieving equity and equal opportunity for African Americans with disabilities (Alston, Russo, & Miles, 1994). The five major provisions in the ADA prohibit discrimination against people with disabilities in Employment, Public Service and Transportation, Public Accommodations, Telecommunication Relay Services for the Deaf, and Activities of State and Local Governments.

TITLE I: EMPLOYMENT—prohibits discrimination in hiring, employing, promoting, and training qualified workers with disabilities and requires reasonable accommodation, if it does not result in undue hardship to employers. The following terms in the statement require further explanations:

Qualified means an individual with a disability who, with or without reasonable accommodation, can perform the essential functions of the job held or sought. Consideration is given to the employer's judgment about which functions of a job are essential. The employer's written job description prior to advertising and recruiting applicants is considered evidence of the essential functions of the job.

Medical examination and inquiries: Pre-employment medical examinations can be required if they apply to all entering new employees to determine the ability to perform job-related functions, and only after an offer of employment has been made to the applicant. The employer should not conduct a medical examination or make inquiries about the type, nature, or severity of disability until after the offer of employment. Results of the medical examinations and disability information must be kept confidential and in separate medical files.

Reasonable accommodation may include making existing facilities readily accessible; job restructuring; modifying work schedules; reassignment to a vacant position; acquiring or modifying equipment or devices; adjusting or modifying examinations, training materials, or policies; providing readers for persons who are visually impaired or interpreters for persons who are hearing impaired.

Undue hardship means significant difficulty or expense to the employer in making reasonable accommodation. The following factors are considered in determining undue hardship to employers: the nature and cost of accommodation; the overall size, type, and financial resources of the facility; the overall size of the business, in terms of number of employees and number of facilities; and the employer's type of operation, including composition, structure, and function of its workforce, and geographic separations.

Employers are not obligated to hire employees who pose a direct threat to the health or safety of other individuals in the workplace. Drug testing is permitted and will not be considered a medical examination. The law does not protect current illegal drug users and alcoholics who cannot safely perform their job functions. Protection is provided to those who are, or have been, participating in a supervised rehabilitation program. People who are HIV-positive, have AIDS, or have other infectious and communicable diseases are protected. However, employers may transfer or reassign employees from food-handling jobs if the danger to possible health and safety cannot be eliminated by reasonable accommodation (Gamble, 1990). In 1991, the Secretary of Health and Human Services published a list of infectious diseases that are transmitted through handling foods.

TITLE II: PUBLIC SERVICES AND PUBLIC TRANSPORTATION—prohibits discrimination from participation in services, programs, or activities of any public entity. The majority of the provisions of this title emphasize public transportation systems available to the general public, such as bus, train, taxi, and limousine. This excludes air travel, which is covered by the Air Carriers Act. New buses, rail cars, or other passenger-transporting vehicles purchased or leased by public entities, as well as remanufactured public transport vehicles, must be accessible and useable by people with disabilities, including wheelchair users. A public entity operating a fixed route system must provide para-transit or other special transportation services to individuals with disabilities that are comparable in service level and response time, without imposing an undue financial burden. Existing rail systems must have one accessible car per train. For wheelchair users, there must be space to park and secure wheelchair, transfer to seat, and fold wheelchair. Existing "key stations," and alterations to them, must be accessible. New bus and rail stations in intercity rail and commuter rail systems must be made accessible within two years of the date of enactment. Two-thirds of the key stations must be made accessible within 20 years. If expensive structural changes are required, then extension may be granted up to 30 years. Individuals may file complaints about violations with the Department of Transportation and bring private lawsuits (National Council on Disability, 1990; U. S. Department of Justice, no date).

TITLE III: PUBLIC ACCOMMODATIONS AND SERVICES OPERATED BY PRIVATE ENTITIES —the major focus of this title is mainstreaming, integration, and fuller participation in all walks of life in the society. The title prohibits discrimination on the basis of disability in the full and equal enjoyment of the goods, services, facilities, privileges, advantages, or accommodations of any place of public accommodation and services operated by private entities. Goods, services, facilities, and privileges must be provided in the most integrated settings appropriate to the needs of the individual. Private clubs and religious organizations are exempted, however. Private entities providing transportation services (bus, rail, or any other conveyance excluding aircraft) must be accessible so that people with disabilities receive services equivalent to people without disabilities. All new vehicles purchased or leased must be accessible in fixed route system if they carry more than 16 passengers including the driver. Operators of public accommodation may not impose application of eligibility criteria that screen out, or tend to screen out, individuals with disabilities from full and equal enjoyment of goods, services, facilities, privileges, advantages, or accommodations. Auxiliary aids, such as readers, interpreters, taped texts, or similar services, must be provided to individuals who are vision or hearing impaired. Other individuals with disabilities must be given an equal opportunity to participate or benefit as do the non-disabled, unless such would result in an undue burden. All new construction and alterations in public accommodations and commercial facilities must be accessible. It is discriminatory to fail to remove architectural and communication barriers in existing facilities, or transportation barriers in existing vehicles and rail passenger cars, if the modification is readily achievable.

TITLE IV: TELECOMMUNICATIONS—This title amended Title II of the Communications Act of 1934 and added requirements that telephone companies must provide telecommunication relay services for hearing impaired and speech impaired individuals who use TDD (Telecommunication Device for the Deaf) or other non-voice terminal devices. Both interstate and intrastate telecommunication relay services must be available 24 hours and charges should not be greater than the charges paid for functionally equivalent voice communication services with regard to the day, time, duration, place, and distance called. The law prohibits the relay operators from keeping records and/or disclosing relayed conversations, altering, refusing, or limiting the length of calls. The title also requires that television public service announcements produced or funded by federal agencies be closed-captioned.

TITLE V: MISCELLANEOUS PROVISIONS—This title explains the relationship to other laws; prohibits state immunity; deals with insurance coverage; delineates implementation procedures and enforcement authorities; and provides congressional inclusion and dispute resolution. The ADA does not minimize the standard of the Rehabilitation Act of 1973 and its subsequent amendments, or invalidate any state or local laws in providing equal protection to persons with disabilities. States are not immune from violation of this Act and are subjected to the same remedies as are available to any public or private entity. Insurers may not refuse, continue to underwrite, classify, and administer risks consistent with state laws. Retaliation is prohibited against an individual who has made a charge, testified, assisted, or participated in an investigation, proceeding or hearing under this Act. Interference, coercion, or intimidation against an individual's exercising his/her rights, or encouraging others to exercise his/her rights, is also prohibited. According to the ADA, homosexuality and bisexuality are not impairments, hence not disabilities. The definition of disability does not include transvestism, transsexualism, pedophilia, exhibitionism, voyeurism, gender identity disorders not resulting from physical impairments, or other sexual behavior disorders; compulsive gambling, kleptomania, or pyromania; or psychoactive substance use disorders resulting from current illegal use of drugs. The Senate, the House of Representatives, and the agencies of the legislative branch are prohibited from discrimination in hiring, discharging, promotion, compensation, or privileges of employment on the basis of age, color, race, national origin, sex, religion, or physical handicap. The ADA encourages voluntary/alternative means of dispute resolution, including settlement negotiations, conciliations, facilitation, mediation, fact finding, mini trials, and arbitration.

The **Individuals with Disabilities Education Act (IDEA**: Public Law 101-46) reauthorized and renamed the Education for All Handicapped Children Act of 1975 (previously discussed). Although revisions were made in both 1990 and 1991, the first significant changes to IDEA since its inception in 1975 occurred in 1997. Not only was IDEA reauthorized in 1997, but also changes were enacted to strengthen the bill. Parental involvement in eligibility and placement decisions and inclusion of children with disabilities into the general classroom and curriculum, which is to be emphasized in the IEP, were increased; local and state assessments were insured; transition planning for teenagers, starting at the age of 14, became a focus; the use of mediation over litigation for disputes between parents and educators was emphasized; and safety and learning environment conditions were emphasized.

IDEA was reauthorized in 2004 (Public Law 108-446). Under these most recent revisions, IDEA has been closely aligned with the No Child Left Behind Act (NCLB) and now includes new standards to ensure accountability and equity in education. The act addresses the need for clearly defined measurable goals for the IEP, and for progress reports on these goals to be made quarterly to parents; a greater need to focus on establishing educational practices that are based on peer-reviewed research; the manner in which learning disabilities are to be defined, releasing schools from earlier provisions in which the child must demonstrate a significant difference between intellectual ability and achievement in order for a learning disability to be diagnosed; parental rights to initiate requests for evaluation. It strengthened previous provisions that precluded educators from classifying a child as disabled if it was determined that the child's educational difficulties were a result of inappropriate instruction as identified in the NCLB act.

In addition to these changes, one of the most significant revisions to the 2004 IDEA, in terms of minorities, concerned the overrepresentation of minority students in special education classes. By the 2004 revisions, it had become clear that, in some cases, students were being inappropriately assigned to special education classes largely based upon racial or ethnic criteria (Boehner & Castle, 2005). Congress mandated that states and schools take positive action to ensure that this practice is eliminated. States are now required to develop specific policies that address this issue, and collect and report data on the presence of minority students in special education classes. This revision went so far as to potentially require educators to use early intervention funds to address the overrepresentation of minorities.

Technology-Related Assistance for Individuals with Disabilities Act Amendments (Tech Act: Public Law 103-218) updated the 1988 Tech Act (Public Law 100-407), authorized the **National Institute on Disability and Rehabilitation Research (NIDRR)** to fund initiatives in each of the 50 states and U.S. territories that would result in the delivery of assistive technology (AT) services and devices to individuals with disabilities. Toward this end, states and territories are provided federal grants to develop programs such as equipment loan libraries and information resources necessary to meet any of the primary goals of the Tech Act (Day & Edwards, 1996). These goals include providing greater access to AT by individuals with disabilities, addressing AT funding, increasing consumer involvement, coordinating activities among the various state agencies, overcoming barriers for timely delivery of services, increasing advocacy for AT services and programs, and reaching out to underrepresented individuals.

In line with this last goal, the 1994 revisions of the Tech Act specifically address the funding and recruitment of minority service providers and institutions. Grant and contract agencies or organizations must now demonstrate that they have a specific strategy to recruit and train individuals with disabilities and/or minority group members who will then provide technology-related assistance. A portion of the grants provided under the Tech Act are reserved for historically Black colleges and other universities whose minority student enrollment is at least 50%. As a criterion for receiving federal grants, state "lead" agencies must demonstrate an ability to implement "effective strategies for capacity building, staff and consumer training, and enhancement of access to funding for assistive technology devices and assistive technology services across agencies" (Public Law 103-218, section 102).

The **Rehabilitation Act Amendments of 1992** (Public Law 102-569) updated and revised the previous Rehabilitation Act of 1973 and made significant changes to the manner in which rehabilitative services are provided

(Button, 1993). The impetus for such changes directly developed out of the ADA of 1990 and focused on providing a vehicle for helping individuals with disabilities gain more choice and assistance in finding and maintaining meaningful employment and full integration into the workforce and community.

In line with the ADA, the Rehabilitation Act Amendments of 1992 clearly articulate that disability is a "natural part of the human experience" and should in no way diminish the rights of disabled individuals in any aspect of their life (Button, 1993). Furthermore, the 1992 amendments highlighted the changing perception of disabilities, from that of un-abled to one of presumed ability. In other words, the bill is predicated on the idea that irrespective of the severity of disability, individuals can achieve meaningful employment and integration, provided the appropriate services and supports are supplied.

The overriding effect of such a change essentially switched the burden of proof from the individual to the rehabilitative system, so that in order to deny services, vocational rehabilitative services had to convincingly demonstrate that an individual is incapable of gaining any benefit from vocational services. In addition, the amendments placed considerable focus on rehabilitative technology and disability representation in the vocational rehabilitative process.

REHABILITATION CAPACITY BUILDING

In recognition of the disproportionate distribution of disabilities, pattern of inequitable treatment, and quality of vocational rehabilitation outcomes of culturally diverse groups reported by contemporary research (Atkins & Wright, 1980; Danek & Lawrence, 1982; Rivera, 1974; Rehabilitation Services Administration, 1993), Section 21 of the 1992 Amendments was promulgated as one of the most powerful pieces of legislation of the 1990s. This legislation represented the first concerted effort to address *the concept of cultural diversity in rehabilitation.* It set aside 1% of all the funds appropriated for programs authorized under titles II, III, VI, and VII, to conduct minority outreach programs and capacity enhancement. Section 21 provided several modalities for addressing the above exigency: (1) funds were provided to minority entities and American Indian tribes for the conduct of research, training, technical assistance, or related activities geared to improve services to minorities, (2) state-federal vocational rehabilitation must focus on recruiting professionals from diverse backgrounds, (3) the Rehabilitation Services Administration (RSA) must provide scholarships to prepare students in vocational rehabilitation and related service careers at the bachelor's, master's, and doctoral levels at minority institutions of higher education, i.e., Historically Black Colleges and Universities (HBCUs), Hispanic Serving Institutions

(HSIs), Tribal Colleges and Universities (TCUs), and other institutions with at least 50% minority enrollment, and (4) the Commissioner of RSA shall develop a plan to provide capacity building and outreach services in order to increase the participation of minority entities in competition for grants, contracts, and cooperative agreements.

Section 21 paved the way for the preparation of qualified rehabilitation counselors of culturally diverse backgrounds, and the enhanced provision of quality services to minorities leading to long-term employment outcome. As a direct result, the number of bachelor's and master's level programs in minority institutions increased from a mere 9 in the early 1990s (Kundu & Dutta, 1995; Kundu & Dutta, 2000) to about 30 in 2006. Despite significant improvements in the participation of culturally diverse groups in vocational rehabilitation, a study of 4,710 state-federal professionals found that 70% were Caucasians, 16% have documented disabilities, about 34% had degrees in rehabilitation, and only 10% were Certified Rehabilitation Counselors (CRCs) (Kundu, Dutta, & Walker, 2006). It is imperative, therefore, that continued and intensive federal efforts are provided for introducing minorities in the mainstream of vocational rehabilitation.

National Institute on Disability and Rehabilitation Research (NIDRR) has taken steps to implement multidimensional aspects of capacity building philosophy in incorporating its Long Range Plans (1999-2004 and 2005-2009) at individual and systems or organizational levels. The scope of its capacity building activities has been expanded to (a) provide advanced training in disability research (both qualitative and quantitative methodologies) for scientists, those with disabilities, and minorities; (b) train at the pre-service, graduate, and in-service levels in application of research findings to improve the quality of lives for people with disabilities; (c) develop capacity of researchers to conduct investigations focusing on the new paradigm as a contextual phenomenon, i.e., disability should be viewed as a function of the interaction between impairments and other personal characteristics and the larger physical, social, and policy environments; (d) train the researchers to conduct holistic and interdisciplinary studies on cultural context of disability; (e) develop capacity of the researchers to conduct studies at homes, work places, schools, recreational facilities, and community support programs; (f) train consumers and family members to be involved in the Participatory Research and become advocate for review, evaluation, interpretation, and dissemination of research findings; and (g) strengthen research portfolio by increasing the partnerships with federal and non-federal research and development agencies. The above objectives are being implemented through Rehabilitation Research and Training Centers (RRTCs), Advanced

Rehabilitation Research Training Centers (ARRTCs), Mary Switzer Fellowships, New Scholars Program, Minority Enhancement Programs, and Disability Rehabilitation Research Projects (DRRPs) (Federal Register 1998 & 2006).

The **School to Work Opportunities Act of 1994 (STWOA**: Public Law 103-329) was created to assist students in making the transition from school to the workforce. In essence, the goal of STWOA is to increase education and career opportunities by promoting business and education collaboration. Federal venture capital grants are provided to state and local agencies to help restructure educational systems, and to establish school-to-work systems. Although there are a variety of grants available under STWOA, all school-to-work systems must include school-based learning that includes career counseling and career major exploration; work-based learning that includes job training, workplace mentoring, paid work experience, or instruction in workplace competencies; and connecting activities that incorporate both employers and educators, which not only can include matching students to job-based training, but also specialized training for those participating in the program (i.e. educators, counselors, work-place mentors).

The act makes explicit mention of students with disabilities, minority students, and women, with a focus on increasing work place opportunities that would be considered outside of those traditional for gender, race, or disability. STWOA also provides specific funding for technical assistance, capacity building, outreach, and research and evaluation.

The **Health Insurance Portability and Accountability Act of 1996** (HIPAA: Public Law 104-191) was established to increase health care access and security. The most widely recognized components of HIPAA revolve around the privacy and security standards enacted by the bill. HIPAA's privacy rule created more stringent standards for the sharing and release of patient medical records. More specifically, HIPAA addressed the need for client consent before releasing information, the need for separate authorization for non-routine disclosures, the right of the patient to request a disclosure history, client access to their own medical records, limits of how information can be shared, standards that require the sharing of only the minimal amount of information necessary, and accountability and establishment of penalties for mishandling patient information.

As important as its security and privacy aspects, HIPAA also focused on improving access to health care through its patient protection and portability standards. HIPAA set new rules governing pre-existing conditions, discrimination based on health-status related factors, the creation of special enrollment privileges, and the purchasing clout of individuals and small companies (U.S. Department of Labor, 2004). In an effort to reduce the rising administrative cost of medical care, HIPAA established national standards for electronic health care transactions to process claims and share information (U.S. Department of Health and Human Services, 2003). Combined, HIPAA's standards have been purported to increase the quality of patient care by ensuring increased security and accessibility, while at the same time lowering costs by establishing unified processing standards.

The **Workforce Investment Act** (WIA: Public Law 105-220). The Workforce Investment Act of 1998 consolidated a variety of employment and training programs into cooperative statewide systems. WIA supersedes the Job Training Partnership Act and subsumes the Rehabilitation Act. The ultimate aim of WIA is to promote employment, job retention, and increased earning potential (Employment Development Department, no date) by providing a wide range of workforce development activities and services. These services include, but are not limited to, basic skills assessments; advice, counseling, and support that includes access to labor market information, job search tools, and educational resources and guidance; literacy training; skills training; leadership development; job mentoring and workplace exposure; unemployment assistance; and on-the-job training programs.

In addition, WIA aims to connect the community, employers, and the workforce, and provides measures that allow local employers increased influence over local employment policies. In this manner, WIA serves job seekers, the unemployed, youth, incumbent workers, new entrants, veterans, individuals with disabilities, employers, and the community as a whole.

A significant portion of WIA is the Rehabilitation Act Amendments of 1998. These amendments focus on increasing consumer choice by mandating that consumers are provided with information and support services that allow them to make informed decisions throughout the VR process; linking services together under umbrella systems (such as staff training sessions, technical assistance, telephone hotlines), and forming cooperative arrangements between VR agencies and other public agencies to provide more efficient services; providing individuals with disabilities access to electronic and information technologies to the level of access afforded those without disabilities; and assisting educational institutions in identifying and implementing, including fiscal support, transitional programs and services for those with disabilities.

The Rehabilitation Act also renamed the State Rehabilitation Advisory Council to the State Rehabilitation Council, renamed the Individualized Written Rehabilitation Program to the Individual Plan for Employment, and relabeled individuals with the most severe disabilities.

An important part of WIA, and the subsumed Rehabilitation Act Amendments of 1998, is its focus on minority employees and groups. As outlined in the bill, WIA mandates specific funds for programs that address American Indian and migrant worker needs. In line with the basic tenets of WIA, programs for these minority populations focus on devolving academic, occupational, and literacy skills to make these populations more competitive. WIA established the **Native American Employment and Training Council** and set aside specific money for migrant worker services that provide for English language training, worker safety training, housing, support services, dropout prevention, and follow up services.

WIA also specially addressed the racial inequities found within the vocational rehabilitation system. The Rehabilitative Act Amendments of 1998 states:

> Patterns of inequitable treatment of minorities have been documented in all major junctures of the vocational rehabilitation process. As compared to white Americans, a larger percentage of African-American applicants to the vocational rehabilitation system are denied acceptance. Of applicants accepted for service, a larger percentage of African-Americans' cases are closed without being rehabilitated. Minorities are provided less training than their white counterparts. Consequently, less money is spent on minorities than on their white counterparts.

WIA provisions, therefore, highlight minority recruitment and outreach needs.

Section 121 (changed from Section 130) of Title I and Part C re-authorized RSA to make grants for the establishment of American Indian Vocational Rehabilitation Service projects for the provision of services to American Indians and Alaska Natives with disabilities. With assistance from RSA funded rehabilitation capacity building projects, the number of Section 121 projects has increased from 14 in 1991 (Guy, 1991) to 76 in 2006, located in 23 states. The states of Oklahoma and Alaska have the highest number of Section 121 programs at this time.

The **Ticket to Work and Work Incentives Improvement Act** (TWWIIA: Public Law 106-170). This Act was signed into law by President Bill Clinton in 1999 as a means of removing Social Security and Medicare/Medicaid disincentives to employment (WorkWorld, 2006). Specifically, TWWIIA expanded Medicare and Medicaid coverage for those with disabilities by extending premium-free coverage for most disability beneficiaries who are employed, by permitting certain working individuals to purchase Medicaid coverage, and facilitating the Medicaid and Medicare reinstatement process.

In addition, TWWIIA established the Ticket to Work and Self-Sufficiency Program. Under this program, individuals with a disability are provided with a "ticket," with which they can obtain vocational rehabilitation services and support services from an employment network of their choice. In this way, TWWIIA, as with previous legislation, focused on consumer empowerment by allowing the beneficiary more choice in the VR services that they obtain.

IMPLICATIONS

The essence of all rehabilitation efforts is to gain independence, improve quality of life, mainstream into the society, earn a full economic wage, and empower consumers with disabilities to exercise their rights. Therefore, it is imperative that rehabilitation professionals be familiar with all legislation in rehabilitation and related fields. Besides federal laws and state-federal programs, each state may have special state and local laws, enactments, service provisions and facilities for citizens with disabilities. Familiarity with such local provisions will help immensely in the quest to become an effective counselor or placement specialist in directing, guiding, and efficient placing of clients in jobs in greater numbers.

Throughout this chapter, emphasis has been placed on civilian vocational rehabilitation acts and amendments over the last 80 years for individuals with physical and mental impairments in general. However, future rehabilitation counselors, placement specialists, and students need to become familiar with the laws, acts, and amendments related to specialized populations, such as persons who are blind and visually impaired, deaf and hearing impaired, developmentally disabled, veterans, and the aged.

The need to find jobs for individuals with disabilities in the future will increase rather than decrease in importance. Vocational rehabilitation, as has been pointed out, is not a social welfare program. It is a cost-effective program that places or returns people with disabilities to the world of work. When people work, their tax dollars return to the government coffers.

The emphasis in the future will be on each American doing his/her share; contributing and working to overcome inflation and recession. There is a greater necessity for rehabilitation counselors, placement specialists, and other professionals to help people with disabilities find jobs than in the last century. Only in this way can individuals who are disabled do their share and become fully functional working Americans. This chapter has attempted to identify some of the significant sociopolitical trends and legislative provisions impacting the quality outcomes for people with disabilities. The following chapters will investigate other relevant issues and provide a holistic overview and understanding of the unique field of rehabilitation.

REFERENCES

Alston, R. J., Russo, C. J., & Miles, A. S. (1994). Brown v. Board of Education and the Americans with Disabilities Act: Vistas of equal educational opportunities for African Americans. *The Journal of Negro Education, 63*(3), 349-357.

Atkins, B. J., & Wright, G. N. (1980). Vocational rehabilitation of Blacks. *Journal of Rehabilitation, 46*, 42-46.

Bitter, J. A. (1979). *Introduction to rehabilitation.* St. Louis: C. V. Mosby.

Blackwell, H. (October 27, 1945). To NAACP Secretary of Veterans Affairs, NAACP Papers, Manuscript Division, Library of Congress, Washington, D.C.

Boehner, J., & Castle, M. (2005). Individuals with Disabilities Education Act (IDEA): Guide to "Frequently asked questions." Committee on Education and the Workforce. Retrieved April 11, 2006, from http://www.house.gov/ed_workforce/issues/109th/education/idea/ideafaq.pdf

Bowe, F. (1985). *Black adults with disabilities: A statistical report drawn from Census Bureau data.* President's Committee on Employment of the Handicapped.

Button, C. (1993). Reauthorized Rehabilitation Act increases access to assistive technology. *A.T. Quarterly, 4.* Retrieved April 11, 2006, from http://www.resna.org/taproject/library/atq/rehbact.htm

Danek, M. M., & Lawrence, R. E. (1982). Client-counselor racial similarity and rehabilitation outcomes. *Journal of Rehabilitation, 48*(3), 54-58.

Day, S. L., & Edwards, B. J. (1996). Assistive technology for postsecondary students with learning disabilities. *Journal of Learning Disabilities, 29,* 486-492.

Department of Labor. (1975). Affirmative action obligations of contractors and subcontractors for handicapped workers. Employment Standards Administration. *Federal Register, 40*(169).

Federal Register. (1998). National Institute on Disability and Rehabilitation Research; Notice of Proposed Long-Range Plan for Fiscal Years 1999-2004, *63*(206), 57215-57218. Washington, DC: US Government.

Federal Register. (2006). National Institute on Disability and Rehabilitation Research; Notice of Proposed Long-Range Plan for Fiscal Years 2005-2009, *71*(31), 8192-8194. Washington, DC: US Government.

Gamble, B. S. (1990). *Analysis and Reports.* Washington, DC: Bureau of National Affairs, 138(C1 through C4).

Graves, W. H., Coffey, D. D., Habeck, R., & Stude, E. W. (1978). NCRE Position Paper: Definition of the Qualified Rehabilitation Professional. *Rehabilitation Education, 1*(1), 5-6.

Guy, E. (1991). Vocational rehabilitation services for American Indians. *OSERS News in Print. 3*, 10-15.

Jefferson, R. F. (2003). "Enabled courage": Race, disability, and Black World War II veterans in postwar America. *Historian, 65*(5), 1102-1124.

Jenkins, W. M. (1980). History and legislation of the rehabilitation movement. In R. Parker and C. Hansen (Eds.), *Rehabilitation Counseling.* Boston: Allyn and Bacon.

Jones, A. (1986). *Detailed Survey of the Rehabilitation Amendments of 1986, Public Law 97-506.* Dunbar, WV: West Virginia Research and Training Center.

Kundu, M. M., Dutta, A., & Walker, S. (2006). Participation of Ethnically Diverse Personnel in State-Federal Vocational Rehabilitation Agencies. *Journal of Applied Rehabilitation Counseling, 17*(1), 30-36.

Kundu, M. M., & Dutta, A. (2000). Rehabilitation capacity building project Inclusion, empowerment, and integration. *Rehabilitation Education, 14*(4), 345-357.

Kundu, M. M., & Dutta, A. (1995). Implementation of rehabilitation counselor training programs at Historically Black Colleges and Universities. *Disability and Diversity: New Leadership for a New Era* (pp. 45-52). Washington, D.C.: The President's Committee on Employment of People with Disabilities and Howard University Research and Training Center.

Lee , J. C. (October 27, 1948). To NAACP Executive Secretary Walter White, Group II, Box G 18, VA Hospital Discrimination, 1945-1948, Veterans Affairs File, 1940-1950, NAACP Papers, Manuscript Division, Library of Congress, Washington, D.C.

McGowan J., & Porter, T. (1967). *An introduction to the vocational rehabilitation process.* Washington, DC: U.S. Department of Health, Education and Welfare, Vocational Rehabilitation Archives.

National Council on Disability. (1990). *The Americans with Disabilities Act.* Washington, DC: Author.

Oberman, C. E. (1965). *A history of vocational rehabilitation in America.* Minneapolis: T. S. Deurson & Co., Inc.

Rehabilitation Act of 1973, Public Law 93-112. (1973). Washington, DC: U. S. Government.

Rehabilitation Act Amendments of 1984, Public Law 83-565. (1984). Washington, DC: U.S. Government.

Rehabilitation Act Amendments of 1986, Public Law 99-506. (1986). Washington, DC: U. S. Government.

Rehabilitation Comprehensive Services and Developmental Disabilities Act Amendments of 1978, Public Law 95-602. (1978). Washington, DC:U. S. Government.

Rehabilitation Services Administration. (1993). *Training on 1992 Amendments to the Rehabilitation Act*. Washington, DC: U.S. Department of Education.

Rivera, O. A. (1974). Vocational rehabilitation of disabled Hispanics (Doctoral dissertation, University of Utah). *Dissertation Abstracts International, 35*(4-A), 2059-2060A.

The Americans With Disabilities Act of 1990, Public Law 101-336. Washington, DC: U. S. Government.

Thoben, P. J. (1975). Civil rights and employment of the severely handicapped. *Rehabilitation Counseling Bulletin, 18(4),* 240-244.

U. S. Department of Justice. (no date). *Americans with Disabilities Act, Requirements in Public Accommodations Fact Sheet*. Washington, DC: Author.

U. S. Department of Health and Human Services. (2003). *Administrative simplification under HIPAA: National standards for transactions, privacy, and security*. Retrieved April 12, 2006, from http://www.hhs.gov/news/press/2002pres/hipaa.html

U. S. Department of Labor. (December, 2004). The Health and Insurance Portability and Accountability Act (HIPAA). Retrieved April 12, 2006, from http://www.dol.gov/ebsa/newsroom/fshipaa.html

Wilkerson, D. A., & Penn, L. A. (1938). The participation of Negroes in the federally-aided program of civilian vocational rehabilitation. *The Journal of Negro Education, 7*(3), 319-330.

WorkWorld. (2006). Ticket to Work and Work Incentives Improvement Act of 1999. Retrieved April 13, 2006, from http://www.workworld.org/wwwebhelp/ticket_to_work_and_work_incentives_improvement_act_of_1999.htm

The authors gratefully acknowledge the contributions of Nancy Hurley for editing; Todd Pietruszka and Katherine Hiestand for research; and Emer Broadbent and Alo Dutta for thoughtful comments and critiques.

CHAPTER 3

ETHICAL ISSUES IN DIVERSITY

JEANNE B. PATTERSON
JANET SPRY

Chapter Highlights

- Revised code of ethics

- The counseling relationship

- Assessment in rehabilitation

- Rehabilitation interventions and Placement

- Research, teaching, and supervision

- Summary

- Appendix

$\mathcal{A}$ culturally competent rehabilitation counselor must have knowledge and skills in both ethics and diversity. Noting the interrelationship between ethics, education, and diversity, many individuals (e.g., McGinn, Flowers, & Rubin, 1994; Wright, 1988)) called for an increased focus on ethics and diversity preceding the 2001 *Code of Professional Ethics for Rehabilitation Counselors* (hereafter referred to as *Code*) (Commission on Rehabilitation Counselor Certification, 2001. Moreover, Harley, Feist-Price, and Alston (1996) and Middleton, et al., (2000) noted shortcomings in the 1987 *Code of Professional Ethics for Rehabilitation Counselors* (CRCC, 1987) that could actually promote unethical behavior with culturally diverse individuals with disabilities. Because the 2001 *Code* addressed many of these concerns, the purpose of this chapter is to discuss the application of specific diversity references in the 2001 *Code* to the rehabilitation process and rehabilitation education, using illustrative case studies.

THE REVISED CODE OF ETHICS

A new standard specific to diversity was an important addition to the 2001 *Code*. In Section A: The Counseling Relationship, Standard A.2 Respecting Diversity requires:

- Respecting Culture. Rehabilitation counselors will demonstrate respect for clients' cultural backgrounds.
- Interventions. Rehabilitation counselors will develop and adapt interventions and services to incorporate consideration of clients' cultural perspectives and recognition of barriers external to clients that may interfere with achieving effective rehabilitation outcomes.
- Non-Discrimination. Rehabilitation counselors will not condone or engage in discrimination based on age, color, culture, disability, ethnic group, gender, race, religion, sexual orientation, marital status, or socioeconomic status.

p. 1

The other references to culture and diversity in the 2001 *Code* include (1) the consideration of culture, along with other characteristics of individuals with disabilities in evaluating career and employment needs (A.1.c); (2) the importance of professional competence and continuing education related to diversity issues (D.1.h and D.1.a); (3) the demonstration and importance of cultural sensitivity in assessment, including the diagnosis of mental disorders (F.3.b), the selection of tests (F.6.c), and the interpretations of tests (F.8.b); (4)

the design, conduct, and reports of research involving human participants (H.1.a) and research issues (H.1.f); and (5) representation of diverse individuals in graduate programs in Rehabilitation Counseling (G.2.g).

These standards are direct attempts to respond to Harley et al.'s (1996) assertion that "a counselor who is attempting to provide services to culturally diverse groups for which he or she does not have adequate skills to do so, is engaging in unethical behavior" (p. 204). To behave ethically, counselors should demonstrate the following three dimensions of multicultural competence: (1) awareness of own values, biases, preconceived notions, and assumptions about human behavior; (2) understanding of the world's views of culturally different consumers; and (3) development and practice of appropriate relevant, sensitive, and ethical intervention strategies and skills for working with culturally different consumers (Arredondo, et al., 1996; Arredondo, 1999).

THE COUNSELING RELATIONSHIP

The relationship between consumer and counselor is one that undergirds the entire rehabilitation process. This relationship can be compromised when counselors lack cultural competence, defined as the ability of the counselor "to relate to the individuals receiving services in a meaningful manner, without distorting the information conveyed or received as a result of cultural differences" (Thomas, Banks, Schroeder, Radtke, & Menz, 2002, p. 1).

Rehabilitation counselors are required to "demonstrate a commitment to gain knowledge, personal awareness, sensitivity, and skills pertinent to working with a div client population" (D.1.a, *Code*, p. 6). To develop meaningful relationships with dive individuals counselors must (1) examine both their beliefs and behaviors, and (2) acc and appropriately utilize information on other cultures. If a counselor does not posses the knowledge, awareness, sensitivity, and skills of another's culture, a meaningful counseling relationship cannot occur. As Rubin, Pusch, Fogarty, and McGinn (1995) noted,

> Counselor insensitivity to cultural differences, such as different language, habits, personality characteristics and values, can lead to diminished counselor empathy, misunderstandings with their clients, and misdiagnosis, thus interfering with the establishment of rapport and trust with clients.

p. 256

46

ISSUES IN TRADITIONAL COUNSELING

Counselors must understand and be sensitive to the multiple ways in which "traditional" counseling approaches can fail individuals from other cultures. Examples of unethical behaviors related to diversity that can prevent or undermine the counseling relationship include:

- Equating the intelligence of an individual with his/her command of the English language or language style.
- Treating an individual as representative of a particular culture, based on the counselor's stereotype of that culture.
- Discounting consumers' experiences with racism.
- Failing to recognize sub-cultures within various cultures.
- Subscribing to a counseling theory that focuses on insight obtained through expressions (i.e., verbal, emotional, behavioral), when showing emotion may be contrary to an individual's culture.
- Encouraging individuals to discuss intimate details, including family matters, without approval from the family.
- Emphasizing "talk therapy," which is contrary to some cultures that are more action-oriented?
- Using English, when the benefit is questionable for individuals for whom English is a second language and their English is not proficient.
- Adhering to counseling theories that focus on long-range goals for individuals whose culture focuses on the "here and now."
- Separating physical and emotional components of an individual, when the culture views the two as inseparable.
- Discounting folk medicine when it is an integral part of a particular culture.
- Using written contracts with individuals whose culture relies on verbal contracts
- Adhering to only one treatment modality.
- Blaming the consumer for problems encountered in counseling

(Bryan, 1999; Chapman, 1988; Chung & Bernak, 2002; Parker, 1988; Pederson, 1988)

LANGUAGE AND ELECTRONIC COMMUNICATION

Language is particularly crucial, since counseling cannot occur without it. Yet Taylor (1987) noted that (1) people do not generally know their feelings about language until they interact with individuals who have a different language, (2) one's language is usually viewed as superior, and (3) to understand a culture in-depth, one must know the language. When counselors lack language skills, the services of an interpreter are frequently employed; however, counselors must remain cognizant of the amount of actual communication that can be lost, even when an interpreter is present.

The Internet and e-mail are widely used in many rehabilitation offices; however, language issues can be intensified when electronic communication is inappropriately used. Not only must counselors explain possible misunderstandings that can occur in e-mail, which lacks visual and auditory cues (Code, Section I.2.j.), Gary and Remolino (2000) noted that some individuals have difficulty expressing themselves in writing and text communication can be an issue when English is a second language. Therefore, electronic communication is not recommended, unless both the counselor and consumer are comfortable and competent with the same written language.

EVALUATING ONE'S CULTURAL COMPETENCE

Developing cultural competence is a life-long process (Taylor, 1987); however, Quiñones-Mayo, Wilson, and McGuire (2000) noted, "counselors in a genuine attempt to address the customer's needs often overlook themselves as part of the counseling process" (p. 22). One approach counselors can use to ensure that they are continuing to develop skills, remind them of the importance of skills, and periodically assess their attitudes and behaviors is to use an inventory such as the *Cross-Cultural Counseling Inventory-Revised* (LaFramboise, Coleman, & Hernandez, 1991) or the *Cultural Competence Self-Test* (Goode, 2000), which is reprinted at the end of this chapter.

Individuals are encouraged to use multiple methods to assess their cultural competence. In addition to inventories that can be used as both a check and reminder, professionals can have a peer or supervisor observe one or more counseling sessions, use consumer satisfaction surveys, or evaluate their caseloads in terms of the representation of diverse individuals, number of services provided, amount of funds expended, and closure statuses of various ethnic groups.

CASE STUDY

John Flatmouth is a Crow American Indian who is seeing an addictions counselor. He has been late for three of five appointments, uses minimal eye contact with his counselor, and though verbally agreeing with treatment goals, has not followed through as planned. Mr. Flatmouth appears withdrawn and participates minimally in the counseling sessions.

Counselor A views Mr. Flatmouth as exhibiting classic denial of his addictions problems, disinterest in counseling, and low commitment to the treatment plan. If the counselor's planned confrontation does not work, the counselor will recommend that Mr. Flatmouth discontinue counseling.

Counselor B views Mr. Flatmouth's tardiness and lack of eye contact as cultural-specific behaviors, which place less emphasis on time and eye contact. Mr. Flatmouth's noninvolvement is viewed as his attempt to avoid attention-seeking behavior. Recognizing that Mr. Flatmouth may nod in agreement to treatment goals with which he does not agree, Counselor B is going to discuss possible involvement of the tribal Medicine Man. Counselor B knows that confrontation could reinforce Mr. Flatmouth's perceptions of the dominant culture. [For additional information on issues in this case study, see Chapman, 1988; Marshall, 2002; Thomason, 1996]

ASSESSMENT IN REHABILITATION

Over the years, testing has had multiple purposes (e.g., school placements, psychological and clinical diagnoses, military services, employment selections, employment promotions, job placement, and career planning) and is now provided to an increasingly diverse population in terms of race, age, gender, sexual orientation, religion, and socioeconomic status. In rehabilitation, assessment results frequently form the basis for the identification of rehabilitation goals and services. Assessments may cause a life-altering process, since they influence an individual's future in terms of lifestyle, economic status, career options, self-esteem, personal success, and job satisfaction.

In recognition of this impact, the *Code* includes a number of standards related to assessment and diversity, including the impact of socioeconomic and cultural experience on vocational outcomes and test selection for culturally diverse populations. It also emphasizes the importance of taking precautions when using assessment instruments, interpretation of performance by populations not represented in norm groups, and recognition of the effects of multicultural deficiencies on socioeconomic status in test administration and interpretation. Collectively, these represent the three major areas in which ethics may be compromised in assessment: test development, test selection and administration, and test interpretation (Austin, 1999).

TEST DEVELOPMENT
Counselors frequently overlook the biases encompassed in test development. Because most test developers lack a multicultural perspective, tests are frequently developed from a Eurocentric perspective and normed on non-diverse groups (Sedlacek & Kim, 1995). If diversity is not addressed in test

development, the tests can perpetuate barriers and inappropriate labeling when they are used with other groups. Test developers have, historically, not addressed culturally specific behaviors, or issues related to ethnic identity or acculturation (Padilla (2001).

Even when test developers include diverse groups in the norming process, they typically fail to include sufficient numbers of individuals representative of within-group differences. For example, they may include American Indians; however, the Bureau of Indian Affairs recognizes 339 American Indian tribes that speak 250 languages within the U.S., as well as 227 Native entities in Alaska (Sanderson, 2001). Generalization of test results is, therefore, still an issue, given the cultural differences between tribes (Hood & Johnson 1997).

TEST SELECTION AND ADMINISTRATION

The Code reminds counselors that when selecting tests, they should "avoid inappropriateness of testing that may be outside of socialized behavioral or cognitive patterns or functional abilities (F.6.c). In selecting tests, counselors should consider (a) language issues (e.g., test instructions, as well as the language of test items), (b) conceptual issues (whether the test concepts are similar across cultures), (c) scale issues (the response formats that are used—true/false vs. Likert scales), and (d) interpretative issues (norms for particular cultural groups) (Austin, 1999). Each of these areas can significantly impact the results of the assessment. It is critical that the test administrator first understand the culture of the individual undergoing assessment, prior to test selection.

Test administrators or counselors should explain the evaluation process and answer any questions that may evolve pertinent to the instruments used and their results. Test administrators should strive to identify if there is a relationship between the instruments used and cultural values, patterns, and/or the functional impact of disability.

TEST INTERPRETATION

Standard F.8.b requires counselors to "place test results and their interpretations in proper perspective considering other relevant factors including age, color, culture, disability, ethnic group, gender, race, religion, sexual orientation, marital status, and socioeconomic status."

As Gainor (2003) noted, even with all we know about the ways that historical and cultural factors affect people of diverse cultural groups, counselors and psychologists continue to interpret assessment results without a clear cultural context for their interpretation. The cultural context should include not only individual differences, but also intracultural variations (Welfel, 2002).

Other areas of bias in testing include (1) items favoring one group over another, and (2) test-related factors (e.g., the individual's motivation, stress level, or test sophistication). Using the example of the word "toboggan," Hood and Johnson (1997) noted that "many sociocultural factors—ethnicity, socioeconomic class, region, and situation—contribute to mismatches between the language of test takers and that of test makers" (p. 298).

Standard F.5.1 of the *Code* summarizes many of the assessment issues by requiring that counselors "recognize the limits of their competence and perform only those testing and assessment services for which they have been trained." Hood and Johnson (1997) remind us that "it is a general rule that the less the counselor knows of the client's culture, the more errors the counselor is likely to make" (p. 299). Incompetence in assessment means that barriers and discriminatory practices toward individuals from diverse groups are perpetuated.

CASE STUDY

Keith, a 24-year-old African American male, received a comprehensive vocational evaluation, which resulted in the following outcomes: (1) his highest interest was recorded in the area of computer technology and repair and (2) based on Wide Range Achievement Test (WRAT) results, he obtained a math level of 4.6 and a reading level of 4.5. Prior to testing, Keith shared with both his advocate and counselor that he wanted to continue with his education in order to achieve a good status in life.

Counselor. Keith's counselor, a white female with 3 months experience following her college graduation, immediately dismissed the possibility of Keith receiving training or returning to school. Based on his test scores, she recommended they develop a plan for direct job placement. Not understanding his options, Keith accepted the judgment of his counselor that his test scores were insufficient to qualify him for any further education or training and considerations.

Advocate. Keith's advocate, a previous supervisor at the agency where his counselor was employed, had over 25 years of extensive experience in testing evaluation, assessment, and working with multicultural populations. When Keith told his advocate about the meeting, the advocate recommended scheduling another meeting with the counselor for the three of them to further discuss Keith's evaluation results and vocational future.

Outcome. Keith's advocate recommended a specialized reading and math assessment to measure his reading and math aptitudes using a different test from that used during his original assessment and to assess his potential to increase his levels. Additionally, a situational assessment was recommended and arranged by the advocate at a school offering a program in Keith's area of interest. Finally, it was recommended that Keith receive an eye examination and eyeglasses as appropriate to address his concerns with the impact of his vision on test results.

Results. As a result of his additional testing, Keith was recommended for individual remediation and a tutorial program where he raised his math and reading levels to over 9th grade, which surpassed the required levels for training. Also, he participated in a one-month situational assessment. When Keith was tested at the completion of his assessment he received a perfect score of 100%, and the school accepted him for training. Keith went on to pass all of his class examinations and the program with an "A" average. He passed all of his certification exams on his first try and is currently furthering his education in his field.

If Keith had accepted the recommendations of his counselor who had limited training, did not take the time to learn about and understand his culture, and did not appear to understand the impact that culture can have on testing and vocational success, his outcome would have been completely different.

REHABILITATION INTERVENTIONS AND PLACEMENT

The demographics of the labor force continue to reflect greater diversity. By 2010, increases are projected for Asian and other non-Hispanic groups (37%), individuals of Hispanic origin (36%), and Black, non-Hispanic (17%) (Staff 2001). The extent to which this labor force will include greater representation of diverse individuals with disabilities is unknown, but can be greatly influenced by rehabilitation counselors.

The standards in the *Code* directly address interventions and placement: Standard A.1.c requires counselors to consider "employment that is consistent with the overall abilities, vocational limitations, physical restrictions, psychological limitations, general temperament, interest and aptitude patterns, social skills, education, general qualifications, and cultural, and other relevant characteristics and needs of clients," and Standard A.2.b requires counselors to "develop and adapt interventions and services to incorporate consideration of client's cultural perspectives and recognition of barriers external to clients that may interfere with achieving effective rehabilitation outcomes." Despite these standards, research on rehabilitation outcomes (e.g., Bellini, 2003) suggests inequities in placement that may, in fact, represent unethical conduct. For example, Bellini (2003) found that European American counselors provided fewer vocational training services to African American and Hispanic/Latino consumers than their European American counterparts. Olney and Kennedy (2002) found that Hispanics and African Americans were more likely to receive on-the-job training or training in job seeking skills, instead of the college or university training received by European Americans and other racial minorities. The results of both of these studies translate into lower salaries in employment for African Americans and Hispanic/Latinos.

Studies also suggest that services (or lack thereof) impact culturally diverse individuals with particular disabilities. For example, Moore, Feist-Price, and Alston (2002) found that race and job placement services were related to the closure status of individuals with mental retardation and Moore (2001) found that African Americans with mental retardation received fewer job placement services and had less successful closures than European Americans. Moore, Feist-Price and Alston theorize that "as mental retardation becomes more severe, so does the negative impact of race on achieving closure success" (p. 166). Also, job placement is a direct result of being accepted for services. Yet most of the research (e.g., Feist-Price, 1995; Wilson, Harley, & Alston, 2001) shows that African Americans have significantly lower acceptance rates than European Americans.

Stereotypes related to suitable occupations for ethnic minorities and myths regarding variables related to the career and educational status of various ethnic groups impede the successful placement of qualified minorities into promising employment opportunities. Some of the barriers that may impact diversity in the workplace and present unfair discrimination include job demands, under utilization, job stress, non-acceptance into organizational culture, attitudes, and stereotypes. The counselor must understand the differences between external and personal barriers and work with the consumers to identify and develop interventions to cope with, and in some cases overcome, those barriers. The counselor should begin by preparing the culturally diverse consumer to effectively approach common workplace barriers, since an individual who is prepared, resilient, and confident has a greater opportunity for success and can more effectively overcome external barriers.

Counselors should recognize that the rehabilitation process itself is eurocentrically based and may conflict with the values and beliefs of diverse individuals. The focus on the individual and the need for dates and timelines within the rehabilitation plan are not consistent with all cultures. Brown (1997) noted that some cultures are less oriented to dates and future time orientations, which must be considered by the counselor in identifying a vocational goal, developing the plan, and assigning any homework.

Marshall, Leung, Johnson and Busby (2003) encouraged counselors to both (1) help consumers preserve their culture and (2) advocate with employers "to find creative methods by which they can communicate with and support the culturally diverse individuals joining their work force" (p. 63). There are tools that may ultimately assist counselors in providing more ethical job placement. Thompson and Berven (2002) reported on the Individualism-Collectivism Vocational Attitudes Questionnaire (ICVAQ), which still needs refinement. They believe this instrument will promote "a better understanding of the ways in which I/C (individualism-collectivism) cultural differences can affect attitudes and beliefs about achievement and competition at work, respect and duty toward authority, independent choice making, and support sharing among family and associates" (p. 85). They believe that an instrument such as this could assist counselors in identifying interventions that are more consistent with one's cultural orientation.

CASE STUDY

Tamyra, a 27-year-old Hispanic woman who lives with her parents, earned an A.A. degree in Food Management Services. With the assistance of her rehabilitation counselor, Tamyra is now working as a management trainee for a local restaurant. Although Tamyra is in her fifth year of English as a Second Language classes, she is very insecure when communicating in the workplace. Tamyra's supervisor, who has been very supportive and who worked closely with Tamyra and her counselor, was recently promoted and moved to a new location. Tamyra's new supervisor has little experience working with diverse populations and individuals with disabilities. Tamyra's new supervisor is overwhelmed with the responsibilities of the position and was not able to work closely with Tamyra's counselor to address her special needs. Although Tamyra had the knowledge, skills, and abilities for the position, her communication skills were clearly a barrier. Therefore, her new supervisor placed her in a position requiring virtually no communication with the public or co-workers. Tamyra initially accepted the change, but after three months she decided to meet with her counselor about her concerns. Her counselor discussed the language barrier with her as well as the need for increased classes and efforts to improve her language and communication skills. She also developed a list of techniques to address and overcome some of the external and personal barriers with which Tamyra was faced. Tamyra explained her plans to her supervisor, who agreed to reconsider Tamyra's duties as her language skills improved.

3

RESEARCH, TEACHING, AND SUPERVISION

Ethical issues related to diversity can occur in research, teaching, and supervision. Although some of these issues parallel those related to counseling, these standards highlight other relationship issues.

RESEARCH

Two standards specifically address diversity. Counselors must "plan, design, conduct, and report research in a manner that reflects cultural sensitivity, is culturally appropriate, and is consistent with pertinent ethical principles (Standard H.1.a) and "be sensitive to diversity and research issues with culturally diverse populations" (Standard H.1.f).

Four practices that can compromise these standards include (1) generalizing research findings to multicultural groups that may not have been adequately represented in the sample, (2) relying on easily accessible research participants who do not represent the larger minority group (e.g., college students), (3) using research paradigms that focus on deviance or cultural deficiencies, and (d) failing to recognize intracultural differences (Howard-Hamilton, 1997; Ponterotto & Casas, 1991). Uswatte and Elliott (1997) recommended that researchers should specify the individual ethnic compositions represented in any research sample rather than just separate groups on the basis of minority/majority. Also, they indicated that any analyses based on race should include "an *a priori* rationale… for such analyses" (p. 68), which is consistent with Howard-Hamilton's beliefs that:

> There has been overemphasis on simplistic client/counselor process variables and disregard for significant cultural and culture-specific psychosocial variables that might impact counseling. … Most research has not considered or incorporated the heterogeneity extant in multicultural populations, a tact which has fostered and perpetuated ethnic stereotypes and negative perceptions.
>
> pp. 31-32

Both the National Institutes of Health (NIH), which includes the National Institute of Mental Health (NIMH), and the American Psychological Association (APA) have attempted to address diversity issues. NIH (2001) requires grant applicants to include women and diverse racial and ethnic groups in clinical research. APA and NIHM identified the following ethical dilemmas and considerations in research with ethnic-minority children and youth:

- Different cultural conceptions of privacy, research risk and benefit, and the roles of parents and communities in permitting child and adolescent research participation;
- Historical and cultural reasons for resistance to research participation;
- The possibility that in poor communities, payment for research participation may be seen as coercive;
- The extent to which ethnic-minority communities will actually benefit from the research in which they participate;
- The degree to which research is likely to stigmatize individuals, families, or communities;
- Factors that may compromise the validity of measures used in research. For example, using arrest records as a measure of aggressive behavior among ethnic-minority youth might bias study results because such records may reflect unfairness in the criminal justice system.

Carpenter, 2001, pp. 2-3

The same cultural sensitivity and cultural knowledge described for culturally competent counselors are also necessary for culturally competent researchers.

TEACHING AND SUPERVISION

Rehabilitation counselor education (RCE) programs are responsible for producing culturally competent counselors. Researchers (e.g., D'Andrea, Daniels, & Heck, 1991; Dixon & Wright, 1996; Leong & Kim, 1991; McRae & Johnson; 1992; Rubin et al., 1995; Schaller & DeLaGarza, 1994) identified four major areas that should be included in counseling programs. Students should have the opportunity to (1) develop self-awareness, identify one's attitudes, beliefs, and values; view one's self as a cultural being; (2) learn about other cultures and their values; (3) develop communication skills appropriate to other cultures and understand the impact of counselors and consumers with different values; and (4) demonstrate the use of multicultural skills, typically in practicum and internship settings. The acquisition of this knowledge and these skills is usually accomplished through infusion of multicultural knowledge and activities throughout the RCE curriculum (Marshall, Johnson, & Johnson, 1996; Schaller & DeLaGarza, 1994) or infusion accompanied by a separate multicultural course (Wehrly, 1991). Because the acquisition of multicultural skills is a developmental process comparable to learning basic counseling skills, one course is not sufficient for students to attain the necessary competencies. The keys to infusion reside with the commitment and the knowledge and skills of the faculty in RCE programs.

56

Ethical issues are inherent in teaching multicultural skills. The situations described by Mpofu and Harley (2000), in using tokenism theory (e.g., numerical skewedness) to explore work-related stress have parallels in higher education and RCE programs. The *Code* (2001) requires diversity in both faculty and students (Standard G.2.g.); however, in many RCE programs culturally diverse individuals are underrepresented, thus more highly visible. The visibility can result in these students being more closely observed by faculty members, which in turn can lead to both performance pressure and social isolation for diverse students. Culturally diverse individuals may feel that they have to conform to the values of the majority group (assimilation) or may be called upon to speak on behalf of a larger cultural group than they represent (role encapsulation). Similarly, diverse students may experience "contrast effects," where their "work contributions…are prejudged to be of a lower quality" than the majority students or they may be assigned to team or role-play with another minority individual" (p. 50).

Similar issues can arise in practicum and internship supervision, although the research in this area is more limited (Fong, 1994). For example, Leong and Wagner noted that race can influence the student's expectations (e.g., support, empathy) of the supervisor.

Some "best practices" that have been identified to counter the effects of tokenism and enhance the supervision process include:

- Pairing a majority and minority person in any teams that are used;
- Addressing the supervisor's and student's cultural backgrounds and expectations for supervision;
- Discussing the power differential, evaluation criteria, and perceptions of fairness;
- Incorporating participatory appraisal procedures that use the students' self evaluations as a basis for discussion of the supervisor's evaluations.

Fong, 1994; Mpofu & Harley, 2000

In addition, Fong recommended that:

> All supervisors-in-training should work with supervisees from racial-ethnic groups other than their own and receive supervision of multicultural supervision. Likewise, experienced supervisors will need to seek continuing education, consultation, and focused supervision of supervision with a multicultural emphasis to meet gaps in experience and education.

p. 3

3

CASE STUDY

After completing two semesters in a graduate counseling program, John Banks, a 27-year old African American male, is considering dropping out of the program. There are only two minority individuals in the program, and the other is a woman who is Chinese. Last semester he was paired with her for both a class project and the pre-practicum role-playing. The Office of Multicultural Affairs has suggested that he meet with the professor before dropping out of the program.

Professor A, a white male, states that John is being overly sensitive and seeing prejudice where none exists. He notes that John is not a strong student, but could make it through the program if he tried harder. He only paired the two minority individuals, because they would have more in common.

Professor B, a white male, thanked John for sharing his concerns. He indicated that he paired the two at the request of the minority female; however, he did not know that the two had been paired in another class. Recognizing the power differences and past experiences that John had likely experienced with tokenism, the professor asked John if they could meet weekly to discuss John's experiences and plan for his practicum experience through discussions of their roles, John's evaluation, and John's expectations of supervision.

SUMMARY

There are a number of ethical issues specific to diversity that must be considered by rehabilitation students and professionals. This chapter highlighted the revised _Code_ and issues related to (1) counseling, (2) assessment, (3) rehabilitation interventions and placement, and (4) research, teaching, and supervision.

To ensure ethical behavior, counselors must commit themselves to life-long learning related to diversity and continually evaluate their values and beliefs. As Marshall et al., (2003) suggested:

> We need to embrace fully the diversity that comes with a multicultural society. We need to celebrate the cultures that make us a diverse people…it is imperative that rehabilitation counselors learn to delve into the lived realities of individuals—into their cultures—if we are to help them make meaningful employment and life choices.

p. 62

58

REFERENCES

Arredondo, P. (1999). Multicultural counseling competencies as tools to address oppression and racism. *Journal of Counseling & Development, 78,* 102-109.

Arredondo, P., Toporek, R., Brown, S. P., Jones, J., Lock, D. C., Sanchez, J., & Stadler, H. (1996). Operationalization of the multicultural counseling competencies. *Journal of Multicultural Counseling & Development, 24,* 42-78.

Austin, J. T. (1999). Culturally sensitive career assessment: A quandary. ERIC Clearinghouse on Adult, Career, and Vocational Education. Available online at http://icdl.uncg.edu/ft/062000-05.html.

Bellini, J. (2003). Counselors' multicultural competencies and vocational rehabilitation outcomes in the context of counselor-client racial similarity and difference. *Rehabilitation Counseling Bulletin, 46,* 164-173.

Brown, D. (1997). Implicationsn of cultural values for cross-cultural consultation with families. *Journal of Counseling & Development, 76,* 29-35.

Bryan, W. V. (1999). *Multicultural aspects of disabilities.* Springfield, IL: Charles C. Thomas.

Carpenter, S. (2001). Experts weigh ethical issues in research on ethnic-minority youth. *Monitor on Psychology, 32*(8), 1-4.

Chapman, R. J. (1988). Cultural bias in alcoholism counseling. *Alcoholism Treatmen Quarterly, 5,* 105-113. Available online at: http://www.lasalle.edu/~chapman/essays/bias.htm

Chung, R. C., & Bernak, F. (2002). The relationship of culture and empathy in cross-cultural counseling. *Journal of Counseling & Development, 80,* 154-159.

Commission on Rehabilitation Counselor Certification (2001). *Code of professional ethics for rehabilitation counselors.* Rolling Meadows, IL: Author.Available online at: http://www.crccertification.com/pdf/code_ethics_2002.pdf

Commission on Rehabilitation Counselor Certification (1987). *Code of professional ethics for rehabilitation counselors.* Rolling Meadows, IL: Author.

D'Andrea, M., & Daniels, J. (1991). Exploring the different levels of multicultural counseling training. *Journal of Counseling and Development, 70,* 78-85.

Dixon, C., & Wright, T. (1996). Service delivery to African Americans with disabilities: How to best train rehabilitation professionals. *Rehabilitation Education, 10,* 139-150.

Feist-Price, S. (1995). African Americans with disabilities and equity in vocational rehabilitation services: One state's review. *Rehabilitation Counseling Bulletin, 39,* 119-129.

Fong, M. (1994). *Multicultural issues in supervision.* ERIC #ED372346. Greensboro, NC: ERIC Clearinghouse on Counseling and Student Services. Retrieved 12/12/02 from ttp://ericcass..uncg.edu/super/fong.html

Gainor, K. A. (2003). Vocational assessment with culturally diverse populations. In L.A. Suzuki, J. G. Ponterotto, & P. J. Metter (Eds.). *Handbook of multicultural assessment* (2nd ed., pp. 169-190). San Francisco: Jossey-Bass.

Gary, J. M., & Remolino, L.(2000). Online support groups: Nuts and bolts, benefits, limitations and future directions. *ERIC/CASS Digest*, EDO-CG-00-7. Retrieved from http://ericcas.uncg.edu/digest/2000-07.html

Goode, T. (2000). *Promoting cultural and linguistic competency.* Retrieved 3/15 from: http://www.georgetown.edu/research/gucdc/nccc/nccc11.html.

Harley, D. A., Feist-Price, S., & Alston, R. J. (1996). Cultural diversity and ethics: Expanding the definition to be inclusive. *Rehabilitation Education, 10,* 201-210.

Hood, A. B., & Johnson, R. W. (1997). *Assessment in counseling: A guide to the use of psychological assessment procedures* (2nd ed.). Alexandria, VA: American Counseling Association.

Howard-Hamilton, M.F. (1997). Research in multicultural counseling. In L.C. Loesch & N.A Vacc (Eds.), CASS Capsules: Research in Counseling and Therapy (pp. 31-34). Greensboro, NC: ERIC Clearinghouse on Counseling and Student Services.

LaFramboise, T. D., Coleman, H. L. K., & Hernandez, A. (1991). Cross-cultural counseling inventory- revised (CCCI-R): Development and factor structure of the cross-cultural counseling inventory-revised. *Professional Psychology: Research and Practice, 22,* 380-388.

Leong, T. L., & Kim, H. H. (1991). Going beyond cultural sensitivity on the road to multiculturalism: Using the intercultural sensitizer as a counselor training tool. *Journal of Counseling and Development, 70,* 112-118.

Leong, F. T. & Wagner, N. M. (1994). Cross-cultural supervision: What do we know? What do we need to know? *Counselor Education & Supervision 34,* 117-131.

Marshall, C. A. (2002). *Rehabilitation with American Indians with disabilities: A handbook for administrators, practitioners, and researchers.* Athens, GA: Elliott & Fitzpatrick.

Marshall, C. A., Johnson, M. J., & Johnson, S. R. (1996). Responding to the needs of American Indians with disabilities through rehabilitation counselor education. *Rehabilitation Education, 10,* 185-199.

Marshall, C. A., Leung, P., Johnson, S. R., & Busby, H. (2003). Ethical practice and cultural factors in rehabilitation. *Rehabilitation Education, 17,* 55-65.

McGinn, F., Flowers, C. R., & Rubin, S. E. (1994). In quest of an explicit multicultural emphasis in ethical standards for rehabilitation counselors. *Rehabilitation Education, 7,* 261-268.

McRae, M., & Johnson, S. (1992). Toward training for competence in multicultural counselor education. *Journal of Counseling and Development, 70,* 131-141.

Middleton, R. A., Rollins, C. W., Sanderson, P. L., Leung, P., Harley, D. A., Ebener, D., & Leal-Idrogo, A. (2000). Endorsement of professional multicultural rehabilitation competencies and standards. *Rehabilitation Counseling Bulletin, 43,* 219-240.

Moore, C. L. (2001). Disparities in closure success rates for African Americans with mental retardation: An ex-post-facto research design. *Journal of Applied Rehabilitation Counseling, 32*(2), 31-36.

Moore, C. L., Feist-Price, S., & Alston, R. J. (2002). VR services for persons with severe/profound mental retardation. *Rehabilitation Counseling Bulletin, 45,* 162-167.

Mpofu, E., & Harley, D. A. (2000). Tokenism and cultural diversity in counselors: Implications for rehabilitation education and practice. *Journal of Applied Rehabilitation Counseling, 31*(1), 47-54.

National Institutes of Health. (2002, November). *Sex/gender and minority inclusion in NIH clinical research.* Retrieved March 3, 2003 from: http://grants1.nih.gov/grants/funding/women_min/training

Olney, M. F., & Kennedy, J. (2002). Racial disparities in VR use and job placement rates for adults with disabilities. *Rehabilitation Counseling Bulletin, 45,* 177-185.

Padilla, A. M. (2001). Issues in culturally appropriate assessment. In L. Suzuki, J. Ponterotto, & P. J. Meller (Eds.). *Handbook of multicultural assessment* (2nd ed., pp. 5-27). San Francisco: Jossey-Bass.

Parker, W. M., (1988). *Consciousness-raising.* Springfield, IL: Charles C.Thomas.

Pedersen, P. (1988). *A handbook for developing multicultural awareness.* Alexandria, VA: American Association for Counseling and Development.

Ponterotto, J, & Cases, M. (1987). In search for multicultural competence within counselor education programs. *Journal of Counseling and Development 65,* 430-435.

Quiñones-Mayo, Y., Wilson, K.B., & McGuire, M. V. (2000). Vocational rehabilitation and cultural competency for Latino populations: Considerations for rehabilitation counselors. *Journal of Applied Rehabilitation Counseling, 31*(1), 19-26.

Rubin, S. E., Pusch, B. D., Fogarty, C., & McGinn, F. (1995). Enhancing the cultural sensitivity of rehabilitation counselors. *Rehabilitation Education, 9,* 253-264.

Sanderson, P. L. (2001). American Indians: An overview of factors influencing health care, disability, and service delivery. In C. Marshall (Ed.). *Rehabilitation and American Indians with disabilities: A handbook for administrators, practitioners, and researchers* (pp. 27-41). Athens, GA: Elliott & Fitzpatrick.

Schaller, J., & DeLaGarza, D. (1994). Infusion of culture and gender issues in rehabilitation counselor education curricula. *Rehabilitation Education, 8,* 166-180.

Sedlacek, W. E., & Kim. S. H. (1995). Multicultural assessment. *Eric Digest,* ED391112. Available online at: http://www.ericfacility.net/ericdigests/ ed391112.html

Staff. (2001). Labor force. Occupational Outlook Quarterly Online, 45(4). Available online at: http://www.bls.gov/opub/ooq/2001/winter/art06.htm

Taylor, O. (1987). *Cross-cultural communication: An essential dimension of effective education.* Chevy Chase, MD: The Mid-Atlantic Equity Center. Available online at: http://www.nwrel.org/cnorse/booklets/ccc/

Thomas, D. F., Banks, M., Schroeder, M., Radtke, J., & Menz, F. E. (2002, September*). Cultural Diversity in Community-Based Rehabilitation Programs (CRPs).* Paper presented at State-of-the-Science Conference, Washington, D.C. Abstract available online at: http://www.cec.svri.org/State%20of%20Science%20Conference/SOS%20 Abstracts/Diversity%20abstract.htm.

Thomason, T. C. (1996). Proposed competencies for counseling Native Americans. In J. W.Bloom (Ed.), *Credentialing professional counselors for the 21st century* (pp. 9-10). Greensboro, NC: ERIC/Cass. Available online at: http://ericcass.uncg.edu/creden/thomason.html

Thompson, V., & Berven, N. (2002). Development of an instrument to measure cultural attitudes and behaviors affecting vocational rehabilitation. *Rehabilitation Counseling Bulletin, 45*, 76-86.

Uswatte, G., & Elliott, T. R. (1997). Ethnic and minority issues in rehabilitation psychology. *Rehabilitation Psychology, 42*, 61-71.

Wehrly, B. (1991). Preparing multicultural counselors. *Counseling and Human Development,24*(3), 1-24.

Welfel, E. R. (2002). *Ethics in counseling and psychotherapy: Standards, research, and emerging issues* (2nd ed.). Pacific Grove, CA: Brooks/Cole.

Wilson, K. B., Harley, D. A., & Alston, R. J. (2001). Race as a correlate of vocational rehabilitation acceptance: Revisited. *Journal of Rehabilitation, 67*(3), 35-41.

Wright, T. (1988). Enhancing the professional preparation of rehabilitation counselors for improved services to ethnic minorities with disabilities. *Journal of Applied Rehabilitation Counseling, 19*(4), 4-10.

3

APPENDIX

PROMOTING CULTURAL AND LINGUISTIC COMPETENCY:
SELF-ASSESSMENT CHECKLIST FOR PERSONNEL PROVIDING PRIMARY HEALTH CARE SERVICES

Directions: Please enter A, B or C for each item listed below.

A = Things I do frequently
B = Things I do occasionally
C = Things I do rarely or never

Physical Environment, Materials, and Resources

_____ 1. I display pictures, posters, artwork, and other decors that reflect the cultures and ethnic backgrounds of clients served by my program or agency.

_____ 2. I ensure that magazines, brochures, and other printed materials in reception areas are of interest to and reflect the different cultures of individuals and families served by my program or agency.

_____ 3. When using videos, films or other media resources for health education, treatment, or other interventions, I ensure that they reflect the cultures and ethnic background of individuals and families served by my program or agency.

_____ 4. I ensure that printed information disseminated by my agency or program takes into account the average literacy levels of individuals and families receiving services.

Communication Styles

_____ 5. When interacting with individuals and families who have limited English proficiency, I always keep in mind that:

_____ 6. Limitations in English proficiency are in no way a reflection of their level of intellectual functioning.

_____ 7. Their limited ability to speak the language of the dominant culture has no bearing on their ability to communicate effectively in their language of origin.

_____ 8. They may or may not be literate in their language of origin or English.

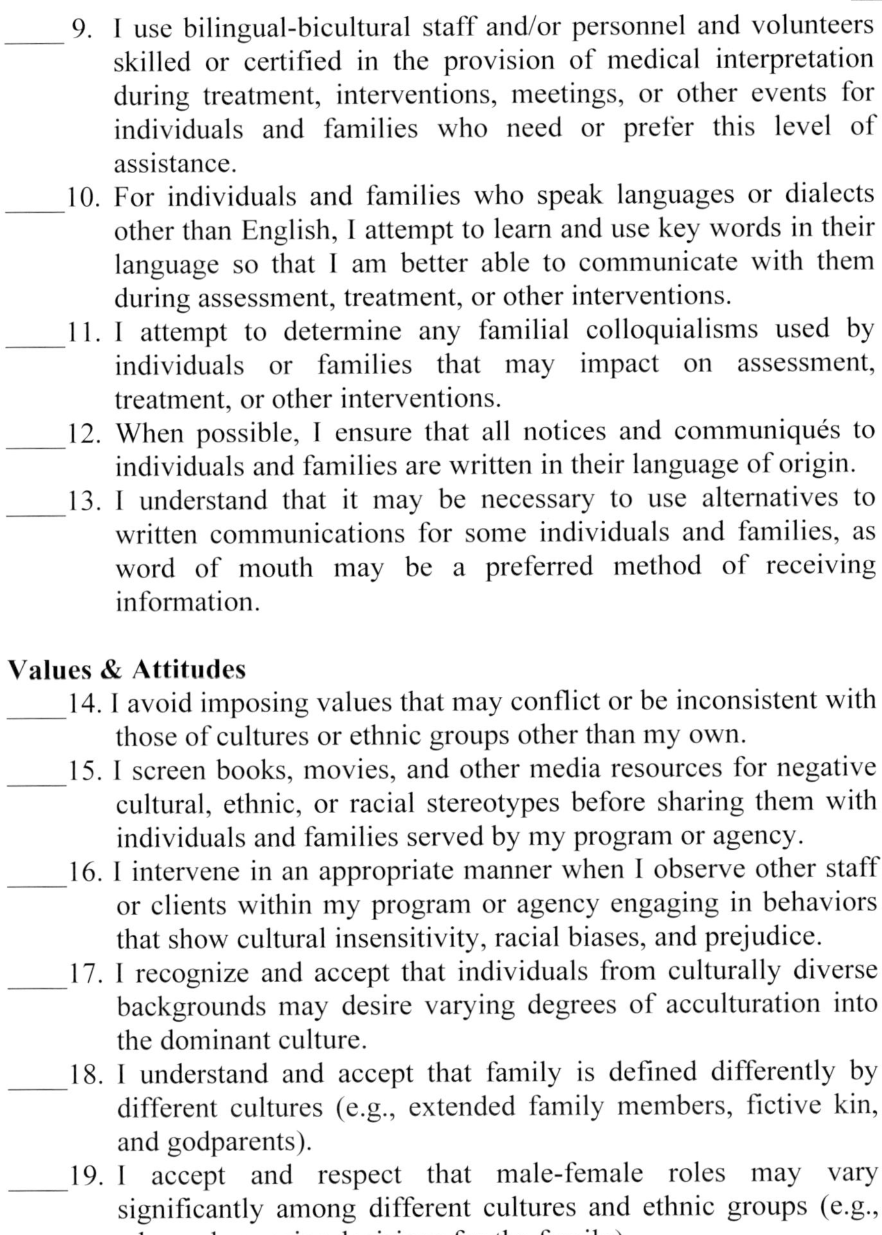

_____ 9. I use bilingual-bicultural staff and/or personnel and volunteers skilled or certified in the provision of medical interpretation during treatment, interventions, meetings, or other events for individuals and families who need or prefer this level of assistance.

_____10. For individuals and families who speak languages or dialects other than English, I attempt to learn and use key words in their language so that I am better able to communicate with them during assessment, treatment, or other interventions.

_____11. I attempt to determine any familial colloquialisms used by individuals or families that may impact on assessment, treatment, or other interventions.

_____12. When possible, I ensure that all notices and communiqués to individuals and families are written in their language of origin.

_____13. I understand that it may be necessary to use alternatives to written communications for some individuals and families, as word of mouth may be a preferred method of receiving information.

Values & Attitudes

_____14. I avoid imposing values that may conflict or be inconsistent with those of cultures or ethnic groups other than my own.

_____15. I screen books, movies, and other media resources for negative cultural, ethnic, or racial stereotypes before sharing them with individuals and families served by my program or agency.

_____16. I intervene in an appropriate manner when I observe other staff or clients within my program or agency engaging in behaviors that show cultural insensitivity, racial biases, and prejudice.

_____17. I recognize and accept that individuals from culturally diverse backgrounds may desire varying degrees of acculturation into the dominant culture.

_____18. I understand and accept that family is defined differently by different cultures (e.g., extended family members, fictive kin, and godparents).

_____19. I accept and respect that male-female roles may vary significantly among different cultures and ethnic groups (e.g., who makes major decisions for the family).

_____20. I understand that age and life-cycle factors must be considered in interactions with individuals and families (e.g., high value placed on the decision of elders, the role of eldest male or female in families, or roles and expectation of children within the family).

_____21. Even though my professional or moral viewpoints may differ, I accept individuals and families as the ultimate decision makers for services and supports impacting their lives.

_____22. I recognize that the meaning or value of medical treatment and health education may vary greatly among cultures.

_____23. I accept that religion and other beliefs may influence how individuals and families respond to illnesses, disease, and death.

_____24. I understand that the perception of health, wellness and preventive health services have different meanings to different cultural or ethnic groups.

_____25. I recognize and accept that folk and religious beliefs may influence an individual's or family's reaction and approach to a child born with a disability, or later diagnosed with a disability, genetic disorder or special health care needs.

_____26. I understand that grief and bereavement are influenced by culture.

_____27. I seek information from individuals, families, or other key community informants that will assist in service adaptation to respond to the needs and preferences of culturally and ethnically diverse groups served by my program or agency.

_____28. Before visiting or providing services in the home setting, I seek information on acceptable behaviors, courtesies, customs, and expectations that are unique to the culturally and ethnically diverse groups served by my program or agency.

_____29. I keep abreast of the major health concerns and issues for ethnically and racially diverse client populations residing in the geographic locale served by my program or agency.

_____30. I am aware of the socioeconomic and environmental risk factors that contribute to the major health problems of culturally, ethnically, and racially diverse populations served by my program or agency.

_____31. I am well versed in the most current and proven practices, treatments and interventions for major health problems among ethnically and racially diverse groups within the geographic locale served by my agency or program.

_____32. I avail myself to professional development and training to enhance my knowledge and skills in the provision of services and supports to culturally, ethnically, racially, and linguistically diverse groups.

_____33. I advocate for the review of my program or agency's mission statement, goals, policies, and procedures to ensure that they incorporate principles and practices that promote cultural and linguistic competence.

Adapted with permission from _Promoting Cultural Competence and Cultural Diversity in Early Intervention and Early Childhood Settings_ and _Promoting Cultural Competence and Cultural Diversity for Personnel Providing Services and Supports to Children With Special Health Care Needs and Their Families_ (June 1989; latest revision July 2000).

How to use this checklist

This checklist is intended to heighten the awareness and sensitivity of personnel to the importance of cultural and linguistic competence in health and human service settings. It provides concrete examples of the kinds of beliefs, attitudes, values, and practices that foster cultural and linguistic competence at the individual or practitioner level. There is no answer key with correct responses. However, if you frequently responded "C," you may not necessarily demonstrate beliefs, attitudes, values, and practices that promote cultural and linguistic competence within health care delivery programs. Self-assessment developed by Tawara D. Goode, Georgetown University Child Development Center-UAP.

CHAPTER 4

PREPARING CULTURALLY COMPETENT PRACTITIONERS FOR REHABILITATION AND ALLIED HEALTH

WILLIAM TALLEY
CHANDRA DONNELL

Chapter Highlights

➡ Evidence of a paradigm shift

➡ The language of cultural competence: The nature of culture

➡ Cultural identity development

➡ Multiculturism and diversity

➡ Power, privilege, and oppression

➡ Context and cultural counseling

➡ Preparing culturally sensitive/competent counselors

➡ Counseling models designed to work with diverse populations

$\mathcal{R}$ehabilitation counseling, counseling psychology, and related helping professions are always evolving. Research often fosters changes, brings about new discoveries, and changes perceptions. Some changes are more dramatic. A discovery or series of discoveries can result in a significant change in the way that people think. Such changes are known as paradigm shifts.

The field of human behavior has experienced a number of paradigm shifts, beginning with Freud's introduction of psychoanalysis to his colleagues in 1895. For the next eight decades, psychotherapists, psychologists, counselors, rehabilitation counselors, and other helping professionals embraced this paradigm that inherently ignored the role that culture plays in shaping human behavior. As counseling theories have evolved, however, the helping professionals have begun to see evidence of a gradual move to acknowledge the role that culture plays in shaping human behavior.

Wrenn (1962) initially described the culturally encapsulated counselor and laid the framework for what has come to be one of the most discussed issues of the day. This latest paradigm shift notes the critical importance that cultural variables, such as ethnicity, religion, sexual orientation, and age, play in the counseling process. Today, given the impact of this critical paradigm shift, it would be thought nearly implausible to ignore the relevance of culture to the process of counseling.

Some authors (Lewis, Lewis, Daniels, and Andrea, 2003) feel "there is considerable reason to believe that a new paradigm shift is, in fact, currently taking place in counseling" (p. 5). Counseling may be taking the next step up the evolutionary ladder, so to speak, by shifting from seeing culture as one of many variables which should be incorporated into existing theoretical approaches, to recognizing the need to develop counseling approaches which address culture as the core issue behind their design. These changes continue to highlight the importance of cultural competence to the counseling profession.

EVIDENCE OF A PARADIGM SHIFT

The importance and necessity of training rehabilitation professionals, counselors, psychologist and others, who are sensitive to culture, as well as competent to work with today's changing client populations, has been highlighted within the fields of rehabilitation, psychology and counseling for the past several decades. So significant has this been to counseling that Pederson (1990) hailed it to be the "fourth force in counseling." In 1992, Sue, Arredondo, and McDavis identified thirty-one proficiencies that were necessary for counselors to work with a culturally diverse clientele. Three broad categories or domains were identified: cultural self-awareness and other awareness, knowledge, and skills. A comprehensive definition proposed by Pope-Davis and Dings (1995, p. 288) further explains that:

> [M]ulticultural counseling competencies are centered on: (a) understanding the different experiences of members of various cultural groups, (b) understand the barriers to communication across cultures that exist as a result of these differences and (c) possessing a specific set of abilities that can potentially make a counselor culturally skilled.

The generally accepted understanding of cultural competence refers to a counselor's preparedness to effectively serve the needs of clients from differing cultural backgrounds by illustrating sensitivity and respect for the cultural norms, values, and mores upheld by the client. The literature in the fields of rehabilitation, psychology, counseling and related helping professions increasingly refers to the need for counselors to pursue and maintain cultural competence. In recent years, the literature has illustrated the enhanced interest and more concerted efforts to address the issue of cultural competence (Corey, 2006; Slattery, 2004; Lum, 2003; Pope-Davis, Coleman, Liu, & Toporek, 2003; Bellini, 2002; Fuertes, Bartholomeo, & Nichols, 2001; Leal-Idrogo, 1997; Okun, Fried, & Okun, 1999; Cross, 1989; Sue et al. 1998). As the discourse on culture, multiculturalism, diversity, and related issues propels forward, the discussion of cultural competence and the need for counselors to pursue it has also been fused into the literature. Most practitioners today would consider it unethical for counselors who lack cultural competence and the characteristics inherent therein to attempt to provide counseling for those clients who are culturally different from themselves. This is a clear departure from practices of the past and an indication of the growth that has occurred in the helping professions.

Diller (1999) notes, "in its broadest context, cultural competence is the ability to effectively provide services cross culturally" (p. 10). Lum (2003), on the other hand, suggests that cultural competence "is a measurable professional standard that evaluates the incorporation of the differential historical, political, socioeconomic, psychophysical, spiritual, and ecological realities, their interaction, and its impact on individuals or groups" (p. 8). Definitions of cultural competence have taken very different approaches, as different researchers and practitioners define culture, multiculturalism, transculturalism, and diversity differently.

As this process has evolved, what appears to have emerged as the most viable standard is the definition proposed by Sue et al. (1999) that was accepted by the American Psychological Association, the American Counseling Association, and the Association for Multicultural Counseling and Development. According to Sue (1998), attaining multicultural counseling competence means that the individual must work to minimize the far reaching influence which results from the socialization we experience in our personal and professional development. To do so effectively, we are encouraged to address what they have described as three Dimensions of Cultural competence, which are:

- Counselors' need to be aware of their culture, values, assumptions, and biases;
- The ability to understand the worldview of culturally different clients; and
- Developing appropriate intervention strategies and techniques for use with different cultural populations.

THE LANGUAGE OF CULTURAL COMPETENCE
THE NATURE OF CULTURE

Developing a framework for a dialogue regarding cultural competence requires that we first understand the language of cultural competence. Terms such as culture, multiculturalism, bias, prejudice, discrimination, oppression, acculturation, and diversity are commonly used, and yet there is substantial debate regarding the meaning of these terms.

CULTURE

Culture impacts all aspects of our lives from the way we perceive ourselves, others, and our environment, to the way that we assess and choose to respond to the situations and individuals that we encounter. Despite the fact that culture permeates every aspect of our daily lives, satisfactorily explaining "what culture means" from a counseling perspective is a unique challenge. The root of that challenge is the fact that culture means different things to different people. Historically, race and ethnicity have been used as virtually synonymous terms for *culture*. Okun (1999), however clearly states that

> [R]ace and ethnicity are both social constructs. Social constructs are categories created by a culture or a society to serve the needs of that society. What this means, for the purpose of our discussion, is that we should recognize that often, who belongs to, or who does not belong to a category is determined by society. For example, in the United States,

> anyone with African ancestry is labeled African American, and
> in Brazil, anyone with white ancestry is labeled white.

(p. 3)

Despite the artificial nature of its origins, as the discussion of culture evolved in the fields of rehabilitation, counseling, and psychology, race is often seen as a critical variable. Membership in one of the racial groups defined by America was viewed as the determining factor for one's values, beliefs, and perceptions. In contrast to race, Diller defines ethnicity as "any distinguishable people whose members share a common culture and see themselves as separate and different" (1999, p. 4). As the discussion of culture has evolved, so has our understanding of race and ethnicity and their relevance to culture. While still seen as a critical component of culture, it is now more practical to include race and ethnicity as variables that should and have been joined by a number of other variables. To accurately reflect the way that culture is treated in the field today, Sue et al. (1998) appropriately point out that "culture is not synonymous with 'race' or 'ethnic group'" (p. 7).

Most importantly, race is an artificial construct that has been used to classify or lump individuals into groups that they may or may not share much in common. Recent developments in genetics suggest that there is as much within-group difference as there is between-group difference among members of various racial groups. As aforementioned, this "artificial construct" has had, and continues to have, major implications in regard to social justice and equity.

Culture, broadly defined, includes variables such as race, disability status, social class, gender, age, spirituality, and sexual preference. Slattery (2004) includes race, ethnicity, class, gender, age, religion, affectional orientation, and ability in his definition of culture, while Ivey (1997) includes age, ethnicity/race, gender, geographical location or community, language, sexual orientation, spiritual/religious beliefs, socioeconomic situation, and trauma.

As Sue (1998) stated, "there are many definitions of culture," (p.7) many of which seem quite viable. As you examine the various definitions available in the literature, the process of considering which definition fits best with your worldview can, in itself, provide a perspective toward greater cultural awareness.

Even those who devote considerable time to the discussion of the subject disagree over whether it should be defined narrowly or from a broader perspective. A historical and somewhat narrow definition of culture promotes a view of race and ethnicity as the key variables to be considered. The argument for defining culture in this manner is that "doing so helps the term maintain integrity and meaning" (Skoyhold and Rivers, 2004, p. 25). When culture is defined more broadly, race and ethnicity are still considered, but in conjunction

72

with variables such as gender, disability status, age, social class, spirituality, and sexual orientation. The latter, broader definition tends to complicate our ability to understand culture and its impact at the individual level, but it also allows for a more comprehensive reflection of culture. Additionally, the broader definition, in a sense, allows for a multi-level examination of the societal and psychological impact of diversity when considering both social and policy-related ramifications. This broader definition is discussed frequently in the fields of rehabilitation, psychology, counseling, and other helping professions. For the purpose of our discussions, the broader definition will be applied.

CHARACTERISTICS OF CULTURE

We should recognize that, as a matter of course, culture is passed on to us from the moment we are born. It is instilled in us through the first human interactions that we have, and it is imprinted on us through countless repetitive exposure. Gollnick (2004) describes culture as the "natural and only way to learn and to interact with others" (p. 6). While Erickson (1997) notes "culture is in us and all around us, just as the air we breathe" (page 33). Culture is not to be considered as a part of our biological makeup. Culture is neither fused into our genetic makeup nor somehow mysteriously passed on to us at the moment of conception. It is the very nature of culture, that it is *learned*. Culture is passed on to us as a part of an ongoing process or more accurately, two similar processes known as socialization and enculturation. Socialization is defined as "the process through which a child learns the rules and norms of a society" (Gladding 2001, p. 112). One example might occur within the realm of religious identity. Children born to parents who are perhaps devout Catholics, are typically taught at a young age the values, mores, and social norms of the religion. Throughout their childhood development, they practice rituals, attend events, and engage in other practices that support these beliefs. They are socialized in the way of being a Catholic.

As a part of this process, we learn how a member of our group is expected to behave. So as we encounter situations that require us to assume different roles such as son, daughter, brother, sister, husband, wife, we have a frame of reference on which we might rely. As we interact with others, our behavior towards them may be influenced by our interpretation of how well they fit with our cultural notion of how someone should behave as a spiritual leader, friend, teacher, politician, or lover.

Enculturation describes the process through which we internalize the characteristics of a culture. Through exposure to that culture, we learn its language, its behaviors, and its nuance. While we are typically born into a culture, what we are at birth grows in relevance when you also consider socialization and enculturation. It is the combined impact of socialization and enculturation that shapes us into members of our respective cultures.

CULTURAL IDENTITY DEVELOPMENT

As you may have suspected, just as there are various ways of explaining culture there are also a number of models to explain how cultural identities develop.

Table I
CULTURAL IDENTITIES MODELS

Authors	Model	
Downing and Roush	1985	Feminist Identity Development for Women
Trosden	1989	Ideal Typical Model of Homosexual Identity Formation
Helm	1990	Racial Identity
Cross	1991	Nigresance Theory
Sellers et al.	1998	The Multidimensional Model of Racial Identity
Sue and Sue	2003	Racial Cultural Identity

Skyhold and Rivers (2003) explain that identity development models attempt to offer a plausible explanation of how individuals "grow, see the world, develop and change attitudes, and relate to other people and groups" (p. 367). As we attempt to understand ourselves, our clients, and the world that we live in, identity development models can serve as useful tools. Because they recognize the disparate variables that influence our development, they can help us see and understand how our cultural experiences with power, privilege, oppression, and other variables influence our behavior and shape our identities as unique cultural individuals.

MULTICULTURALISM AND DIVERSITY

In general, the term multicultural relates to the idea that there is more than one viable cultural group and that all cultures have value to their respective members. Multiculturalism also recognizes that race, gender, disability status, sexual orientation, religion, and social class are categories that can be used to define and understand the cultural perspectives of individuals. As suggested by Sommers-Flanagan and Sommers-Flanagan (2004), the discussion of culture and the meaning of the term may take on a slightly different meaning depending upon who is framing the discussion.

Currently, multicultural counseling is considered the phrase of choice when describing counseling scenarios that involve individuals from differing cultural backgrounds. There is, of course, no universally accepted definition for multicultural counseling, but there are a number of definitions that are commonly accepted. Consider, for example, the following definition offered by Sue (2003). Multicultural counseling refers to a helping role and process that uses approaches and defines goals consistent with the life experiences and cultural values of clients, balancing they importance of individualism versus collectivism in assessment, diagnosis and treatment.

According to Corey (2005), "Multicultural counseling focuses on understanding not only racial and ethnic minority groups (African Americans, Asian Americans, Latinos, Native Americans, and white ethnics) but also women, gay men and lesbians, people with physical disabilities, elderly people, and a variety of special needs populations" (p. 15). As we define multicultural counseling and consider its relevance to our work, we must bear in mind that it refers to both the helping role and the process that we choose, as well as the various modalities that we employ. It is also shaped by the cultural values of consumers, and it should promote the application of strategies that are designed to be compatible with those we serve.

Multicultural counseling may be alternately described as cross-cultural, intercultural, culturally sensitive, culturally competent, or culturally aware counseling. Given the diverse nature of the world today, when the categories gender, race, disability status, sexual orientation, religion, and social class are considered to be elements of an individuals culture, it is difficult to imagine any counseling session that would not involve multicultural counseling.

While *transculturalism* is a term that appears less frequently in the literature, it is useful to point it out its meaning differs slightly from that of multiculturalism. While multicultural approaches give equal consideration to both the differences and the similarities that exist between cultures, the term

Transculturalism has as its sole focus, the discovery of those elements that are common to all cultures. Unlike multicultural approaches and related research, the focus of transcultural approaches and research is on exploring those variables which all cultures share in common.

ASSIMILATION AND ACCULTURATION

Assimilation and acculturation are terms that have been used to provide an explanation of the changes that individuals experience as cultures collide. Brammer (2004) suggest that as the fields of counseling and psychology discovered the relevance of culture to the practice of counseling, they sought ways to explain it. Initial suppositions relied heavily on the assumption that indigenous cultures were inferior to the dominant culture. Since the dominant culture was superior by definition, it was only natural to assume that those from inferior cultures would either simply be overwhelmed by it or willingly give into it. Assimilation and acculturation offer slightly different explanations of what actually takes place when cultures come into contact with each other. The underlying assumption behind assimilation is that when two separate and distinct cultures come together, the dominant culture would, and from the counselors' perspective, should absorb the members of the non-dominant culture. In that process, members of the non-dominant culture would be transformed to fit into the dominant cultural structure. Here again, the assumption is that this process would be healthier for the client.

There are, of course, several problems with this concept; starting with the flawed assumption that one culture is superior to another. What seems unlikely is that the members of any culture would willingly give up their values for those of another culture. The implication that members of the culture that by definition must be seen as lesser will give up their cultural identity in preference for becoming a member of the dominant culture, seems unlikely. Even if the members of the lesser culture intended to divest themselves completely from their old culture it seems impractical, to say the least, to think that they could. A third assumption, which seems unlikely, is that the members of the dominant culture would remain relatively unchanged by this interaction.

Assimilation soon proved to be a flawed and ineffective means of describing what happens when cultures collide. Brammer (2004) and Jackson (2001) noted the even if it were possible for individuals to "assimilate," the harmful effects that they would experience far outweighed any potential benefit that they would derive through the counselors efforts to facilitate their assimilation. Acculturation was thus proposed as an alternative means of explaining what should take place when members of different cultures come into contact with each other.

Acculturation is similar in nature to assimilation in that it too infers the existence of lesser and greater cultures. Unlike assimilation, acculturation implies that members of the presumed lesser cultures can be merged and integrated into the greater culture. As the two cultures come into contact, the members of the lesser culture find a means of grafting themselves onto the second (dominant) culture. This adaptation to the dominant culture, supported by the counseling professional, is supposed to assist clients to make a healthy transition from their inferior culture, to the dominant culture. It should be noted that assimilation and acculturation are concepts that were developed and practiced in the US as conceptualized by practitioners that, for the most part, thought of themselves as members of this superior culture. While acculturation is a well known and commonly used term, its application, much like other terms used to frame discussions concerning culture, is still being debated.

Diller, (1999) notes, "researchers have long argued over how best to conceptualize the process of acculturation. Is it one-dimensional or multidimensional? That is, does acculturation, exist on a single continuum ranging from identification with the indigenous culture at one end to identification with the dominant culture at the other? Or does it make more sense to conceive of an individuals attachment to the two groups as independent of each other, with the possibility of simultaneously retaining an allegiance to ones traditional culture as well as to the dominant American culture?" (p. 96). The debate regarding the conceptualization of acculturation, like the debate over culture, multiculturalism, and diversity is quite likely to linger for some time.

Assimilation and acculturation are useful concepts in that they offer some insight into the thinking that was historically prevalent in the field of counseling. Assimilation and acculturation, however, share a common flaw. They are based on the premise that members of non-dominant or indigenous cultural groups would be agreeable to supplanting portions of their cultural underpinnings, in part or wholly, in favor of elements that would be derived from the culturally dominant group. While plausible under some circumstances, it would not seem that such an assumption would be viable or healthy for most people. Brammer (2004) suggested, "there is a growing awareness that people remain distinct and maintain primary friendships within various cultural groups. Rather than form a single shared culture, multifarious societies seem to exist as a collective of distinct components" (p. 4). Recently, the model of acculturation has given way to that of cultural pluralism. Cultural pluralism is an approach that recognizes that cultures tend to maintain their integrity even as they are mixed together in what Pope (1995) refers to as the salad bowl effect. While assimilation and acculturation suggest the existence of a dominant culture which might absorb or convert those from other, inferior cultures, cultural pluralism suggest that all cultures tend to maintain their identities even when exposed to other cultures. Cultural pluralism is built on the assumption that the world is comprised of a number of separate and distinct cultural groups that for practical reasons maintain a degree of separation from other cultures. It is also built on the assumption that while differences may exist between cultures, all cultures are, relatively speaking, equal, and valued by the individuals who belong to them. As cultures come together, they simply add their unique flavor to the existing group.

The fact remains, however, that when cultures interface, people change. How they change, what factors influence the ability and extent to which an individual may change, and how those changes impact the individuals who change is still a matter of some debate, but that they change seems evident. When the interface between cultures is sudden and the individuals involved do not have adequate time to prepare for the interface or the interface is too prolonged or intense, the phenomena known as culture shock takes place. Culture shock describes the anxiety, disorientation, and fear that occur when an individual from one culture is abruptly immersed in a second, unfamiliar culture (Lum, 2003). Take for example how an individual from an agrarian based, technologically unsophisticated, rural culture might respond if some disaster forced them to relocate to a country where a different language is spoken and they find themselves in a large, modern, technologically advanced, urban setting. The cultural mechanisms that they have employed to survive and prosper in their old environment would no longer apply, and they would, in all probability, find it difficult to adapt to the new environment.

POWER, PRIVILEGE, AND OPPRESSION

As we attempt to understand oppression from a counseling perspective, it is important to place it in its proper context. People often struggle to explain the cause of oppression, and of course, we can explain it from various theoretical perspectives. Using a behavioral model, for example, we could say that the behavior *oppression* exists because the individual or group exhibiting the behavior receives a reward or positive reinforcement that perpetuates the behavior. Those who are rewarded by increased access to jobs, educational opportunities, membership in social groups or organizations, or simply peer approval, will tend to persist in that behavior as long as the reinforcement carries sufficient weight.

There seems to be no simple answer to the question: Why do people discriminate? One plausible explanation is that people in power, the privileged, tend to want to stay in power, and simply take those actions needed to keep themselves and their group in power, thus retaining their privilege. Another explanation could be that people simply discriminate against those that their peers and other situational pressures place outside of their group. When Muslims in Saudi Arabia discriminate against Christians, it could be because their peers drive them to do so. The discrimination could also be rooted in the perceived inferiority of the group being discriminated against. You may find that people without disabilities, or those temporarily able-bodied, will discriminate against persons with disabilities because of a perception of the person with the disability being "less than" or "beneath" the person who is able bodied. This treatment could also be attributed to our society's values of strength, the body beautiful and perfection; variables that some perceive persons with disabilities to not have.

For the purpose of our discussions, the criteria for determining oppression rest in the consequences of that behavior, and not the cause. After all, as health care professionals, we must find a means of addressing, and when possible, **ameliorating** the consequences regardless of the cause. Ridley (2005) agrees that "the criteria for determining racism, lie in the consequences of behavior, not the causes." Racism is not determined by the causes of behavior, because good intentions often lead to bad interventions. As culturally competent practitioners, the question we need to respond to is not whether someone intends to oppress, but whether the consequences of their behavior has the effect of oppressing.

Most people like to think of themselves as fair and unbiased, and yet we are generally not. Bias is simply another part of the human condition that exists in all of us. Consider what it means to be biased. According to Gladding, it means, "To have a negative attitude toward an individual, an idea or a group" (Gladding, 2001, p. 18). Each time we express a preference or dislike for something or someone, we flirt with bias, because if we prefer something do not we also prefer something else less? Bias, however, is not the problem. We can like or dislike a person, group, or thing, or be prejudiced in our opinions because we hold some stereotype of a group. If we do not act or if we cannot act on those feelings; if we fail to discriminate against or in favor of someone or some group, then what harm has been done? As rehabilitation professionals we should, at the very least, endeavor to make ourselves aware of any bias or preconceived attitude that we may hold.

Consider for a moment what it is like to be a member of a privileged group or, for that matter, its polar opposite, an oppressed group. Can you be a member of an oppressed group and not be harmed by it? Can you be a member of a privileged group and not benefit from it? As you consider your answers, consider this. Those who have privilege and choose to act to ensure that they retain that privilege obviously do so to their advantage, and if it is to their advantage does that not also imply that it is to the injury of someone else? Of course, there are those who, in their estimation, do nothing to discriminate against others, but simply choose not to give up their privilege. If they do not actively participate in the effort to bar the door for some racial, ethical, religious, disability, or gender group, are they still acting in an oppressive manner? The same simple question would seem to apply in this situation as well. Do those with privilege benefit from the situation?

We should also acknowledge that systemic oppression or discrimination continues to exist today. It too is the legacy of decades of racial, gender, ability, and age bias that existed, unchecked in our society. As a consequence of these years of oppression, today's systems are often set up in ways that continue to discriminate against many of these same groups. Even though the discrimination may be unintentional, it is harmful nonetheless. A system that is set up from a monoculture perspective is unlikely to be responsive to the needs of those who fall outside of that culture.

Notwithstanding the fact that we live in one of the most enlightened democracies on the planet, privilege, much like oppression, continues to permeate the fabric of our daily lives. It is our legacy from the racist, sexist, ability biased, age biased, society that serves as the foundation of what exists today.

Having a meaningful discussion about privilege and who is or is not the beneficiary of privileged status can be challenging, to say the least. One of the most difficult aspects of having an equitable dialogue about privilege is related to the deep feelings many people have on the matter. Many African Americans, for example, feel that they continue to be victimized because of the privileges enjoyed by whites in the United States. On the other side of the issue, many whites feel that America is no longer a racist society, and they, in turn, feel victimized by affirmative action. Race, of course, is not the only factor to be considered where privilege is concerned. Individuals with disabilities are often bothered by the privileges they see afforded to the able, and women express frustration with a system that offers so much privilege to men.

The underlying problem in discussing privilege was aptly pointed out by Slattery (2004) as he states "Becoming aware of privilege, is often difficult because it requires that we give up the Just World Hypothesis" (Slattery, 2004, p. 71). The central belief in the Just World Hypothesis is that we have all that we have because we have earned it, and of course, we deserve it. To acknowledge that we are members of a privileged class means that we must acknowledge that we have, at times, benefited from that privilege. If we have benefited, then others have been victimized. It brings us face to face with the issue of discrimination, and more importantly, the fact that we may have discriminated against others, or at the very least, allowed surrogates to discriminate against them on our behalf.

If the privileged exist, then so do the oppressed. Hays (1995) viewed oppression in terms of the actions taken by the privileged that excluded or marginalized groups of people. Those who had their ability to participate in any of the daily acts of living negatively impacted by their group membership were then, by definition, oppressed. Unless it is an extremely obvious example of discrimination, it is often difficult to see and understand oppression. Slattery (2004) notes that "Most of us would recognize a lynching as a racist act; however, most oppression is much more difficult to see" (pg. 67). Because privileges attributed to gender, race, class, ability et cetera have evolved as integral parts of our respective cultures; they are often so subtle that they are simply taken for granted. The interplay of several dimensions, race and class or gender and disability, also present challenges for understanding the impact of oppression and limits one's ability to decipher the roots of any subtle or overt experiences of discrimination.

BIAS OR PREJUDICE
Bias is defined by Gladding (2004, p. 18) as "prejudice or a negative attitude toward an individual, idea or group." Prejudice, on the other hand, is defined as "Preconceived opinions or judgments about someone or something formed without just grounds or sufficient knowledge" (Gladding, 2004 p. 94). A male may be prejudice, for example, if he judges all women to be too emotional to participate in a debate. A heterosexual who assumes all homosexuals are sexually promiscuous also shows prejudice. The existence of prejudice or bias does not necessarily lead to discrimination. Nor does it always do harm to the person toward whom the bias is directed. While difficult, it is possible that a person with a bias or prejudice could refrain from acting on said bias and, therefore, avoid harming the party toward which the prejudice is directed. Of

course, if you are unaware that you have a bias, it seems unlikely that you could avoid acting on it.

Unlike prejudice, stereotypes can be either positive or negative. Gladding describes a stereotype as "a fixed image or thought of people, things, and places that is oversimplified, rigid, and often prejudice (2004, p. 115). Some common stereotypes might be "all persons with disabilities are mild mannered;" "all African American men are naturally good athletes;" "all Asians are good in math;" and "all those of Jewish decent are good managers of money." Bias, prejudice, and stereotypes do exist where discrimination is found, but the existence of bias does not always result in discrimination. For discrimination to exist, people must not only have a prejudice, but also they must act in a discriminatory manner. People will usually act in what they see as their own self-interest, so if social edicts indicate that acting in a discriminatory manner will produce results they do not desire they will tend to refrain from discriminating. Of course, when a society provides rewards for acting in a discriminatory manner, people will tend to discriminate.

There are people who will simply choose not to discriminate because they feel it is the right thing to do. People do not always realize or acknowledge that they have a bias, or that they themselves are members of some privileged group. Knowingly or not, people are likely to act on their prejudices, and such action by definition is discrimination and does cause harm.

CONTEXT AND CULTURAL COUNSELING

It is a simple matter to recognize that behavior does not occur in a vacuum. That people differ in the way that they perceive, assess, and react to others is obvious: the question is, why? What shapes the behavior of a client, or the way that the client responds to a given situation? For that matter, what shapes the way that the client perceives an individual or a situation in the first place? To understand why people perceive people and circumstances as they do we must understand the context in which their perceptions and behaviors take place. As we learn to understand the cultural context within which behavior takes place, we move closer to understanding the individual. Understanding who people are and why they behave as they do requires that we consider them and their behavior from a cultural context. The individual's behavior can then be understood by considering how the various elements of their culture, language, race, disability status, gender preference, spirituality, et cetera contributes to their perception of their environments, and shapes their response to that environment. We must learn to look at others and ourselves from a cultural context. As we noted, culture shapes our perceptions, views, and behaviors across a number of dimensions such as spirituality, gender preference, locus of control, individuation, gender roles and much more. To the extent that we understand how these variables impact us, we develop a keener self-awareness and we develop a broader framework from which to consider the behavior of others.

Consider the relative value you assign to your independence. This is represented by a cultural dimension referred to as individuation. Individuation is one of the cultural variables that are frequently used to differentiate one cultural group from another. Cultures that are highly individualistic place a high value on personal independence, and on having autonomy. On the other end of the spectrum, you have cultures that are collectivist in nature. These cultures place a high value on the needs and desires of the group. Cultures that are considered more collectivist include African Americans, Asian Americans, First Nation Peoples, and Latino Americans. European Americans, on the other hand, are considered to be relatively more individualistic in nature. If you understand how this impacts individuals from their respective cultures, it may help you place the behavior of a client in its proper context, giving you greater insight into the person. Take a moment to consider your own orientation toward individuation. If you are a European American (white), chances are that you are relatively individualistic in nature. Consider this bit of information as a piece of a larger puzzle. The more pieces you fill in, the more of the puzzle you get to see. To better understand clients from a cultural context, you must understand how they are impacted from a cultural context.

PUTTING CULTURE IN CONTEXT

Knowing that a person is Hispanic American or African American may tell you something about their culture, but their disability status, gender, sexual preference, social status, country of origin, or religion might tell you just as much. Where you begin your discussion of culture often influences where you end up. Worldview is a concept that is used to encompass individuals' understanding and perception of their world based on their upbringing, disability status, gender, parental relationships, spiritual beliefs, education, sexual orientation, socioeconomic status, heritage, and ethnic group membership, to name a few.

According to the literature, (Okun, 1999; Ibrahim, 1985: Sue & Sue, 1990) the term worldview refers to "one's basic perceptions and understandings of the world" (Okun, 1999, p. 12). An individual's worldview develops as a consequence of their life experiences. Individuals have a worldview that is shaped by these variables as well as many others that can impact persons during their lives. It is the very nature of culture that ensures that it touches virtually every aspect of our lives. It is a complex multifaceted construct, which shapes the way we view and interact with our environment, while it in turn is shaped by that environment.

For the purpose of our discussions, let us consider the definition of culture provided by Gladding (2001), who describes culture as the "shared values, belief, expectations, world views, symbols, and appropriate behaviors of a group that provides its members with norms, plans, and rules for social living (pg, 34). As the definition implies, culture shapes individuals' perceptions of the world they live in and the way they interact with the various elements of that world. "The philosophy underlying the MCCs is as follows: All counseling is multicultural in nature; sociopolitical and historical forces influence the culture of counseling beliefs, values, and practices, and the worldview of clients and counselors; and ethnicity, culture, race, language, and other dimensions of diversity need to be factored into counselor preparation and practice" (Arredondo and Arciniega, 2001, p. 266).

PREPARING CULTURALLY SENSITIVE/
COMPETENT COUNSELORS

Achieving some degree of cultural competency is a process. One that, in order to be effective, must be preceded by the struggle to understand one's personal cultural beliefs, values, and attitudes. A counselor seeking to develop culturally sensitive and competent counseling skills will need the ability to both acknowledge and accept the similarities and differences that exist between themselves and their clients. Bellini, (2002) asserts that skilled multicultural counselors understand that helping styles and intervention strategies may be culture bound, and they seek to adjust their counseling approaches to the culture, values, and needs of the individual. In rehabilitation counseling, it can be argued that historical indifference to the significance of racial/ethnic diversity on issues affecting clients with disabilities may be attributed not only the low numbers of racially/ethnically diverse populations participating in rehabilitation, but also the documented differential treatment they encounter in the system (Watson & Collins, 1993 as seen in Middleton, et. al, 2000). The process of striving toward cultural competence is pertinent to the process of effective counseling and service provision.

Corey (2001) states, "first, effective counselors have moved from being culturally unaware to ensuring that their personal biases, values, or problems will not interfere with their ability to work with clients who are culturally different from them" (pg 26). Counselors are faced with the challenge of finding a means of moving toward this state of cultural awareness in a way that is consistent with their needs. Because we are the unique beings with cultures, personalities, and theoretical orientations that are our own, our routes to obtaining cultural competence will also be uniquely our own.

CHARACTERISTICS OF CULTURALLY COMPETENT COUNSELORS
Culturally competent counselors should value the beliefs of the clients that they serve. They should at once be capable of having knowledge of the clients' culture and of respecting the clients' beliefs, even when they differ from their own. Culturally competent counselors do not assume that their culture is superior to that of their clients, nor do they attempt to persuade the client that they should abandon their cultural beliefs in preference for those of the counselor. Assistance should be provided to the client within a cultural context that works best for the client.

Culturally competent counselors strive to understand how the dynamics of bias, prejudice, racism, oppression, stereotyping, and discrimination impact relationships. Understanding how concepts such as racism and oppression impact counseling can be difficult enough in and of itself, considering the possibility that you as a counselor may have acted as an oppressor in the past, or that you may be racist, can be very difficult indeed. Meier (1989) notes, "Every beginning counselor will eventually confront difficult questions about her or his personal issues. Answers to these questions may not be readily apparent. Your issues, however, do influence how you counsel" (p. 55).

There are a number of variables that make it more or less likely that a student will begin to master the knowledge, skills, and abilities that they will need to become an effective, culturally sensitive counselor. However, not one exceeds the need for students to have the ability and temperament to look critically at their lives, their cultures, and the variables that shape and influence their behavior towards others. Before counselors attempt to understand why others think and behave as they do, they should carefully examine the assumptions that underpin their own thoughts and behavior. This is especially true where matters of culture are involved. As they describe the personal qualities of a counselor, Gillard, James (1998) note that "unless counselors can work vigorously and systematically on self evaluation, and the solution to their own problems, much of the therapeutic value of their contact with clients will be lost" (p. 8). The popular opinion of traditionally trained psychotherapists proposes that a prospective therapist should undergo therapy and self-evaluation.

Who we are as individuals will invariably impact who we are as counselors. Therefore, the counseling approach and the techniques used within that approach must be seen in light of how they relate to the personality, character, and culture of the counselor. While there is, perhaps, no ideal set of traits that are best suited for counselors to have; there are some personal characteristics that can have a definitively positive impact on the counseling process by the mere virtue of their presence or absence.

To begin with, the culturally competent counselor should believe in the value of both the process of counseling and the critical role that culture plays in that process. It is, after all, their conviction in the process that will serve as the anchor for their belief that the approach that they are using has the actual potential to help those they are serving. It is the counselors' faith in the value of the process that should allow them to bring certain energy to that process which they can pass on to their client.

Counselors who can exhibit *allegiance* (Bordin, 1983) by effectively communicating their honest and sincere belief in counseling, and who can cultivate a strong working alliance (Bordin) by illustrating their cultural awareness and a sincere value of the client, can thus devote more of their energy to the process of helping. Genuineness implies that the counselor is willing to share who they are with the client and to interact with the client based on a genuine respect for both the client and their culture. Counselors' sincere interest in the client and their genuine respect of the client's cultural values are the essential building blocks for the culturally competent counselor. They serve to both lay the foundation for understanding the client and demonstrate the counselors' unconditional positive regard for the client. One factor allows the counselor to consider the client's behavior in its proper context, the other supports the counselor's effort to establish rapport.

Counselors need to be able to rely on the security of being solidly grounded in their own cultural identity. They should have a solid understanding of who they are, what they value, what they believe in, and how these factors impact their relationship with others. They should be comfortable enough with their own cultures to allow them to easily and honestly respond to questions about themselves that may arise during a counseling session. Corey, (2006) suggests that among other characteristics, counselors should be enthusiastic about the counseling process, have the courage not to hide their true selves from their clients, and possess a willingness to confront themselves. In short, counselors' ability to help clients understand their strengths and weakness, or the things that truly make them happy, angry, or sad, as well as those things that introduce anxiety and fear into their lives, centers on counselors' ability to understand and confront these things in their own lives.

One aspect of self-awareness relates to counselors' knowledge of their role as counselor, and the authority, power, and responsibility imbedded in that roll. Clients and others often credit counselors with a great deal of personal power. Counselors should respect the nature of their relationships and exercise caution so that they do not abuse their power. This is particularly relevant when working with clients for whom there exists a perceived social power differential (e.g., able-bodied counselors and clients with disabilities; male counselors and female clients, or chronologically older counselors and clients who are younger in age).

COUNSELOR BELIEFS AND ATTITUDES

Counselors have numerous opportunities to validate the clients' efforts to preserve their cultural identities and respect for their cultures. They also have the opportunity to foster in a client circumstances that could lead the client to have a diminished view of the significance of the cultural values and practices held by that client. It is an awesome responsibility to shoulder and one that counselors would be well advised to carefully prepare themselves to address.

Counselors should give considerable thought to the principles they will use to guide themselves through the complex minefield of issues associated with counseling individuals across cultures. The relevance of racism, bias, and prejudice can be difficult issues to fully understand or navigate through in counseling, but no more so than oppression, acculturation, assimilation, or culturally bound behaviors. Counselors who desire to effectively serve clients from diverse backgrounds need to carefully consider the principles that will be used to guide their efforts.

We offer the following statements as considerations that prospective culturally competent counselors should keep in mind as they attempt to enhance their competency in counseling multicultural clients.

- Culture is difficult to rigidly define, as are the boundaries of its influence.
- Culture is and should be treated as a fluid, not as a static influence on behavior.
- The culture of those you serve has value to them, and as such deserves your respect.
- Clients come to you to acquire the help they need to live their lives within their own unique cultural realities.

- Counselors should attempt to understand their own cultures and master whatever cultural issues they have prior to attempting to help others master theirs.
- Counselors should acknowledge, understand, and respect connectivity to their own culture as an important part of the process of becoming culturally competent.
- Counselors should consider it their duty to help clients maintain their cultural values so long as they can do so while maintaining their identity, their ethical standards, and their objectivity as a counselor.
- What you come to consider as the normal cultural behavior for someone from a particular group may be accurate in general terms, but quite inaccurate in specific, individual cases.

SKILLS ASSOCIATED WITH CULTURAL COMPETENCE PRACTICE
Counselors will need to develop a number of skills if they are to practice culturally competent counseling. Many of these skills are simply related to good counseling practices. To accurately reflect the knowledge, skills, and abilities that the culturally competent practitioner is expected to possess as it relates to the fields of rehabilitation, counseling, psychology, and related health care professions, we have relied heavily on the cultural competencies described by Sue (Sue et al., 1998). The following list of knowledge, skills, and abilities are paraphrased from those competencies. The culturally competent practitioners should

- Recognize that there are too many culturally distinct groups in existence to allow them to know all there is to know about each one. They acknowledge their limitations and attempt to be knowledgeable of the cultural information relevant to the clients they serve most frequently.
- Be aware that all cultures have strengths and weaknesses, and that it is possible and desirable to seek out the resources of a culture, which can be employed to assist the client.
- Approach all counseling situations with respect for the culture(s) of the individual(s) involved.
- Consider the impact of the intersection of various cultural variables on the lives of their clients (e.g., race and socio-economic status; disability and race; or gender and socio-economic status).

- Have expended considerable time and energy to develop awareness of self and of the cultural self. This awareness includes, but is not limited to, an awareness of culturally based beliefs, biases, prejudices, attitudes, behaviors, and stereotypes, and they work diligently to comprehend how these circumstances might impact their interactions with and behavior toward others.
- Be capable of using their knowledge of cultural matters (race, culture, prejudice, oppression, et cetera), their knowledge of culturally appropriate practices, and their knowledge of a genuine rapport with clients from other cultures.
- Be capable of effectively communicating that, while they are secure in their own values, they are mindful that the client can hold different values and that neither is superior to the other.
- Make themselves aware of the myriad problems that can result from privilege, oppression, and discrimination, and be open to considering how such concerns factor into the counseling process.
- Make every effort to discover culturally relevant material that may impact counseling, but remain aware of the fact that there could be other reasonable explanations.
- Be aware of the potential for culturally based assumptions to be formed by either themselves or their clients, and consider potential for such an occurrence to either negatively or positively impact the counseling relationship or process.

COUNSELOR KNOWLEDGE

- Have developed sufficient knowledge regarding their cultural heritage and how it may impact both the counselor and the counseling relationship.
- Have amassed knowledge related to the manner in which bias, prejudice, discrimination, and stereotyping influences them. This knowledge, in turn, allows them to develop further knowledge of how their beliefs, attitudes, biases, prejudices, et cetera, may have resulted in discriminatory acts that were targeted toward racial groups, individuals with disabilities, members of one gender or the other, the elderly, or members of other diverse groups.

- Have acquired knowledge relevant to the cultural group, or groups that they serve.
- Have developed knowledge regarding the manner in which variables such as race, ethnicity, disability status, culture, language group, gender, et cetera, may subsequently impact matters such as identity formation, self esteem, vocational aspiration, propensity to seek help, and the relevance of counseling techniques and approaches.
- Have developed knowledge that facilitates their understanding of the various socio-political forces, such as sexism, ableism, racism, poverty, stereotyping, and oppression that may impact the development and behavior of clients.
- Have extensive knowledge regarding the various theories and techniques of counseling, and how respective approaches may conflict with the cultural vales of some groups.
- Have developed knowledge regarding the existence of institutional barriers that inhibit the ability of some cultural groups to access healthcare services.
- Have acquired knowledge regarding assessment instruments to the extent that they understand that bias exists in the development, administration, and interpretation of these instruments.
- Have developed knowledge regarding the family and community structure that exists within the cultural group(s) that they serve, and they are knowledgeable of the resources that exist.
- Are knowledgeable of the discriminatory or oppressive practices that exist in the communities they serve.
- Have knowledge of the models of identity that apply to majority and minority cultural populations.
- Are familiar with various models of psychosocial adaptation to disability and understands the impact of race/ethnicity on adaptation.

BELIEFS AND ATTITUDES

Culturally competent practitioners should

- Value other cultures and have moved from being relatively culturally unaware to being relatively culturally aware, and also be aware of the attitudes, biases, prejudices, and negative reactions that they may have toward other cultural groups.

- Understand the potential for bias, attitudes, experiences, and values that impact behavior, believe that as practitioners they should be aware of their own cultural values experiences and attitudes, and the potential for these to impact their behavior.
- Be aware of their cultural competencies and their limits.
- Be aware of the differences that exist between cultures, understand the differences that exist between themselves and members of other cultures, and feel comfortable and not threatened by these differences.
- Be aware of the stereotypes and attitudes that exist. Be aware of those that they hold and how they may impact the counseling process.
- Be aware of the spiritual beliefs of clients and acknowledge and respect those beliefs.
- Be aware of the salience of disability for clients and the variance of this salience across individuals and disability groups (e.g., the Deaf culture).
- Be aware of traditional and nontraditional helping practices that exist in certain cultures and believe that it is appropriate to incorporate those practices into the helping process.
- Appreciate bilingualism, understand the differences that exist between language groups, and do not regard language as a barrier to effective counseling.

TRADITIONAL COUNSELING THEORIES

Historically, the traditional counseling theories were validated on and practiced from a mono-cultural perspective. The culturally competent practitioner should consider how specific critiques relate to their application to diverse client populations. Many theories have been revised to acknowledge and address the impact of culture in the counseling relationship. In the chart that follows, we have attempted to provide a brief overview of widely used traditional models that are thought to have some potential for use with multicultural populations. This overview includes reference to key characteristics that each theory/model may offer, which may make them more or less suitable for utilization with specific populations.

Table II

TRADITIONAL COUNSELING THERAPIES AND MULTICULTURAL STRENGTHS

Theoretical System	Founder/Major Contributors	Key Characteristics	Multicultural Focus
Person Centered	Carl Rogers	Humanistic, self-theoretical, unconditional	Promote under standing, accepting and valuing diversity. Promotes cross-cultural empathy.
Gestalt	Frederick Perls	Existential, here-and-now oriented, confrontational	The primary focus on **what** (process) is happening to client vs. content is an advantage to diverse clients. Can be empowering to those with gender issues by focusing on self-awareness.
Psychoanalytic	Sigmund Freud	Deterministic, historical, insightful, unconscious	Importance placed on family history is appealing to various cultural groups. Symbolic work alleviates reluctance some diverse clients feel about sharing/talking in therapy.
Adlerian	Alfred Adler	Holistic, Phenoma-logical,	Historically focused on equality and sensitivity. Driving

Table II (Continued)

Theoretical System	Founder/Major Contributors	Key Characteristics	Multicultural Focus
		socially oriented	force is social involvement and equitable participation of everyone.
Behavioral	B. F. Skinner	Behavioristic, pragmatic, learning theoretical, goal-oriented	Focus on modification of behavior is appealing to diverse clients. Straightforward steps and application make sense to people from various walks of life.
Trait-Factor	E. Griffin Williamson U. of Minnesota	Rational problem-solving, non-pathological maladjustment, unique traits	Person X environment fit. Focus on choice vs. change and approach appears less threatening. May have intrinsic appeal due to time-limited and goal-oriented attributes.
Solution Focused Brief Therapy	S. de Shazar Insoo Kim Berg	Positivistic, focuses on client strengths, here-and-now	Focus on client strengths is appealing to some diverse clients. Construction of solutions also resonates with some diverse clients who are goal orient

(table continues)

Table II (Continued)

Theoretical System	Founder/Major Contributors	Key Characteristics	Multicultural Focus
Existentialism	Karl Jaspers J. P. Satre	Philosophical orientation toward human existence and decision.	Promotes individuals' unique set of choices. Moves away from deterministic and genetically bound outcomes.
Reality	William Glasser	Present focused, strong counselor-client working alliance	Supports strong, trusting relationship between counselor-client to promote allegiance and adherence to counseling treatment plan.
REBT	Albert Ellis	Action-oriented, cognitive, emotive, philosophical	Promotes potential to understand emotional relation-ship to behavior and need for balance.
Cognitive Behavioral	A. Beck, D. Meichenbaum	Cognitive, rational, mental and emotive, perceptual	Initiates a relationship of mutual trust and promotes appreciation of the client's point of view.

Many of the other modern models of psychotherapy have been updated to address multicultural issues. Although these models have been updated to address some aspects of culture, their beginnings were not predicated on the consideration of cross-cultural interactions. They were not designed with counseling persons from diverse backgrounds in mind. Due to this oversight, there were movements to develop models that focused on working with diverse populations.

4

COUNSELING MODELS DESIGNED TO WORK WITH DIVERSE POPULATIONS

There are literally hundreds of counseling models in existence today, many of which can be used effectively with diverse cultural populations. It is not our intent to tell the reader what theory is "the best" approach to use; that is a personal decision that should rest with the reader. Instead, we provide a brief summary of key counseling models with observations regarding their relative strengths and weaknesses when applied to selected cultural groups.

Unlike our predecessors, today's counselors and psychotherapists have access to a wide variety of counseling models, and many of these more effectively address the issue of diversity in counseling. Counseling models, such as Multicultural Counseling and Therapy (MCT), Respectful, and Adressing have been developed with the understanding that culture is a critical element of counseling. Below, we briefly discuss these models that have been designed to effectively serve culturally diverse client populations.

MULTICULTURAL COUNSELING AND THERAPY

Multicultural Counseling and Therapy (MCT) is considered to be the first counseling model to use culture as a core concept (Nystul 1999, Sue, Ivey, and Pederson 1996). MCT is based on six basic assumptions:

- MCT can be used to provide an organizational framework for understanding Western and non-Western theories and methods of helping.
- Counselors' and clients' identities are reflected in various levels of human experience (individual, group, system, and universal). Contextual issues in treatment must, therefore, be addressed as necessary.
- Cultural identity development affects how the counselor and the client view the self and others and how they formulate counseling goals and interventions. It is, therefore, important to be cognizant of how cultural identity development is impacting the counseling process, including an awareness of the different socio-cultural forces that influence its development.
- The efficacy of MCT is enhanced when counselors use procedures congruent with the values and experiences of the client. Counselors are encouraged to broaden their helping

responses so that they demonstrate multicultural sensitivity throughout the counseling process.

- MCT encourages counselors to expand their helping roles to include conventional and alternative methods of helping necessary to meet the cultural needs of clients.
- A fundamental goal of MCT theory is the liberation of consciousness from a relation-contextual perspective. In this regard, MCT attempts to provide opportunities to promote an awareness of how cultural and relationship issues impact present concerns.

A detailed account of this theory can be found in "*Introduction to Counseling: An Art and Science Perspective*" (Nystul, 1999).

RESPECTFUL COUNSELING MODEL

The respectful counseling model, which shares some points in common with MCT, was developed by D'Andrea and Daniels in the late 1990's. The authors (Lewis, Lewis, Daniels & D'Andrea 2003) describe the model as follows: "The RESPECTFUL counseling framework (a) recognizes the multidimensional nature of human development and (b) addresses the need for a comprehensive model of human diversity that has practical utility for the work of mental health professionals" (pg 8). The model is comprised of 10 factors, which D'Andrea and Daniels selected in an effort to comprehensively list those factors which impact "psychological development and personal well being" (Lewis, Lewis, Daniels and D'Andrea 2003, p. 9).

The specific factors that the RESPECTFUL counseling framework directs attention to include

R	religious/spiritual identify
E	economic class background
S	sexual identity
P	level of psychological maturity
E	ethnic/racial identity
C	chronological/developmental challenges
T	various forms of trauma and other threats to one's sense of well-being
F	family background and history
U	unique physical characteristics
L	location of residence and language differences

4

ADRESSING MODEL

Another culturally based approach to counseling is the Adressing model developed by P. A. Hayes. This model was designed to systematically consider the influence that culture has in counseling. In the Adressing model, each letter represents a different cultural factor to be considered during the counseling process. The factors included in this model include

A	age and generational influences
D	disability related issues
R	religious and spiritual issues
E	ethnicity and race
S	social status
S	sexual orientation
I	indigenous heritage
N	national origin
G	gender

The Adressing counseling model is considered trans-cultural in nature and "places a high value on culture-specific expertise" (Hayes 1996, p 334).

These models rest on the foundation of multicultural counseling and multicultural counseling competency. They assert that you must comprehensively consider the diverse aspects of your individual clients. By doing so, you must have a basic knowledge of the diverse variables, an awareness that this diversity exists, and a skill base to address these variables as they mediate the clients' experience.

OTHER CULTURALLY SENSITIVE APPROACHES

Counselor Wisdom Paradigm	Hanna, Bemak & Chung	(1999)
Multicultural Model of Psychotherapy	Ramirez	(1999)
Model of Multicultural Understanding	Locke	(1998)
Coping with Diversity Counseling Model	Coleman	(1997)
Perspectives in Internalized Culture	Ho	(1995)
Cross Cultural Specifio Model	Herring & Walker	(1993)
Multicontextual Model	Steenbargers	(1993)

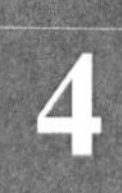

OUTLINING A PROCESS OF BECOMING

Becoming a culturally competent counselor is a process, not an event. There are several steps that individuals may take to move themselves forward from a state of being less culturally competent to a state of being more culturally competent. Those who wish to become culturally competent should begin that process by taking actions that will allow them to facilitate that process. Those who wish to be culturally competent counselors should

- Seek to become culturally aware,
- Avoid the temptation to supplant the clients cultural values with their own,
- Accept the impact that culture has had on the development of your life related behaviors,
- Recognize how little you may actually know about other cultures and work to improve your knowledge of cultures other than your own, especially those of the clients you serve,
- Recognize stereotypes when they exist and avoid them,
- Consider whether your approach to counseling is culturally sensitive,
- Be aware of the culturally valid or invalid assumptions that exist within counseling theories,
- Commit to taking active steps to continue learning about and interacting with diverse cultures,
- Select interventions that are culturally appropriate.

Becoming aware of your culture does not suggest that you are free of negative attitudes or bias. It does, however, make it more likely that you will be cognizant of whatever culturally based biases or prejudices that you do have. Culturally aware counselors should be sensitive to the culturally based concerns of others. The experience of exploring your culture, what it is, what it means to you, and how it has shaped you, should provide you with a framework from which to explore the culture of those with whom you come into contact. A benefit of exploring your culture is that it also has the potential of providing you with insight into the process that clients go through as they attempt to explore their own. You should also learn to acknowledge any negative or overly positive reactions that you experience toward individuals from cultures other than your own. Once counselors develop sensitivity to cultural variables, they are better equipped to monitor their reactions to certain clients and behaviors which may be generated as a result of their culturally influenced view of the world.

Because becoming a culturally competent practitioner is a process, you must understand that the process may take considerable time, thought, and energy. To minimize the potential for encountering problems, counselors should develop a planned approach to assist their efforts to become culturally competent.

There is no one route that we or anyone else have discovered that can direct you to cultural competence. It does seem logical and practical to suggest that if you intend to pursue becoming a culturally competent practitioner, you do so as a part of a larger, structured, and diverse group. Your results will be dependent on the makeup of your group, who leads the process, and the circumstances surrounding the group process. Joining a group that is more heterogeneous should enhance your chances of having a successful experience; just as joining a group dominated by one specific group (race, gender, et cetera) is likely to limit your growth potential. As you consider what may happen, do not confuse the degree of comfort you have with any given group with your potential of improving cultural competence. Look for group experiences that give you the opportunity to have new experiences with those who differ from yourself. If you are uncomfortable around those who differ from yourself, consider what this means, both to you and for anyone you might counsel that could also be different.

As you consider the group process, discuss the intent of the group and the reason for the steps that make up its process. Make certain that you are comfortable with the desired focus of the group. Remember that groups that are dominated by one group or another may tend to make it difficult for the minority members' point of view to he heard. This is as true for those who are traditionally in the majority as it is for those who are traditionally thought of as minorities. The steps we recommend that you consider as a part of your group process are

- Start by participating in a process designed to facilitate self-analysis.
- Complete a cultural biography for yourself.
- Develop a cultural ethnograph.
- Develop a community ethnograph.
- Review the major assumptions, values, and attitudes affiliated with your cultural group.
- Discuss how your culture impacts your view of the world and your interactions with it.
- Using the information that you have collected so far, interview someone from a culture not your own.

- Discuss the treatment of culture in counseling theory, both historically and currently.
- Review the literature and discuss which theories (both traditional and culturally sensitive) most effectively address the needs of diverse client populations.
- If you have not already done so, consider and select the theory that will guide your approach to counseling, and consider its strengths and weaknesses.
- Study the issues involved in working with special populations.
- Pay special attention to barriers to effective cultural counseling.
- Develop a working definition of culture, and the related terms.
- Put what you have learned into practice.
- Refine your practice base of experience and research.

An important part of this process centers on your choice of a theoretical foundation for your practice. When selecting a counseling theory to serve as the underpinning for your practice as a counselor, you should take the time to answer several critical questions about the theories that you consider. Is it a system that is compatible with your personal beliefs? Does it offer a satisfactory explanation of human behavior and personality? Is the approach advocated one that you can comfortably and consistently apply? Is it a good personal fit? Will it (as it is or could it be with the addition of other techniques) meet the needs of the client populations that you plan to work with?

To effectively serve you, the theory that you select should be one that you can live by. It should be a comfortable fit and give you clear guidance in your interpersonal interactions. It should also allow some flexibility with appropriate application of techniques from other theoretical approaches that may be better suited to individual clients' needs. Counselors should take great care when selecting the theory of counseling that will serve as the foundation for their orientation to counseling.

BARRIERS TO CULTURALLY COMPETENT COUNSELING.
Despite the emphasis that has been placed on meeting the needs of culturally diverse clients (D'Andrea, Daniels, & Heck, 1991; Sue, D., Arredondo, P., & McDavis, J., 1992; Pope-Davis & Ottavi, 1994; Sodowsky, G. R., Taffe, R. C., Gutkin, T. B., & Wise, S., 1994), there still exists a gap from that point of

100

knowledge to service delivery. Subsequently, one might assume the following barriers still exist:

- Counselor ability to thoroughly assess themselves.
- Counselor educator receptiveness to the concept of multicultural counseling competencies.
- Lack of effective training programs.
- Varying definitions of "multicultural" and the terms that surround it.
- The entrenched nature of monocultural values that remain in some systems.

The ability of counselors to see clients for who and what they are, to objectively assess the client's situation and to realistically interpret how he/she may assist the client are all critical aspects of counseling. Acknowledging and appreciating the worldview of the client is imperative to any counseling relationship. Counselors, who are hampered by the inability to accurately understand clients from a cultural perspective, will be impeded in their efforts to assist their clients.

CULTURE AND THE COUNSELING PROCESS

Some authors (Corey & Corey, 2006, Pedersen, Draguns, Lonner & Trimble, 2002, Ponderotto, Cosas, Suzuki, & Alexander, 2001, Abad, Ramos, & Boyce, 1974, Trimble, 1981, Ruiz and Ruiz, 1983) have suggested that clients may fair better if the counseling process employed is more suitable to their cultural makeup. Rehabilitation counselors must employ multicultural understanding to effectively provide appropriate services to culturally diverse clients, and to begin to combat the inequities that have been previously noted in rehabilitation counselor literature.

Because culture tends to shape the way we perceive our environment, it often impacts us in ways too subtle for us to understand. Our collective experiences have reinforced some negative observations our parents, friends, and peers offered over the years. Which is why we are seldom surprised when African American clients act in a similar manner. In fairness, other studies (Folensbee, Draguns, and Danish, 1986), have noted that they failed to substantiate differences in the preference of clients for one counseling process over another.

Dinkmeyer and Sperry (2000) suggest that people tend to view things a particular way because their culture provides them with a unique way of looking at the issue. Alston and Bell (1997) also purport that historical treatment by government institutions of African Americans and other underrepresented groups in the country, has festered into a huge snowball of distrust for modern-day governmental programs and services.

Working with individuals who have disabilities, their families, and significant others presents the aspiring rehabilitation professional with an additional set of cultural concerns. The well-trained rehabilitation professional must be aware of culture in its traditional sense, and also as it is uniquely impacted by the existence of disabilities. Hearing impaired individuals who identify with the Deaf culture, for example, will have little difficulty in explaining that their culture is unique and one in which they have great pride. There are many ways of considering the nature of the impact that culture has on work that includes individuals who have disabilities. There are the cultural influences associated with selected groups of individuals, the impact of and acceptance of the use of technology, and the nature of the relationships to family members and significant others. Belgrave and Jarma (2000) offer some insight when they state that "Culture influences disability prevalence, the experience of disability, participation in rehabilitation, and one's overall level of functioning and adaptation to a disability" (pg 585).

In the sixties, Wrenns' (1962) suggestion that culture significantly impacted counseling was nothing short of radical. Gradually, a number of scholars (Vontress, 1966, Pederson, Lonner and Draguens 1976, Diller, 1999, Axelson, 2000, and Okun, Fried and Okun, 1999) have highlighted the importance of considering how culture impacts the client, the counselor, and indeed the counseling process. Today it is difficult to imagine that there was ever a time when culture was not seen as an issue that must be considered as a critical element of the counseling process.

Despite the tremendous progress made in this area, multicultural counseling is still an emerging field. This should come as no surprise, however, in view of the huge task at hand. Freud and his peers, in the psychoanalytic congress of Vienna, struggled for decades to build a model of psychotherapy, which began to describe the psychology of man. Considerable research utilizing empirical, qualitative, and narrative story methodologies are examining multicultural competencies, their impact in the field, on counseling outcomes, client satisfaction, and counselor efficacy in serving diverse clients (Ponterotto, 1998). Continued examination and validation of competency scales also promises to further promote the need and true worth of multiculturally competent counselors to the overall mental health of *all* of the individuals we serve.

4

"CULTURE IS THE LENS THROUGH WHICH WE VIEW LIFE."
It may help if you remember that culture tends to act as a lens or filter that colors our perception of life. Because the lens has always been there, we view life through it without considering how it impacts our perception of it. Consider then the impact cultural values have on the way you view families, religion, good food, property, the role of men in society, even something as mundane as what you find acceptable to wear to work. As you do so, remember that your client has cultural values that are just as relevant for them. If you can manage to accomplish this small step, then congratulations, you have taken one of the many steps you will need to complete to move toward becoming a culturally competent practitioner.

REFERENCES

Arredondo, P., & Arciniega, G. M. (2001). Strategies and techniques for counselor training based on the multicultural counseling competencies. *Journal of Multicultural Counseling and Development, 29*, 263-273.

Atkinson, D. R., Morten G., & Sue, D. W. (1997). *Counseling American Minorities: A cross-cultural perspective* (5th ed.). New York: McGraw-Hill.

Brammer, R. (2004). *Diversity in Counseling.* Belmont CA: Thompson/Brooks/Cole.

Bellini, J. (2002). Correlates of multicultural counseling competencies and vocational rehabilitation counselors. *Rehabilitation Counseling Bulletin, 45*(2), 66-75.

Capuzzi, D., and Gross, D. R. (1999). *Counseling & Psychotherapy: Theories and interventions.* Upper Saddle River, New Jersey: Merrill/Prentice Hall.

Coleman, H.L.K. (1997). Conflict in Multicultural Counseling Relationships: sources and resolution. *Journal of Multicultural Counseling and Development, 25*, 195-200.

Corey, G. (2001). *Theory and Practice of Counseling and Psychotherapy* (6th ed.). Pacific Grove, CA: Brooks/Cole.

Corey, G. (2006). *Groups – Process and Practice* (7th ed.). Pacific Grove, CA: Brooks/Cole.

Corey, G. (2005). *Theory & Practice of Group Counseling* (6th ed.). Pacific Grove, CA: Brooks/Cole.

Corey, M. S. & Corey, G. (2003). *Becoming a Helper* (4th ed.). Pacific Grove, CA: Brooks/Cole.

Cross, T. L., Bazron, B. J., Dennis, K. W. and Isaacs, M. R. (1989). *Toward a Culturally Competent System of Care.* Washington, D.C.: Georgetown University Child Development Center.

Cross, W. E., Jr. (1971). The Negro-to-Black Conversion Experience: Toward a psychology of black liberation. *Black World, 20* (9), 13-27.

Cross, W. E. (1987). A Two-Factor Theory of Black Identity: implications for the study of identity development in minority children. In J. S. Phennay and M. J. Rotheram (Eds.)
Children's Ethnic Socialization: Pluralism and development. Nebburing Park, CA: Sage Publications.

Cross, W. E., Jr. (1991). *Shades of Black: diversity in African American identity.* Philadelphia, PA. Temple University Press

Devore, W., & Schlesinger, E. G. (1991). *Ethic-sensitive social work practice* (3rd ed.). New York: Macmillan.

Diller, J. V. (1999). *Cultural Diversity: a primer for the human services.* Toronto, Canada. Brooks/Cole. Wadsworth.

Dinkmeyer, D. & Sherry, L. (2000). *Counseling and Psychotherapy: An integrated, individual psychology approach* (3rd ed.). Upper Saddle River, NJ. Merrill, Prentice Hall

Downing, N. E. & Roush, K. L. (1985). From Passive Acceptance to Active Commitment: a model of feminist identity development for women. *The Counseling Psychologist, 13*, 695-709.

Erickson, F. (1997). Culture in Society and in Educational Practices. In J.A. Banks and C. A. M. Banks (Eds.), *Multicultural Education: classes and perspectives* (3rd ed., pp 32-60). Needham Heights, MA: Allyn & Bacon.

Fuertes, J. N., Bartholomeo, M., & Nichols, M. (2001). Future research directions in the study of counselor multicultural competency. *Journal of Multicultural Counseling and Development, 29*, 3-12.

Gay, G. (2000). *Culturally Responsive Teaching: Theory, research, & practice.* New York: Teachers College Press.

Gillard, B. E., James, R. R. and Bowman, J. T. (1994). *Theories and Strategies in Counseling and Psychotherapy* (3rd ed.) Needham Heights, MA. Allyn & Bacon.

Gladding, S. T. (2001). *Counseling: A comprehensive profession* (5th ed.). New York: Merrill.

Gladding, S. T. (1999). *Counseling: A comprehensive profession* (4th ed.). New York: Merrill.

Gladding, S. T. (2001). *The Counseling Dictionary: Concise definitions of frequently used terms*. Upper Saddle River, NJ. Merrill, Prentice Hall.

Gollnick, D. M. & Chinn, P. C. (2004). *Multicultural Education in a Pluralistic Society* (6th ed.) Upper Saddle River, New Jersey Pearson, Merrill, Prentice Hall.

Hanna, F. T., Bemak, F., & Chi-Ying Chung, R. (1999). Toward a New Paradigm for Multicultural Counseling. *Journal of Counseling and Development*, 77, 125-134.

Helms, J. E. (1984). Toward a Theoretical Explanation of the Effects of Race on Counseling: a black and white model. *The Counseling Psychologist*, *12*(4), 153-165.

Helms, J. E. (Ed.) (1990). *Black and White Racial Identity: theory research and practice*. West Point CT: Greenwood.

Herring, R. D., & Walker, S. S. (1993). Synergetic Counseling: toward a more holistic model with a cross-cultural specific approach. *TCA Journal. 22*(2), 28-53.

Ho, D. Y. F. (1995). Internalized Culture Culturocentrism and Transcendence. *The Counseling Psychologist, 23*, 4-24.

Ibrahim, F. A. (1985). Effective cross-cultural counseling and psychotherapy: A framework. *The Counseling Psychologist, 13*, 625-638.

Ivey, A. E., & Ivey, M. B. (2003). *Intentional Interviewing and Counseling: Facilitating client development in a multicultural society* (5th ed.). Pacific Grove, CA: Brooks/Cole.

Ivey, A. F., Ivey M. B. and Simck-Morgan. (1997). *Counseling and Psychotherapy: a multicultural perspective* (4th ed.) Boston, MA: Allyn & Bacon.

Leal-Idrogo, A. (1997). Multicultural rehabilitation counseling. *Rehabilitation Education, 11*(3), 231-240.

Pope-Davis, D. B., Coleman, H. L. K., Liu, W. M., & Toporek, R. L. (2003). *Handbook of multicultural competencies in counseling and psychology.* Thousand Oaks, CA: Sage Publications.

Lee, C. C., & Richardson, B. L. (1996). *Multicultural issues in counseling* (2nd ed.). Alexandria, VA: AACD.

Lewis, J. A., Lewis, D. L., Daniels, J. A., D'Andrea, M. J. (2003). *Community Counseling: Empowerment Strategies for a Diverse Society* (3rd ed.). Pacific Grove, CA: Brooks/Cole.

Locke, D. C. (1998). *Increasing Multicultural Understanding (2nd ed.). Newbury Park*, CA: Sage.

Lum, D. (2003). *Culturally Competent Practice: a framework for understanding diverse groups and justice issues*. Toronto, Canada. Thompson. Brooks/Cole.

Meir, S. T. (1989). *The elements of counseling*. Pacific Grove, CA: Brooks/Cole.

Nystul, M. S. (1999). *Introduction to Counseling: An art and science perspective*. Needham Heights, MA: Allyn and Bacon.

Okun, B. F., Fried, J., Okun, M. L. (1999). *Understanding Diversity: A learning-as-practice primer*. Pacific Grove, CA: Brooks/Cole.

Parrott, L. (2003). *Counseling and Psychotherapy* (2nd ed.). Pacific Grove, CA: Thompson, Brooks/Cole.

Pederson, P. B. (1990). The Multicultural Perspective of a Fourth Force in Counseling. *Journal of Mental Health Counseling, 12*, 93-95.

Pedersen, P. B., Lonner, W. J., & Draguns, J. G. (eds.), (1976). *Counseling Across Cultures*. Honolulu: University of Hawaii Press.

Pedersen, P. B., Draguns, J. G., Lonner, W. J., & Trimble J. E. (Eds.), (2002). *Counseling Across Cultures* (5th ed.). Thousand Oaks CA: Sage

Ponterotto, J. G. Casas, J. M. Suzuki, L. A. & Alexander, C. M. (Eds.), (2001) *Handbook of Multicultural Counseling*. Thousand Oaks, CA: Sage.

Pope-Davis, D. B., & Dings, J. G. (1995). The Assessment of Multicultural Counseling Competencies. In J. G. Ponterotto, J. M. Casas, L. A. Suzaki, & C. M. Alexander (Eds.) *Handbook of Multicultural Counseling* (pp 287-311). Thousand Oaks, CA. Sage Publishing.

Rahimi, M., Rosenthal, D. A., & Chan, F. (2003). Effects of Client Race on Clinical Judgment of African American Undergraduate Students in Rehabilitation. *Rehabilitation Counseling Bulletin, 46*(3), 157-163.

Ramirez, M., III (1999). *Multicultural Psychotherapy: an approach to individual and cultural differences* (2nd ed.). Boston: Allyn & Bacon.

Ridley, C. R. (2005). Overcoming Unintentional Racism in *Counseling and Therapy: a practitioner's guide to intentional intervention* (2nd ed). Thousand Oaks, California. Sage Publications.

Sellers, R. M., Shelton, N., Cooke, D., Chavous, T., Rowley, S. J., & Smith, M. (1998). A Multidimensional Model of Racial Identity: assumptions, findings, and future directions. In R. L. Jones (Ed.) *African American identity development* (pp 275-302). Hampton, VA: Cobbs & Henry.

Skouhold, T. M., and Rivers, D. A. (2004). *Skills and Strategies for the Helping Professions*. Denver Colorado: Love Publishing Company.

Slattery, J. M. (2004). *Counseling Diverse Clients: bringing context into therapy*. Nelson Caradu. Thompson, Brooks/Cole.

Sommers-Flanagan, J. & Sommers-Flanagan, R. (2004). *Counseling and Psychotherapy Theories in Context and Practice: Skills, strategies, and techniques.* Hoboken, New Jersey.

Steenbarger, B. N. (1993). A Multicultural Model of Counseling: bridging brevity and diversity. *Journal of Counseling and Development, 72,* 8-15.

Sue, D. W., Arrendondo, P., & McDavis, R. J. (1992). Multicultural Competencies/Standards: a pressing need. *Journal of Counseling and Development, 70,* 477-486.

Sue, D. W., Ivey, A., & Pederson, P. (Eds.). (1996). *A Theory of Multicultural Counseling and Therapy.* Pacific Grove, CA: Brooks/Cole.

Sue, D. W., & Sue, D. (1999). *Counseling the Culturally Different: Theory and practice* (3rd ed.). New York: Wiley.

Sue, D. W. & Sue, D. (1990). Counseling the culturally different: Theory and practice, New York: Wiley.

Sue, D. W. et al (1998). *Multicultural Counseling Competencies: individual and organizational development.* Thousand Oaks, California. Sage Publications.

Traden, R. R. (1989). The Formation of Homosexual Identifies. *Journal of Homosexuality, 17,* 43-73.

Wrenn, C. Gilbert (1962. *The Counselor in a Changing World.* Personnel and Guidance Association, Washington DC.

CHAPTER 5

CASE MANAGEMENT AND VOCATIONAL REHABILITATION COUNSELING

KEITH B. WILSON
TYRA N. TURNER WHITTAKER
VIRGINIA BLACK

Chapter Highlights

➡ Introduction

➡ Demographics of people of color with disabilities in the United States

➡ Multicultural counseling techniques

➡ An overview of case management

➡ Models in case management

➡ Case management strategies to assist consumers who are racially diverse

➡ Conclusion

*I*n the United States, minority is a term usually applied to individuals who are persons of color who belong to the four major racial and/or ethnic groups, Black (African American) Asian (Asian American), American Indian (Native American), and Latino/Hispanic (Axelson, 1993; Wilson II & Gutiérrez, 1985). The authors will refer to the aforementioned groups as "people of color" and/or racial and ethnic minority groups. Speaking of people of color, most Hispanics in the VR systems (over 90 %) classify themselves as White/European American, not people of color. This distinction is important because Hispanics are included under the "people of color" category in most demographic studies (Wilson & Senices, 2005). The racial flexibility of Hispanics/Latinos is made more interesting because Hispanics/Latinos will become the largest ethnic minority group in the United States, passing people who classify themselves as African Americans (Sue et al., 1998). Rawlings and Saluter (1994) reported that "Hispanics constitute an ethnic group rather than a racial category, and their members may classify themselves as White, Black, or some other race" (p. xii). As reported by Wilson and Senices, among the four major racial and ethnic groups in the United States, many Hispanics/Latinos may not have as many negative experiences because of their phenotype (i.e., white skin color/hue).

The word *race* includes biological and physical traits used to depict certain people, mainly hue or skin color (Wilson & Senices, 2005). In contrast, ethnicity tends to deal with things like shared cultures, values, and language of a particular population (Dana, 1998). Not withstanding how people who are Hispanic/Latino classify themselves racially, many people who are part of racial minority groups can be characterized by three different qualities: identifiably, differential power, and pejorative treatment (Dworkin & Dworkin, 1999). We will use the terms minority and people of color interchangeably in this chapter.

INTRODUCTION

Case management has been a core function of the rehabilitation professional since the inception of the profession. The concept of case management has evolved greatly in the health and human service profession in general, and the rehabilitation profession in particular. In the beginning, case management was birthed during World War II to outline the extensive services needed for those with psychiatric disabilities (Lee, Mackenzie, Dudley-Brown, & Chin, 1998). In the 1960's, case management was viewed as a systematic method to organize and deliver services without duplicating such services (Giuliano & Poirier, 1991). In the 1970's, as a result of escalating costs for worker's compensation and the passage of the 1973 Rehabilitation Act, the development of a more comprehensive service delivery system in the private rehabilitation sector began to emerge (Shaw, McMahon, Chan, Taylor, & Wood, 2001). In the 80's, we observed a fundamental change in the direction of case management. In particular, case management began to be viewed as case or care coordination where the focus was on client empowerment (Woodside & McClam, 2003). Today, case management is considered a multidimensional role in the rehabilitation counseling process that provides case coordination, monitoring, and follow-up services to persons with disabilities. This chapter provides the reader with an overview of effective case management practices, and culturally sensitive service delivery for racial and ethnic minorities.

DEMOGRAPHICS OF PEOPLE OF COLOR WITH DISABILITIES IN THE UNITED STATES

Evidence suggests that access to Vocational Rehabilitation (VR) services is more difficult for racial minorities than for non-minorities/White Americans in the United States (Wilson, Harley, McCormick, Jolivette, & Jackson, 2001; Wilson, Jackson, & Doughty, 1999; Wilson & Senices, 2005). While access to VR services have been studied for several years (Wilson, 1999; Wilson, 2002), the impact of certain processes has received less attention, such as case management relative to racial and ethnic minorities in the VR system. Given that the process of case management is a primary function of VR counselors, variables affecting case management outcomes, such as the race and ethnicity of a consumer, are not only worthy of examining but also necessary when looking at the changing complexion of consumers in many human service organizations.

With the aforementioned demographic backdrop in motion, Organista, Chun, and Marin (1998) reported that racial and ethnic minorities are approximately 25% of the population in the United States and are projected to become the majority of the United States population by the year 2050 (U.S. Department of Commerce, 2001). The Census also projects that racial and ethnic minorities will become a numerical majority by 2050. According to some private polls, however, White Americans may become the numerical minority by the year 2030 (Sue, 1996). This demographic milieu is helping not only VR agencies, but also human service agencies focus their attention on issues of multicultural concerns that have arisen concerning the lack of diversity issues in many organizations in the United States. Although it is important to acknowledge the increasing numbers of diverse consumers in human service organizations, it is more problematic to address these concerns

110

in the context of how case management services are delivered to diverse populations in the VR system in the United States. In California and Texas, the demographic transformation can be readily observed. It is evident that the complexion of the United States already reflects more racial and cultural diversity than in prior years. In order to successfully serve a more diverse population, human service organizations in general, and VR agencies in particular, must continue to seek new ways of facilitating services to our expanding clientele. If not, these populations will continue to feel isolated and disconnected from many human service organizations.

MULTICULTURAL COUNSELING TECHNIQUES

Because much of case management deals with the VR counselor interacting with both people who are consumers and VR personnel, it is important to advocate for VR counselors to use Multicultural Counseling Techniques (MCT) in their strategies to facilitate services for not only people of color, but for all people with disabilities in the state-federal system. Wilson et al. (2003) reported that:

> The study of multicultural counseling [techniques] (MCT) has continued to grow and become influential in the human services. Early advocates of MCT pointed out that there was little understanding about the history, experiences, life styles, and worldviews of culturally different populations. Furthermore, counseling professionals did not take into consideration the sociopolitical realities of the clients they served. Hence, counselors are less likely to include a systematic approach to address sociopolitical issues when dealing with racial and ethnic minority clients.

(p. 8)

Utilizing MCT in case management with non-White Americans will allow counselors to determine the efficacy of services. Although not recognized earlier by many counselors, MCT continues to gain acceptance within the counseling community to access the history, experiences, life styles, and worldviews of racially and culturally diverse populations (Wilson et al, 2003).

While an exhaustive list of variables need not be addressed when using MCT, it is vital to pay close attention to the consumers' worldview, social class, gender, sexual orientation, and disability status when delivering case management services. For example, let us explore worldview. Because much of what we know about counseling and case management tends to be from a White American perspective (e.g. abstract ideas and linear analytic thinking), many VR counselors may inadvertently harm people of color because they are imposing a worldview on people of color that may be different in many respects (i.e., holistic and none linear thinking). Because many White Americans tend to value decisiveness when making decisions during the case management (intake) process, consumers who delay making a decision to consult with elder family members may be viewed as non-assertive and passive aggressive. When in fact, consulting with family members by some African Americans, for example, may be viewed within the family as a protocol of respect and inclusion. A good MCT would be for the White American VR counselor to allow the African American consumer enough time to consult with family members, if necessary, to facilitate the planning process and goals for the consumer. Locke (1998) states that a holistic approach is valued and Blacks tend to respond to things in sum as opposed to focusing on the parts. In addition, reciprocity and altruism are valued and one's worth is found in what one contributes to the family and/or community (Sudarkasa, 1997). As viewed in the aforementioned example, tension can exist when worldviews are in direct opposition to one another. Not only do human services professionals risk diagnosing undue pathology in racial minorities when worldviews collide, but it is likely that racial minorities will not return to VR or to other human service organizations.

CULTURAL VALUES

Though common cultural values have been reported for each of the four major racial minority groups (e.g., African Americans, Asian Americans, Native Americans, & Hispanics/Latinos) in the United States, it is vital to note that cultural variation exists within each of these groups (Axelson, 1993; Locke, 1998; Ponterotto & Casas, 1991). Because a discussion of intra-group cultural differences is beyond the scope of this book chapter, the reader is referred to other chapters in the text for further explanation of how cultural values impact various racial groups during and after the initial interview process.

INEQUITY OF SERVICE DELIVERY TO PEOPLE OF COLOR

Historically, there has been a discrepancy in services received between people of color and their White American counterparts during the rehabilitation process. People of color have been disproportionately rejected for vocational rehabilitation services and prematurely terminated at a higher rate than their Caucasian counterparts (Dziekan & Okocha, 1993; Wilson, 1999; Wilson, 2002; Wilson, Harley, & Alston, 2001). Further, research conducted by Wilson, Turner, & Jackson (2002) concluded that there were differences in the types of services received by African-Americans and White Americans upon successful closure. They discovered that African-Americans were more likely to receive maintenance, transportation, and adjustment training, whereas their White American counterparts were more likely to receive diagnostic, college training, and physical/mental restoration services (Wilson, Turner, & Jackson, 2002). Several research teams have deduced that racial and ethnic biases within the VR systems is a primary reason why many disparities appear not only in the VR system regarding racial and ethnic minority outcomes, but in the human services as well (Wilson, 2002; Wilson, Alston, Harley, & Mitchell, 2002). In part, these disparities revealed a lack of cultural sensitivity on behalf of the rehabilitation counselor. The lack of cultural sensitivity is a common theme in both the VR and psychology literature. To address the cultural sensitivity issues, or the lack thereof, is constantly under debate.

The authors recognize that increasing one's level of cultural sensitivity can enhance the rehabilitation process and assist the rehabilitation counselor in providing equitable services with noted outcomes for the consumer of color. Because over 93 percent of VR counselors and approximately 92 percent of VR administrators classify themselves as White American in the United States (Whitney-Thomas et al., 1999), the need for cultural sensitivity is not only warranted, but necessary, to begin to address the needs of racial and ethnic minorities in the VR system. How one is perceived when seeking VR services has been and remains an issue in the state-federal system. For example, evidence suggests that people of color may have a more difficult time in the VR system when compared to people who classify themselves as White Americans. More importantly, not all people who classify themselves as racial and ethnic minorities have similar experiences with discrimination. As Wilson and Senices (2005) recently adduced regarding VR outcomes, many forms of discrimination in the VR systems are based on ones color (hue). Vocational rehabilitation consumers with darker hues (e.g., Black, Hispanics/Latinos) are more prone to be discriminated against inside and outside of the VR agency than consumers who classify themselves as White Americas.

AN OVERVIEW OF CASE MANAGEMENT

Within a single lifetime, how many adaptations does an individual make? Individuals change and adapt to their own growth and developmental patterns as well as to the environmental pressures and social situations of a given milieu, such as the VR agency. Persons with physical, intellectual, or emotional disabilities have their own unique way of adapting to the demands of their surrounding environment. The role of case managers and vocational counselors

is to help each individual adapt to one's own particular situation through the use of case management models (Brill, 1998).

If we think of case management as an umbrella, then we are able to tease out the various components involved in this creative and collaborative process, which involves organizing, consulting, counseling, assessing, teaching, monitoring, and advocating (Mullahy, 1998). Case management is generally defined as "a creative and collaborative process, involving skills in assessment, consulting, teaching, modeling, and advocacy that aim to enhance the optimal functioning of the consumer's served" (Mullahy, 1998; p.4). Roessler and Rubin (1992) describe case management in rehabilitation counseling as the counselor's capability to guide the consumer through the rehabilitation process from intake to case closure. Because case management is a process that involves individuals making decisions for VR consumers, VR counselors and administrators must remember to address possible stereotypes that may lead some VR consumers, like African-Americans with disabilities, to not receive the services they need and deserve. To support the stereotype assertion, Rosenthal and Koscuilek (1996), Sue, Arrendondo, and McDavis (1992), and Middleton et al. (2000) all reported that racial and ethnic group stereotypes could lead practitioners to hasty conclusions and unsound postulations about consumers. More specifically, Rosenthal and Berven (1999) reported that counselors in training bring their stereotypes into the counseling session. They also reported that African American consumers might not receive the services they are eligible for because of negative prejudices held against them. Our point is that one must look at both the process of case management and the people who police the process, who are VR counselors, staff, and administrators, to name a few.

Case management is obviously a complex service that is constantly evolving to meet the increasing diversity of consumers and job opportunities. As a case manager, how do all of the various components (e.g., consulting, counseling, assessing, teaching) get addressed, considering the uniqueness of each individual? Case management is viewed as a process for assessing the client's total situation and addressing the needs and problems found in that assessment (Summers, 2006, p.37). To meet the needs of each individual, various models of case management have been introduced over the years. Several models of case management are available, because services need to be delivered in a variety of ways. Case management remains a flexible process in order to meet the unique needs and goals of each individual (Woodside & McClam, 2003). While the process of case management is dynamic, people operating as "gate keepers" may not be flexible enough to adjust to different clientele. Thus, the following models are provided as guides to not only

114

facilitate the case management process for racial and ethnic minorities, but the human service profession in the United States.

MODELS IN CASE MANAGEMENT

Several models of case management exist to enhance the method in which services are delivered in the VR system. We view the following model as salient to facilitating the case management for all VR populations, not just for people of color. Five models of case management will be introduced: the Crux Model, the Broker Model, the Rehabilitation Model, the Assertive Community Treatment (ACT) Model, and the Strengths Model. Information on the advantages and disadvantages and the utility of each model for persons of color is provided to assist human service personnel to achieve productive outcomes for their particular clientele.

THE CRUX MODEL

The rehabilitation counselor's main goal is to promote the quality of life (QOL) of persons with disabilities. One central supporting element of QOL is obtaining and maintaining employment. Rehabilitation counselors prepare individuals to obtain employment by first helping them progress toward personal independence, adjustment, and health. As these three basic requirements gain momentum, rehabilitation counselors can begin assisting persons with disabilities in meeting specific educational standards that conform to the prerequisites of their specified employment interests (Roessler & Rubin, 1998). Matching the individual to a job is one of the core concerns in vocational counseling. With all the extraneous variables, where does the counselor begin? Roessler and Rubin reported back in 1979 that the Crux Model is structured towards bringing in all the relevant variables of the vocational counseling process and organizing them into vocational possibilities.

The Crux Model is divided into an evaluation phase and a planning phase. Within the evaluation phase, the counselor collects information on "the consumer's past, current, and potential capacities in physical functioning, psychosocial functioning, and educational and vocational skill development" (Roessler & Rubin, 1998, p.31). Roessler and Rubin also asserted that assessing the consumer's current economic situation is an important part of the evaluation phase of the Crux Model. They outline a series of factors that might assist in the evaluation phase of the model (physical factors, psychosocial factors, educational and vocational factors, and economic factors), in order to get a broad picture of the consumer.

A culturally sensitive rehabilitation counselor should also obtain information about the consumer's cultural background, including issues with race, ethnicity, and nationality. Information can be obtained through a dialogue with the consumer as rapport is being established and also through personal research of the consumer's particular culture. In fact, it is useful to do additional research on any culture that one is unfamiliar with. While gaining additional information about a particular clientele might be time-consuming, the potential gains, advantages, and positive outcomes will clearly outweigh any possible inconveniences. Collecting culturally sensitive information is also useful in evaluating the material gathered in a cultural context (e.g., To what extent do the family and friends support the rehabilitation process? Does the family have unrealistic expectations of the individual with the disability? Is the community involved in economically supporting the individual?). Many VR counselors and other human services professionals fail to address culture during the case management process.

The evaluation phase of the Crux Model is completed once the rehabilitation counselor obtains adequate information in the four aforementioned areas outlined by Roessler and Rubin (1998). Rehabilitation counselors need to fully utilize all the available information from intake interviews, vocational tests and evaluations, medical evaluations, psychological evaluations, and any other relevant sources. Using a range of information allows the VR counselor to fill in any gaps in the evaluation phase and move smoothly into the second phase of the Crux Model, the planning phase. In the initial steps of the planning phase, the counselor analyzes all the evaluation information. Upon consideration of possible vocational positions, the counselor must remain aware of the consumer's strengths and limitations. Depending on the demands of the potential jobs, the consumer's mental and physical abilities, their socio-cultural background, and their goals and interests, a range of vocational possibilities should be generated incorporating a wide-range of sources. As with the rehabilitation counselor philosophy, this holistic approach is necessary to complete the cultural picture of potential consumers.

During the vocational planning phase of the Crux Model, the rehabilitation counselor and the consumer collaborate on selecting a job that is compatible with the characteristics of the consumer and the job. Once a vocational goal is agreed upon, the steps to getting or maintaining a job need to be addressed. These intermediate steps focus on particular rehabilitation needs that were addressed in the evaluation phase (e.g., level of education, work experience, vocational interests). Fulfilling each need brings the consumer one step closer to becoming a satisfied employee in a suitable environment. Even though the Crux Model focuses on matching an individual to a particular job, the outcome is not obligatory or absolute. Rather, the Crux Model should be used for occupational exploration. The role of the rehabilitation counselor is to help facilitate this exploration and ideally, to help the consumers make their own vocational decision. The role of the rehabilitation counselor not only calls for being a skilled vocational counselor, but also an experienced case manager. Therefore, the process does not end when a vocational decision is reached. Once a vocational decision is reached, the case management process continues into the areas of vocational training, job placement, work accommodations, and eventually, into job analysis and job modifications (Roessler & Rubin, 1998).

The Crux Model is very comprehensive and provides ample opportunity to gain personal information about the consumer's culture. Advantages are apparent when incorporating the cultural background of all VR consumers. By adding a cultural component, the Crux Model provides the foundation for a long-term relationship between the counselor and the consumer. Time and honesty are needed to foster trust within the counselor-consumer relationship. Time and honesty are vital since many consumers of color enter counseling and the VR system with a certain level of cultural mistrust of the counselor. Cultural mistrust is the tendency for a consumer of color, for example, to mistrust Caucasians (European Americans)—especially in the major areas of government (i.e. education, business and work, interpersonal and social relations, and politics and law) (Terrell & Terrell, 1981). Establishing rapport allows the counselor to create a climate of faith that helps to facilitate the rehabilitation process.

One disadvantage of the Crux Model for persons of color is the need for the consumer to be extremely verbal during the rehabilitation process. For example, depending on the value orientation of a specific culture, the consumer may not be as verbal as the counselor expects or even needs. Information must then be gathered through other entities such as family members. Thus, there may be a likelihood of the VR counselor attaching unnecessary pathology to people of color in the VR system.

THE BROKER MODEL

The Broker Model emphasizes assessing the needs of consumers, treatment planning, and ultimately referring the consumer to other agencies (Grech, 2002). The Broker Model considers the case manager as a "broker" or negotiator of services who requires the skills to effectively link a consumer's needs with available resources (Grech, 2002). Once the consumer is connected to needed resources, the case manager's role is completed. In the Broker Model, most of the responsibility is placed on the consumer and the consumer's family. The case manager does not serve in the capacity of an advocate for services.

5

Within this model, the case manager assesses the consumer's needs and identifies what services would be beneficial and available. Ultimately, the Broker Model is very limited in its helpfulness in that a long-term consumer-counselor relationship may not be possible.

Those rehabilitation counselors ascribing to the Broker Model must evaluate this model in a cultural context. For example, a Hispanic consumer may expect the rehabilitation counselor to assume most of the responsibility in the rehabilitation process. The Hispanic consumer may view the counselor as the authoritarian and wait on the counselor to initiate needed activities. Using this example, the culturally sensitive counselor must be aware of language barriers that may exist within the Hispanic population. Bilingual consumers are often prematurely terminated based on language barriers. To support this assertion, Moore (2002) reported that language barriers are important to understand when working with Hispanic consumers. It is obvious that such barriers with any population may impede the rehabilitation process. Therefore, the rehabilitation counselor must be mindful that they may have to assume a more active role with certain populations than what the Broker Model allows.

In 1995, Rapp did an extensive literature review on the use of case management within the mental health field. Rapp reported results from six studies evaluating the Broker Model, which suggested that for the most part, the model produces few positive effects. Since the Broker Model emphasizes a formal relationship between the consumer and the case manager, Rapp found that more consumers relied on hospitals and did not show an increase in quality of life. Holloway and Carson (2001) reported that case managers using the Broker Model were mostly coordinators and brokers of services. These case managers were typically assigned large caseloads, 50:1, and worked a majority of the time directly from their offices. Theoretically, there was a potential strength to this model despite the case manager functioning as a dispassionate broker; the case manager was able to meet the needs of a large population in the most cost-effective way (Holloway & Carson, 2001). Obvious weaknesses arose, however, particularly in the assumption that case managers were effectively connecting consumers to appropriate services without direct contact between the managers and the consumers.

Cultural sensitivity is inherently far removed when using this model with non-mainstream consumers. The Broker Model may not be useful when working with a clientele that relies on personal contact and a personal relationship in order to follow through with services. Some populations may consider the counselor who uses the broker system as another person who is giving them the run-a-round. While this perception may be historical in nature, it is these kinds of perceptions that will likely impede the case management and

118

counseling process of the client. It is also obvious that counselors who use this particular model will have to explain upfront what, why, and who during the initial minutes of the intake process. Though there are never guarantees, it is vital to decrease ambiguity early in the case management process when one uses this particular model.

THE REHABILITATION MODEL

The third model is the Rehabilitation Model (Anthony et al., 1988), which is a consumer-centered model. The case manager is responsible for helping the consumer identify individual strengths and weaknesses and teaches skills that may enhance their quality of life. The Rehabilitation Model works toward enriching the consumer's strengths by using planning programs that evaluate areas where the consumer has skill deficits. With this model, there is a strong emphasis on the consumer's preferences (e.g. the type of job the consumer would like to obtain) (Roessler & Rubin, 1998). The Rehabilitation Model is similar to the Bervin assessment model of case management. Bervin's Assessment Model of case management evaluates assessment data using the following three values: assets, limitations, and preferences. Bervin (1984) defined assets as particular characteristics of the consumer that help facilitate the attainment of future goals. Limitations were defined as any obstacles that could stand in the way of the consumer and the particular goal(s) of the consumer. As Bervin views it, each consumer has preferences (e.g. interests, needs, fears, likes, dislikes) for safely and effectively reaching future goals. Case managers collect assessment data from all the relevant areas (e.g. medical, vocational, psychological, social) and work closely with the consumer to determine whether an area is an asset, a limitation, or a preference. Once each area is broken down and analyzed, the counselor is able to interpret all the parts as a whole to determine the best plan of action for the consumer (Bervin, 1984). The plan should lead to an effective goal attainment if there is good rapport and collaboration between the counselor and the consumer. The critical element is the counselor's ability to analyze, synthesize, and interpret the assessment data in order to accurately recommend what is best for the consumer.

The assessment phase is critical for the rehabilitation counselor in the Rehabilitation Model. Assessment is a continuous process throughout every stage of the rehabilitation process. It is critical for assessment to continue until a case closes (Roessler & Rubin, 1998). The Rehabilitation Model, as well as Bervin's Assessment Model, emphasizes the importance of the consumers clearly defining their goals. For the counselor, it is equally important to continually assess the consumer's rehabilitation process, and work on areas of deficiency. Counselors must also work on linking each consumer to a unique

service within the community while continuing to monitor the progress. Caseloads within both the Rehabilitation and Bervin Models typically range from 20:1 to 30:1 (Holloway & Carson, 2001).

The Rehabilitation Model and the Bervin Model possess great utility in providing rehabilitation counseling services for consumers of color. The two models are sufficiently broad to allow the counselor to focus on consumers' specific strengths and weaknesses that may influence the rehabilitation process, rather than culturally biased evaluation measures. Due to the emphasis on consumer's preferences, the Rehabilitation Model heavily relies on the counselor's knowledge of the consumer's preferences within a cultural context. Consumers of color's preferences may not stem from their individual preferences, but from the preferences of their family and other internal support systems. The culturally sensitive counselor must be aware of and sensitive to the factors surrounding the consumer's preference, or lack of preference.

THE ASSERTIVE COMMUNITY TREATMENT (ACT) MODEL

The fourth model is the ACT Model, which is based on Project ACT in Madison, Wisconsin (Stein & Test, 1980). Work on this model has recently been updated (Thompson et al., 1990; Stein & Santos, 1998). As a backdrop, the ACT Model was developed for individuals who frequently used mental health services. In 1980, Stein and Test sought to empower individuals by moving them out of hospitals and into a supportive local community. Individuals begin to learn and use daily coping skills, which is a strong motivating force in helping consumers form community relationships, live independently, and face daily problems with minimal assistance. In addition, the ACT Model recognizes that circumstances may arise when the individual needs temporary hospitalization (Holloway & Carson, 2001).

ACT is based on the principle that services are delivered by an interdisciplinary team, led by a single case manager that works collaboratively with all their consumers. Meetings are scheduled on a regular basis to discuss and evaluate the progress of each consumer. More important to the title of the model, the team typically spends 80% of their time in the community with their consumers. Most of the services are provided by the ACT team, rather than by outside professionals as we observed in the Broker Model. Caseloads are small in the ACT Model due to the amount of fieldwork expected by the team. An optimal caseload ratio is 10:1 and in some areas 15:1 (Holloway & Carson, 2001).

Several researchers of multicultural counseling emphasize the fact that most people of color ascribe to a "collectivistic" versus an "individualistic" value orientation (Kluckhohn, & Strodtbeck, 1961). Culturally sensitive

120

counselors utilizing the ACT approach may find that they achieve better outcomes because they continuously interface with the consumer's community. Rehabilitation counselors must earn the trust of their consumers of color to be successful. As previously mentioned, many consumers of color enter counseling with a level of cultural mistrust towards the VR counselor. If trust is not perceived, neither the consumer nor the counselor will achieve successful outcomes in the rehabilitation process. To this avail, being a part of the consumer's community allows the counselor to develop better rapport with the consumer, which should lead to better outcomes for both the counselor and the consumer.

THE STRENGTHS MODEL

The final model, the Strengths Model, focuses on the consumer's strengths rather than on the disability. There is a strong importance placed on the counselor-consumer rapport in this model. Initially, counselors work with their consumers to identify their strengths. Next, the counselors create scenarios that the consumer is able to successfully accomplish. This feeling of success boosts the consumer's personal strengths and sense of power and control. As in the role of the rehabilitation counselor, this model seeks to empower consumers with disabilities. Feelings of satisfaction and a sense of power encourage consumers to continue to pursue their goals. The Strengths Model asserts that rehabilitation counselors or case managers must develop four key areas of support: natural, peer, income, and housing (NCDHR, 1990). The focus on the consumer's strengths is a very important key in this model.

The Strengths Model also rests on the premise that a consumer's behavior depends largely on the resources available in the community. It has been stated and mentioned in several publications; individuals with disabilities need equal access to community resources to be successful (Roessler & Rubin, 1998). The Strengths Model has been reviewed in eight studies with consistently positive outcomes in the following areas: hospitalizations, quality of life, social supports, consumer satisfaction, and leisure activities (Marty, Rapp, & Carlson, 2001; Roessler & Rubin, 1998). Interestingly, this model functions dually as a service philosophy and a case management model. Some aspects of the Strengths Model have been used in writing mission statements in several case management centers (Onyett, 1992). According to experts using the Strengths Model, the ideal caseload ranges from 10:1 to 20:1 (Marty, Rapp, & Carlson).

The Strengths Model lends itself to culturally sensitive rehabilitation counseling in that the Strengths Model considers consumers' views of their strengths and goals versus counselors' perception of strengths. In the Strengths Model, the consumer assumes a major role in the rehabilitation process. More specifically, there is ample opportunity for consumers of color to integrate aspects of their culture into the rehabilitation process. The disadvantage of this model in a cultural context is that counselors are not encouraged to assume culturally sensitive skills as they would in other models.

Based on the literature of these five case management models, the relationship between the consumer and case manager is critical, which has always been a fundamental element in traditional rehabilitation counseling. Another essential element in successful case management is the use of teams (Roessler & Rubin, 1998). Rehabilitation counselors should never be expected to take on all the activities involved in rehabilitation counseling. Teams are needed for planning and monitoring a consumer's goals and progress, as well as supporting each other and offering expertise from each member's own background. Finally, teams benefit from diversity, and collaborating with psychiatrists, social workers, rehabilitation counselors, and nurses enriches the assessment process and the lives of the consumers (Roessler & Rubin, 1998).

CASE MANAGEMENT STRATEGIES TO ASSIST CONSUMERS WHO ARE RACIALLY DIVERSE

In observing the Parham (2002) model for African American males, we realize that concepts in this model can also be used for a variety of diverse consumers. We have also modified the therapy/counseling model to include the process of case management. In order to gain a complete understanding of the processes involved with the Parham model, one must first be open to changing and modifying one's behavior to increase the chances of a productive outcome for both the consumer and the VR counselor:

- *Connecting with your consumers*: Because there are several ways to connect with consumers, VR counselors may want to consider creating an atmosphere that would facilitate the client being open during the case management process.
- *Assessment*: As Parham (2002) noted, there are several techniques that contribute to a counselor's ability to assess what is going on with the client. Understanding cultural strengths and using appropriate clinical instruments are only two tools to consider. Many of the tools that are used to assess the strengths and weaknesses of VR consumers use norms that exclude persons of color. Understanding the instrument limitations based on sample representation, for example, could be very helpful when the results of such assessments are used to exclude consumers from receiving certain services.

- *Facilitating Awareness*: Reframing and understanding functional behaviors are two ways to facilitate client awareness during the case management process.
- *Setting Goals*: As Parham (2002) noted, the goals that you have during the case management process will chart the course of healing. It is important to respect the need for client distance and examine the client from a culturally centered theoretical basis.
- *Taking Action and Instigating Change*: Empowering, teaching, and becoming a social advocate and engineer on behalf of clients, can assist clients to confront and handle their circumstances in a productive way.

CONCLUSION

While the models and techniques discussed in this chapter are examples of how to use basic case management measures and procedures with culturally diverse populations, the first action must be the willingness of VR counselors to be open to new ways of performing their job functions. As discussed, there are basic strengths and weaknesses to all models. Based on the changing demographics in the United States population, new ways of approaching case management with diverse populations is not only warranted, but critical in continuing to provide services to groups that have typically been served inadequately for many years. This call to the profession must be understood as a call that will help all people with disabilities in the VR system.

REFERENCES

Axelson, J. (1993). *Counseling and development in a multicultural society* (2nd ed.). Pacific Grove, CA: Brooks/Cole.

Anthony, W.A., Cohen, M.R., Farkas, M. & Cohen, B.F. (1988). Clinical care update: the chronically mentally ill. Case management-more than a response to a dysfunctional system. *Community Mental Health Journal, 24,* 1263-1266.

Bervin, N. (1984). Assessment practices in rehabilitation counseling. *Journal of Applied Rehabilitation Counseling, 15* (3), 9-14.

Brill, N.I. (1998). *Working with people: The helping process (6th edition).* White Plains, NY: Longman.

Burnett, P. C. (1999). Assessing the structure of learning outcomes from counseling using the SOLO taxonomy: An exploratory study. *British Journal of Guidance and Counseling, 27*(4), 567-580.

Burnett, P. C., & Meacham, D. (2002). Learning journals as a counseling strategy. *Journal of Counseling and Development, 80*(4), 410-416.

Cohen, R., Phillips, S., & Swerdlki, M. (1996). *Psychological testing and assessment* (3rd ed.). CA: Mayfield.

Dana, R. H. (1998). *Understanding cultural identity in intervention and assessment. Multicultural aspects of counseling series 9*. Thousand Oaks, CA: Sage.

Dziekan, K., & Okocha, A. (1993). Accessibility of rehabilitation services: Comparison by racial-ethnic status. *Rehabilitation Counseling Bulletin, 36*, 183-189.

Dworkin, A. G., & Dworkin, R. J. (1999). *The minority report: An introduction to racial, ethnic, and gender relations* (3rd ed.). Fort Worth, TX: Harcourt Brace.

Grech, E. (2002). Case management: a critical analysis of the literature. *International Journal of Psychosocial Rehabilitation, 6*, 89-98.

Giuliano, K. K. & Poirier, C. E. (1991). Nursing case management: Critical pathways to desirable outcomes. *Journal of Nursing Management, 22*(3), 52-55.

Holloway, F. & Carson, J. (2001). Case management: an update. *International Journal of Social Psychiatry, 47*(3), 21-31.

Lee, D .T. F.; Mackenzie, A. E.; Dudley-Brown, S., & Chin, T. M. (1998). *Journal of Advance Nursing. 27*(5), 933-940.

Locke, D. C. (1998). *Increasing multicultural understanding: A comprehensive model* (2nd ed.). Thousand Oaks, CA: Sage.

Kluckhohn, F. R., & Strodtbeck, F. L. (1961). *Variations in value orientations*. Evanston, IL: Row Petersen.

Mahoney, M. J. (1991). *Human change processes*. New York: Basic Books.

Marty, D., Rapp, C. A., & Carlson, L. (2001). The experts speak: the critical ingredients of strengths model case management. *Psychiatric Rehabilitation Journal, 24*(3), 214-221.

Middleton, R. A., Rollins, C. W., Sanderson, P. L., Leung, P., Harley, D. A., Ebener, D., & Leal- Idrogo, A. (2000). Endorsement of multicultural rehabilitation competencies and standards: A call to action. *Rehabilitation Counseling Bulletin, 43*, 219-240.

Moore, C. (2002). Comparative competitive employment levels for Latinos and Non-Latinos without 12 years of education. *Journal of Applied Rehabilitation Counseling, 33*(1), 12-18.

Mullahy, C. (1998). *The case manager's handbook.* Gaithersburg, MD: Aspen.

North Carolina Department of Human Resources, Division of Mental Health, Developmental Disabilities, and Substance Abuse Services (1990). *Approaches to case management with adults with severe and persistent mental illness.* Raleigh, NC.

Onyett, S. (1992). *Case Management in Mental Health.* Chapman & Hall, London.

Organista, P. B., Chun, K. M. & Marín, G. (Eds.). (1998). *Readings in ethnic psychology.* New York: Routledge.

Parham, T. A. (2002). Counseling models for African Americans: The what and how of counseling In T. A. Parham (Eds.), *Counseling Persons of African Descent: Raising the bar of practitioner competence* (pp. 100-118). Thousand Oakes, CA: Sage.

Ponterotto, J. & Casas, M. (1991). *Handbook of racial/ethnic minority counseling research.* Springfield, MA: Charles C Thomas.

Power, P. W. (2000). *A guide to vocational assessment* (3rd ed.). Texas: Pro-Ed, Inc.

Rapp, C. (1995). The active ingredients of effective case management: a research synthesis. In L. Giesler (Ed.), *Case management for behavioral care* (pp. 5-46). Cincinnati, OH: NACM.

Rawlings, S. W., & Saluter, A, F. (1994). Household and family characteristics: U. S. Bureau of the Census, *Current Population Reports*, 20-483.

Roessler, R.T. & Rubin, S.E. (1998). *Case management and rehabilitation counseling: procedures and techniques* (3rd edition). Austin, TX: Pro-ed.

Roessler, R.T. & Rubin, S.E. (1992). *Case management and rehabilitation counseling: procedures and techniques* (2nd edition). Austin, TX: Pro-ed.

Roessler, R.T. & Rubin, S.E. (1979). Diagnostic and planning guidelines for the vocational rehabilitation process. *Rehabilitation Literature, 40*(2), 34-37.

Sandhu, D. S. (1995). Pioneers of multicultural counseling: An interview with Paul B. Rosenthal, D.A., & Berven, N.L. (1999). Effects of client race on clinical judgment. *Rehabilitation Counseling Bulletin, 42*, 243-264.

Rosenthal, D. A., & Kosciulek, J. F. (1996). Clinical judgment and bias due to client race or ethnicity: An overview with implications for rehabilitation counselors. *Journal of Applied Rehabilitation Counseling, 27*, 30-36.

Sue, D. W., Arredondo, P., & McDavis, R. J. (1992). Multicultural counseling competencies and standards: A call to the profession. *Journal of Counseling & Development, 70*, 477-486.

Shaw, L. R.; McMahon, B. T.; Chan, F.; Taylor, D., & Wood, C. (2001). Survey of rehabilitation counselor education programs regarding health care case management in the private sector. *Journal of Rehabilitation, 63* (3), 46-52.

Stein, L.I. & Santos, A.B. (1998). *Assertive Community Treatment of Persons with Severe Mental Illness*. Norton, New York.

Stein, L. & Test, M. (1980). *Alternative* to mental hospital treatment. *Archives of General Psychiatry, 37*, 392-397.

Sue, D. W. (1996). ACES endorsement of the multicultural counseling competencies: Do we have the courage. *Spectrum, 57*(1), 9-10.

Sue, D. W., Carter, R. T., Casas, J. M., Fouad, N. A., Ivey, A. I., Jensen, M., LaFromboise, T., Manese, J. E., Ponterrotto, J. G., Vazqueq-Nutall, E. (1998). *Multicultural counseling competencies: Individual and organizational development* (v 11). Thousand Oaks, CA: Sage.

Sudarkasa, N. (1997). African American families and family values. In H. P. McAdoo (Ed.), *Black families* (pp. 9-40). Thousand Oaks, CA: Sage.

Summers, N. (2006). Fundamentals of case management practice: Skills for the human services (2nd edition). Belmont, CA: Brooks/Cole.

Terrell, F., & Terrell, S. L. (1981). An inventory to measure cultural mistrust among Blacks. *The Western Journal of Black Studies, 5*, 180-184.

Thompson, K.S., Griffith, E.E.H. & Leaf, P.J. (1990). A historical review of the Madison model of community care. *Hospital and Community Psychiatry, 41*, 625-634.

United States Department of Commerce. (2001). *Resident population estimates of the UnitedStates by sex, race, and Hispanic origin*. Available: http://www.census.gov/population/estimates/nation/intfile3-1.txt.

Whitney-Thomas, J., Timmons, J. C., Gilmore, D. S., & Thomas, D. M. (1999). Expanding access: Changes in vocational rehabilitation practice since the 1992 Rehabilitation Act Amendments. *Rehabilitation Counseling Bulletin, 43*, 30-40.

Wilson II, C. C. & Gutiérrez, F. (1985). *Minorities and media: Diversity and the end of mass communication*. Newbury Park, CA: Sage.

Wilson, K. B., Harley, D. A., McCormick, K., Jolivette, K. & Jackson. R. (2001). A literature review of vocational rehabilitation acceptance and explaining bias in the rehabilitation process. *Journal of Rehabilitation, 32*, 24-35.

Wilson, K. B., Jackson, R., & Doughty, J. (1999). What a difference a race makes: Reasons for unsuccessful closures within the vocational rehabilitation system. *American Rehabilitation, 25*, 16-24.

Wilson, K. B., Henry, M., Sayles, C., Senices, J., & Smith, D. (2003). Multicultural counseling and counseling competency in vocational rehabilitation. *Journal of the Pennsylvania Counseling Association, 5*, 15-18.

Wilson, K. B. (1999). Vocational rehabilitation acceptance: A tale of two races in a large midwestern state. *Journal of Applied Rehabilitation Counseling 30*, 25-31.

Wilson, K. B. (2002). The exploration of vocational rehabilitation acceptance and ethnicity: A national investigation. *Rehabilitation Counseling Bulletin, 45*, 168-176.

Wilson, K. B., Harley, D. A., & Alston, R. J. (2001). Race as a correlate of vocational rehabilitation acceptance: Revisited. *Journal of Rehabilitation, 67*(3), 35-41.

Wilson, K. B., Alston, R. J., Harley, D. A., & Mitchell, N. (2002). Predicting vocational rehabilitation acceptance based on race, gender, education, work status at application, and primary source of support at application in the United States. *Rehabilitation Counseling Bulletin, 45*, 132-142.

Wilson, K. B., & Senices, J. (2005). Exploring the vocational rehabilitation acceptance rates of Hispanics and non-Hispanics in the United States. *Journal of Counseling and Development 83(1)*, 86-96.

Wilson, K. B., Turner, T., & Jackson, R. J. (2002). Vocational rehabilitation services received after successful closure: A comparison by race. *Journal of Applied Rehabilitation, 33(1)*, 26-34.

Woodside, M. & McClam, T. (2003). *Generalist case management: a method of human service delivery (2nd edition)*. Pacific Grove, CA: Brooks/Cole.

CHAPTER 6

DIVERSITY ISSUES IN PSYCHOLOGICAL ASSESSMENT

CHOW S. LAM
DEBRA B. HOMA
AMY BUSER

Chapter Highlights

➡ Introduction

➡ Multicultural issues in the assessment process

➡ Issues in the assessment process for persons with disabilities

➡ Conclusion

Introduction

*W*hat is *psychological assessment?* According to the Standards for Educational and Psychological Testing (American Educational Research Association, American Psychological Association, & National Council on Measurement in Education, 1999), psychological assessment is:

> A comprehensive examination of psychological functioning that involves collecting, evaluating, and integrating test results and collateral information, and reporting information about an individual. Various methods may be used to acquire information during a psychological assessment: administering, scoring, and interpreting tests and inventories; behavioral observation; client and third-party interviews; analysis of prior educational, occupational, medical, and psychological records.

p. 180

As stated in the above definition, psychological assessment gathers data from multiple sources, and the clinician analyzes these data within the context of the individual's life history, referral records, and behavioral observations (Meyer et al., 2001). The purposes of psychological assessment are varied and often depend on the setting in which they are conducted, the needs of the individual, and information requested by the referral source. In a clinical setting, psychological assessments are typically used to assess the individual's current level of psychological functioning, formulate a diagnosis, assist in treatment planning, and assess progress in therapy (AERA, APA, & NCME, 1999; Meyer, et al., 2001). Psychological assessments may also be conducted to assess cognitive strengths and deficits, diagnose neuropsychological impairment and learning disabilities, assess academic achievement levels, and provide information needed for career decision-making (AERA, APA, & NCME, 1999).

Some of the most common tools employed in psychological assessments include the clinical interview, intelligence and aptitude tests, achievement tests, personality tests, and vocational tests. The clinical interview may be structured, semi structured, or unstructured and is generally the first step in a psychological assessment; the interview allows the clinician to elicit important background information from the client and establish rapport (Berven, 2001). Intelligence tests measure cognitive strengths and limitations as defined by purported constructs of intelligence, often based on theory (AERA, APA, & NCME, 1999). In their broadest sense, most intelligence tests are designed to assess capacity for learning (Power, 2000) and provide a score in the form of the well-known intelligence quotient, or IQ. The most widely used intelligence test for adults in the United States is the Wechsler Adult Intelligence Scale-Third Edition (WAIS-III), considered by Power to be "perhaps the best general adult intelligence test available" (p. 133). Like intelligence tests, aptitude tests are intended to measure an individual's learning potential but are focused on a specific skill, often with the purpose of determining whether an individual would benefit from training in a particular area (Power, 2000).

In contrast, achievement tests assess the knowledge and skills an individual has already acquired through education and training (Power, 2000). Achievement tests typically include assessment of academic skills, such as reading, spelling, vocabulary, and mathematics. Personality inventories are designed to measure personal characteristics, such as individual differences in thoughts, feelings, and behavior, based either on theoretically derived constructs or on empirically based factors that are believed to influence an individual's behavior and functioning in various settings (AERA, APA, & NCME, 1999). While some personality inventories focus on normal personality functioning, others, such as the Minnesota Multiphasic Personality Inventory (MMPI), are designed to assess maladjustment and psychopathology (Power, 2000). Interest inventories assess occupational preferences and are among the most widely used vocational tests. Other types of vocational tests include inventories of work values and needs as well as tests designed to measure career maturity and decision-making (AERA, APA, & NCME, 1999).

Although psychological assessment is conducted in a variety of settings and with a wide range of age groups, this chapter will focus on the psychological assessment of adults in clinical and counseling settings and will provide an overview of diversity issues in clinical diagnosis, vocational assessment, and the assessment process, including the clinical interview and testing.

What is a diverse population? As used here, the term diverse populations refers to individuals who fall outside of the mainstream majority culture in the United States, usually designated as "minority groups," which include persons with disabilities and individuals from racial/ethnic groups other than European American. Although assessment issues regarding ethnic minorities and persons with disabilities will be addressed separately, this division is, to some extent, arbitrary. Persons with disabilities represent the largest minority group in the U.S. and share with other minority groups' experiences of discrimination and stigma. Like racial/ethnic minority groups, they have their own culture (Olkin, 1999). This similarity is especially highlighted by deaf individuals, who possess a unique culture and language.

Poverty and race/ethnicity are inter-related and complicate the assessment process of individuals from diverse populations. For example, the 1995 U.S.

130

Census provides the following data regarding poverty rates in the U.S.: 29.3% were African American, 30.3% were Hispanic, 14.6% were Asian and Pacific Islanders, and 14.3% were American Indians (U.S. Bureau of the Census, 1996, cited by Frisby, 1998b). Race/ethnicity is also associated with disability, lower rates of employment, and low-income levels (Myers & Rodriguez, 2003; Olkin, 1999). National data suggest that African Americans and Hispanics are at greater risk than others of incurring physical disabilities (Elliott & Umlauf, 1995). Assessment issues involving ethnicity and disability are, therefore, likely to overlap.

Recognizing the increasing importance of addressing the needs of culturally diverse individuals in service delivery, the American Psychological Association's Board of Ethnic Minority Affairs established a Task Force in 1988, which developed the American Psychological Association (APA) Guidelines for Providers of Psychological Services to Ethnic, Linguistic, and Culturally Diverse Populations. These guidelines call on psychologists to be culturally responsive to their clients in both assessment and treatment through awareness of ethnic and cultural influences on emotions and behavior and by being respectful of cultural differences in beliefs and worldviews (APA, 1990). The Ethical Principles of Psychologists and Code of Conduct (APA, 1992) stipulate that psychologists be mindful of the impact of race, ethnicity, disability, national origin, and language in both administration and interpretation of assessment results.

MULTICULTURAL ISSUES IN THE ASSESSMENT PROCESS

As mentioned earlier, psychological assessment involves multiple sources from which to gather information on the individual. During the psychological process, attention to special issues is needed when serving persons with a diverse background. The coverage of all areas of assessment issues is beyond the scope of this chapter. We choose several major assessment issues that we believe are essential when considering their application to persons from a diverse background.

CLINICAL INTERVIEW

A most frequent and widely used tool usually is the first step in the assessment process (Berven, 2001; Puente & Perez-Garcia, 2000). Although the interview is an essential element for obtaining case history information and providing contextual data needed to understand persons from diverse cultures, it is subject to bias and errors arising out of characteristics of both the client and the clinician. Clinicians unfamiliar with an individual's culture, worldview, and language may misunderstand and incorrectly record information needed for appropriate diagnosis (Jenkins & Ramsey, 1991). Negative reactions to cultural differences and racial or ethnic stereotypes may also adversely affect clinicians' ability to establish rapport and lead to misdiagnosis. Due to cultural norms, some individuals may be reluctant to divulge personal information to a stranger (Puente & Perez-Garcia, 2000) or may be distrustful of authority figures. Chinese Americans, for example, may be hesitant to initiate conversation out of respect for the clinician's authoritative role and be reluctant to disclose personal difficulties, which should not be misinterpreted as a sign of defensiveness (Chan, Lam, Wong, Leung, & Fang, 1988). To counteract the limitations of the interview, clinicians should obtain information from a variety of sources (Hays, 2001), such as family members, educational and medical records, and persons in the client's community.

When interviewing immigrants, clinicians should obtain information about a number of variables, including age at the time of immigration, generation level, previous occupation, educational background, and acculturation with the new country. Individuals who have recently immigrated experience a period of adjustment, and the process of adapting to a new country may even produce culture shock and a sense of disorientation (Comas-Diaz & Grenier, 1998), which could affect their behavior in the interview. Clinicians must maintain awareness of these issues to help prevent misdiagnosis.

CLINICAL DIAGNOSIS

In a review of the literature, Gray-Little and Kaplan (1998) noted a link between ethnicity and diagnoses, finding that "race and ethnicity are sometimes predictive of diagnosis, independent of symptoms" (p. 142). Studies over a 30-year period indicate that Whites are diagnosed with affective and personality disorders more often than African Americans. Asian Americans are more likely to be diagnosed with affective disorders, and African Americans are more likely to be diagnosed with schizophrenia, even among patients of similar socioeconomic status. The reasons for these findings are not clear. Clinical judgment bias has been implicated as one possible source, though Gray-Little and Kaplan (1998) found inconsistent results in their review of the literature, with some studies indicating that ethnic minorities are sometimes over-diagnosed and sometimes under-diagnosed. They concluded that overall, patients' race or ethnicity had an impact on clinical judgment beyond what would be warranted on the basis of symptoms. In the assessment of persons with disability, clinical judgment may be distorted by prejudices and stereotypes, causing clinicians to assume maladjustment and then elicit

132

information from the client that only serves to confirm their prior assumptions, rather than seeking evidence to the contrary; thus resulting in over-diagnosis. In contrast, under-diagnosis may occur due to a process called diagnostic overshadowing, in which the clinician ignores potential signs of psychopathology because they are overshadowed by characteristics of the disability (Olkin, 1999).

Clinical judgment errors may also be caused by the clinician's lack of knowledge of culturally based behaviors and folk beliefs (e.g., beliefs in the presence of spirits, "evil eye," and hexes), which could be misconstrued as symptoms of psychopathology (Paniagua, 1998; 2000). Hays (2001) maintains that one of the greatest challenges to the clinician in cross-cultural assessment is to differentiate behaviors and ways of thinking that are culturally normal from those that are pathological. Language differences also may complicate the diagnostic process. In a review of the literature, Paniagua (2000) found studies indicating that clients were assigned higher ratings of psychopathology when interviewed in English rather than in their first language.

Numerous studies have also documented cultural variations in how individuals express distress (Westermeyer, 1987), and one of the most robust findings is that Asian Americans and Hispanic patients are more likely to report physical symptoms when they are depressed, as compared to European Americans (Gray-Little & Kaplan, 1998). Research of Asian Americans suggests these patterns become more similar to those of European Americans with increased acculturation (Hall & Phung, 2001). Dana (2001b) describes five types of psychological distress in multicultural populations (1) disorders that are general and correspond to the categories of the Diagnostic and Statistical Manual of Mental Disorders - IV (DSM-IV) (American Psychiatric Association, 1994), such as depression and schizophrenia, though the symptoms may be expressed differently; (2) culture-bound syndromes; (3) everyday living problems; (4) difficulties caused by societal oppression; and (5) symptoms associated with acculturative stress, that is, difficulties in adapting to the mores and worldviews of the new host culture (Marsella & Yamada, 2000). Some racial/ethnic groups have had different experiences of discrimination and prejudice that could influence their expressions of distress. African Americans, for example, have had unique experiences compared to other ethnic groups, with a history of oppression accompanied by violence that has generated coping and adaptation strategies needed for survival within a dehumanizing sociopolitical system (Morris, 2000a).

Implications of these culturally based expressions of symptoms are that the DSM-IV's descriptions of symptomotology according to diagnostic categories may not provide an accurate fit for persons from diverse cultures (Gray-Little &

Kaplan, 1998). The fourth edition of the DSM (1994), however, is an improvement over previous versions in that it provides a description of cultural variations of symptoms for some disorders, a listing and description of culture-bound syndromes, and cultural formulation guidelines to help the clinician take into account the client's cultural context. These cultural formulations comprise five categories: cultural identity; cultural explanation of illness; cultural factors related to psychosocial environment and level of functioning; cultural elements of the relationship between the clinician and the client; and overall cultural assessment for diagnosis and care (Paniagua, 2000).

PSYCHOLOGICAL TESTING

An important issue in testing involves the cultural equivalence of the traits and abilities test instruments are designed to measure. Just as there are cultural differences in expressions of distress, some research suggests that, through a process of learning and adaptation, the environment influences how individuals' abilities develop from one culture to another. As a consequence, cultures may assign different meanings to various traits and do not necessarily share Western notions of what intelligent behavior is (Greenfield, 1997). Sternberg and Grigorenko (2001), for example, noted that their research in Kenya suggested that its inhabitants place more value on social skills as an aspect of intelligence than do individuals in the United States. As Anastasi and Urbina (1997) point out, psychological tests represent a sample of behavior, and since behavior is shaped by the culture in which an individual develops, "cultural influences will and should be reflected in test performance" (p. 342). This implies a reciprocal association in that standardized tests will measure characteristics that are valued by the majority culture in which the tests are developed (Greenfield, 1997; Samuda, 1998) and may not assess behavior that is characteristic of individuals from minority cultures (Smart & Smart, 1993). In addition, the constructs the tests measure may have different meanings among persons of different cultures.

Standardized testing may present concerns for individuals who received their schooling outside the U.S., especially in a developing country. Some immigrants may have received very limited education or their schooling may have differed significantly from that provided in the U.S. These immigrants are less likely to have had experiences with tests designed to measure cognitive abilities and may be unfamiliar with such tasks. When working with these individuals, clinicians should exercise considerable caution in interpreting test results (Scheuneman & Oakland, 1998).

134

TEST BIAS

Given that most commonly used tests are designed on the basis of European American culture, bias in testing is an issue of concern in the psychological assessment of individuals from diverse cultures who differ from the group upon which the tests were standardized (Padilla, 2001). Even when different racial/ethnic groups are included in a test's standardization group, the sample is often too small and lacks controls regarding acculturation level (Dana, 2000). Test bias refers to whether a test is valid for different groups in a differential way; for example, if it underestimates the future performance of a group (Anastasi, 1992; Gray-Little & Kaplan, 1998). Bias may have an impact on test scores in the following ways:

- Construct bias, that is, when a construct has different meanings across cultural groups;
- Item bias, which occurs if individuals respond differently to test items because of cultural variables, even though they have the same amount of the particular trait being measured;
- Method bias, which may be present in test procedures and administration format.

Dana, 2000; Van de Vijver, 2000

Consequences of test bias include diagnostic errors, such as misdiagnosis (Paniagua, 1998), inappropriate educational placements (for example, a disproportionate number of minority students placed in special education programs), and under-prediction of scholastic or occupational potential.

Instruments designed to assess personality and psychopathology have been developed in recent years that include racial and ethnic minorities in standardization samples. The re-standardized edition of the Minnesota Multiphasic Personality Inventory (MMPI-2), for example, was published in 1989 after 10 years of research and gathered a larger normative sample that included proportional representation of diverse populations, based on U.S. Census data (Handel & Ben-Porath, 2000). Due to population changes since that time, Hispanics and Asian Americans are now under-represented (Velasquez et al., 2000). Handel and Ben-Porath (2000), in summarizing studies of the MMPI-2 between 1994 and 1998, find that the MMPI-2 appears to be applicable to African Americans in a variety of settings, but more research is needed for other ethnic groups. Other reviews of MMPI-2 research (Gray-Little & Kaplan, 1998; Velasquez et al., 2000) note a tendency for Latinos to score higher than White respondents on the L (Lie) scale, one of the validity scales designed to assess test-taking attitudes (Greene, 1991). This may be interpreted not as a tendency towards deception, but perhaps to present oneself in a socially desirable manner. Individuals from some Latin American countries

135

may have experienced authoritarian and repressive sociopolitical systems (Dana, 2000; Cuellar, 2000) that, perhaps, could produce a socially desirable response pattern. Clinicians need to be aware that most ethnic groups are not homogeneous (Hall & Phung, 2001) and research on many groups, such as Latinos, should be examined as subgroups, rather than as one large category (Handel & Ben-Porath, 2000). Acculturation may also have an impact on MMPI-2 results (Hall & Phung, 2000; Velasquez et al., 2000). Cuellar (2000) suggests that individuals who are less acculturated, especially when combined with a lower socioeconomic status and education, tend to obtain higher scores on measures of psychopathology.

The MMPI-2 may be problematic for individuals with physical disabilities because some clinical scales comprise questions about physical symptoms, and elevations on these scales may reflect realistic consideration of physical concerns rather than psychological difficulties (Elliott & Umlauf, 1995; Olkin, 1999), though more research in this area is needed (Hays, 2001). Rodevich and Wanlass (1995) investigated the effects of a T-score correction procedure for the MMPI-2 for individuals with spinal cord injury. They found that before using the correction procedure, the average scores of participants reflected varying degrees of maladjustment or other psychological problems. After using the correction procedure, they found that as a group, the participants would now be seen as being emotionally well adjusted. In a review of studies using the MMPI and MMPI-2 for individuals with vision impairment, Harrington and McDermott (1993) noted a tendency toward elevations on Depression and Social Introversion scales that could be attributed to the disability rather than psychopathology, due to bias in test content, and they advised caution in interpreting MMPI results for this population.

The MMPI's usefulness is very limited with deaf individuals because its eighth grade-level reading requirements surpass the reading skills of the average deaf high school graduate, and it has biases in content for deaf examinees (Brauer, Braden, Pollard, & Hardy-Braz, 1998). Translation into American Sign Language (ASL) of critical items of the MMPI has suggested this to be a promising area for further research into the applicability of a translated version of the MMPI-2 (Brauer, 1992). The use of standardized personality tests for deaf individuals is a complex issue, requiring knowledge about deafness, deaf culture, and the individual's case history. Vernon (2001) noted the possibility that deafness may affect environmental experiences and produce "an essentially different organization of personality and make normality for a person who is deaf or hard of hearing different from normality for a person with no difficulty hearing" (p. 389). Brauer, et al. (1998) describe research findings suggesting that clinicians who were not knowledgeable of

136

deafness and who relied on instruments that were not adapted for use with deaf individuals were more likely to incorrectly diagnose personality aberrations than clinicians who were experienced with this population.

The issue of test bias has been especially controversial regarding cognitive ability testing, as research over a period of many years has indicated significant between-group differences among various racial and ethnic groups. East Asian and Jewish examinees are usually at the top, followed by Caucasians, Hispanics, and African Americans, with the latter groups score often falling one standard deviation below that of Caucasians (Suzuki, Short, Pieterse, & Kugler, 2001). The issue has been complicated by the fact that numerous studies to evaluate test bias, usually through regression models comparing intelligence test scores to a criterion such as academic performance, have failed to find evidence of bias. These findings have led many researchers to conclude that, at least on the basis of psychometric data, test bias does not exist because many cognitive ability tests predict various educational and employment performances about equally well for persons from both majority and minority cultures (Cole, 1981; Frisby, 1998a; Hale, 1991).

In some instances, studies have suggested that these tests tend to over-predict future performance of diverse populations (Sirici & Geisinger, 1998). In a literature review of studies examining racial/ethnic differences on intelligence tests, Suzuki and Valencia (1997) noticed a decline in studies of test bias over the years, perhaps due to a belief that the controversy had been settled. They cite mixed results of previous research and suggest that this issue is not yet resolved. The researchers noted that comparisons between racial/ethnic groups are misleading because the within-group differences are usually greater, with socioeconomic status (SES) often being a major factor in these differences (both within and between groups). Since intelligence tests are more likely to tap experiences and values based on middle-class European culture, ethnic minorities who have grown up in a different cultural environment could be expected to be at a disadvantage (Jenkins & Ramsey, 1991). Moreover, the criteria used for assessing predictive validity, such as school performance and occupation may be biased, considering the limitations imposed by society's opportunity structure (Suzuki & Valencia, 1997).

Remedies for test bias will not be easily accomplished. The goal of developing culture-free tests seems elusive thus far and may be impossible to achieve (Janda, 1998; Paniagua, 1998). Test developers have attempted for many years to design tests that minimize the impact of culture, usually in the form of nonverbal measures. Even nonverbal test performance has been found to be influenced by culture, perhaps because nonverbal tests involve abstract reasoning skills that are valued in Eurocentric cultures; while persons from

137

other cultures may favor an approach to problem solving that is more contextually based (Anastasi & Urbina, 1997). Developing culture-specific tests and norms for different ethnic groups is a first step in minimizing test bias but has the disadvantage of preventing comparisons across cultures. Cultures are constantly changing, with differing levels of acculturation, so that norms may soon become outdated (Van de Vijver, 2000). Obtaining norms from different ethnic groups may also be impractical. Asian and Pacific Islanders, for example, represent 28 different countries (Hays, 2001) with marked cultural and language differences between these groups and each having its own unique history (Leung & Sakata, 1988). In recent years, advanced test development methods have sought to minimize bias through using expert panels to examine item content, including different racial/ethnic groups in the standardization sample, and applying statistical techniques to examine test performance and differential responding among groups (Suzuki, et al., 2001).

Criterion-referenced scores may help minimize the impact of test bias by allowing comparison to a performance standard, rather than to a norm group. Criterion-referenced scores would provide a measure of what the individual knows or can do and determine if this matches the performance standard (for example, math skills required in a particular job). Instead of focusing only on prediction of performance, the criterion-referenced approach would allow clinicians to identify deficient areas and recommend strategies for improvement that would enable the individual to meet the performance standard (Samuda, 1998).

Another solution to test bias has been offered by Cuellar (2000) who suggests that data regarding an examinee's acculturation level may be used as a moderator of personality and other psychological assessment measures to correct for test bias. Acculturation data allows the assessor to determine how well psychological test scores predict behavior for persons who are not well represented in standardization samples; using the acculturation score as a moderator, the assessor can raise or lower the individual's score. For example, the Acculturation Rating Scale for Mexican Americans (Cuellar, Arnold, & Maldonado, 1995, cited by Zane & Mak, 2003) has been used to correct the tendency of the MMPI to over-diagnose pathology among Latinos. Cuellar (2000) proposes applying an Index for Correction of Culture (ICC), which is based on the correlation between the examinee's acculturation score and the criterion for a particular group. The ICC shows how different the examinee is from the normative sample, so that the assessor can adjust test scores accordingly. In practice, however, clinicians rarely have the quantitative data needed to apply this correction procedure and must instead rely on clinical judgment. In addition, in a review of 21 instruments designed to measure

138

acculturation, Zane and Mak (2003) remarked that most were for Hispanic Americans, with only a few designed for Asian/Pacific Islanders and African Americans, thereby limiting clinicians' resources for applying a correction for culture to test results.

TEST TRANSLATION

Test translation involves more than an accurate linguistic translation; it requires determining whether and how the psychological construct is understood across cultures. For example, a concept may be understood differently among different cultural groups or may not be meaningful to a group for whom a test is being translated (Arnold & Matus, 2000). To ensure accurate translation, a test should be "back translated," that is, translated back into the original language from the translated version. Achieving high-quality translations can be very costly and, according to Padilla (2001), "few tests are ever translated for use with limited English speakers" (p. 21). An important concept in multicultural assessment is that of "etic" versus "emic" assessment instruments (Dana, 2001a). Etic instruments are those that are developed from outside the culture in which they are being applied; they are often incorrectly assumed to be universally applicable. In contrast, emic instruments are developed from within the culture in which they are being used and, therefore, measure traits that are meaningful to that culture (Lonner, 1985). Instruments must also demonstrate cultural equivalence, which is defined according to four categories (1) functional equivalence, or the role that a behavior or trait plays in different cultures; (2) conceptual equivalence, or the similarities in meaning associated with behaviors and constructs; (3) metric equivalence, a psychometric property requiring that a measurement scale assesses the same trait across cultures; and (4) linguistic equivalence, or appropriate translation of the test (Fouad, 1993; Lonner, 1985).

TEST SELECTION

Before selecting tests or procedures to use in the assessment, clinicians should first obtain thorough background information about the client, including medical information, educational background, level of acculturation, English proficiency, and how recently the client immigrated to the U.S. (Suzuki, et al., 2001). English proficiency by itself may not be sufficient, as clinicians still need to ascertain the client's preferred language for assessment (Velasquez & Callahan, 1992). After gathering this information, they can determine whether or not standardized testing is appropriate. If testing appears to be appropriate, they should proceed cautiously, beginning with a careful reading of the manual for each test being considered. Particular attention should be paid to the examination of norm groups (for example, to see if they include the client's race/ethnic group), and information about validity and reliability. If a test has not been used with diverse populations, clinicians should find out if other tests or procedures would be more suitable (Geisinger, 1998). Clinicians also need to ensure that the test does not require skills or behaviors that the examinee has not had the opportunity to perform or learn (Feist-Price, Harley, & Alston, 1996).

Appropriate test selection is also important in vocational assessment, a common type of psychological testing often used to help individuals make career decisions by providing them with information about their interests, values, aptitudes, and skills (Gainor, 2001). When applied to culturally diverse populations, the counselor needs to keep in mind that vocational counseling is influenced by the values of European American culture with its emphasis on individualism, linear style of decision-making, and success in the competitive labor market (Fouad, 1993). The counselor needs to be aware that these values may be counter to those of clients from diverse cultures and be respectful of these differences.

Vocational tests, such as interest and values inventories, enable counselors to obtain information efficiently and help provide career direction, but they may be subject to bias because they do not represent the experiences of persons from diverse cultures. The career development theories, upon which these tests are based, with their focus on individualism, may not be applicable to persons from collectivistic cultures (Gainor, 2001). Although studies of cross-cultural interest assessment have produced mixed results over the past 20 years (Day & Rounds, 1998), findings in recent years have been positive. In a 1993 review of research on the use of interest inventories across cultures, Fouad (2002) noted that, compared to European Americans, African Americans tended to have more Social-Enterprising-Conventional interests (based on Holland's career development model of six occupational themes). Higher scores in sales, social services, business, and verbal-linguistic areas suggest differences in the development and expression of interests. In contrast, in their large sample size (49,450) investigation of the applicability of Holland's model for five racial/ethnic groups, Day and Rounds (1998) found similar interest structure among the groups, suggesting that it is universal. Using an ethnically diverse sample of both professionals and students who took the Strong Interest Inventory, Fouad (2002) found only a small effect size for race/ethnicity on Holland's occupational themes, with greater within-group differences (due to sex and age) than between-group differences based on ethnicity.

These findings suggested that the Strong Interest Inventory could be useful with diverse populations. In an extensive review of 44 career assessment instruments, including nine interest inventories, Eby and Russell (1998) concluded that most of the inventories could be useful for culturally diverse individuals (including persons with disabilities). They cautioned that few of the instruments reviewed provided reliability or validity information regarding diverse populations. In addition, they recommended that more research was needed to validate career assessment instruments for diverse populations as well as to develop instruments for specific groups. Gainor (2001) likewise advised caution when interpreting results of interest inventories for individuals from diverse cultures. Results need to be viewed within a cultural context, including the impact of acculturation and ethnic identity.

Interest inventories developed specifically for individuals with physical or mental disabilities are lacking (Power, 2000), and few studies have examined the potential impact of a disability on vocational interests. One exception, a 1982 study by Rohe and Athelstan, found that individuals with spinal cord injury tended to have job interests which were inconsistent with their physical limitations, suggesting that clinicians may need to be creative in helping persons with physical disabilities identify vocational options that are congruent with both their interests and capabilities.

TEST-TAKING BEHAVIOR

Cultural factors can influence test-taking behavior (Anastasi & Urbina, 1997) and the clinician should take into account the potential impact of cultural factors on test performance (Morris, 2000b). Test-taking performance may be affected by motivation as well as by culture-related behaviors such as work speed, cooperativeness, familiarity with testing, and a tendency to give socially desirable responses (Lonner, 1985). Individuals who received their schooling outside the U.S. in a developing country, or those who received little schooling, may be unfamiliar with testing expectations and common test formats (Scheuneman & Oakland, 1998) and are likely to be at a serious disadvantage when taking cognitive tests, even those designed to be culture-fair.

Motivation is an important variable in test performance. For many ethnic groups, especially for individuals from a lower socioeconomic level, tests may be seen as a repetition of failure experiences and they may see little likelihood of success (Samuda, 1998). Such expectations may affect motivation to perform well, as research suggests that expectations influence motivation in testing; when individuals believe they have a chance of succeeding if they apply effort, they are more likely to do their best (Katz, 1968, cited by Samuda, 1998). Smart and Smart (1993) suggest that Hispanics may not be acculturated to the assessment process and not understand the relevance of testing, which affects motivation level. Clinicians can promote the motivation of Hispanic clients by explaining the practical usefulness of assessment and its future benefits. Both Hispanics (Smart & Smart) and African Americans (Gainor, 2001) may be distrustful of the assessment process due to prior negative experiences with testing and with public institutions. Clinicians can help reduce distrust by being open about this issue, establishing rapport, and trying to understand Hispanics worldview (Altson & McCowan, 1993). By taking the time to ensure informed consent, clinicians may also alleviate distrust by fully explaining the assessment process so that clients know what to expect and how the test results will be used.

Fear of failure may also occur, resulting in a tendency to avoid challenging situations, or to give up (Alston & McCowan, 1994). Characteristics of the assessment setting itself may have a strong impact on test motivation. Morris (2000b), for example, suggests that if African American clients view the setting or clinician as being antagonistic or intimidating, they may "sabotage their own performance during the assessment process" (p. 577). Compounded by fears of failure and negative past experiences, such a setting can generate feelings of anxiety that impair test performance (Samuda, 1998). Cultural stereotypes may also have an impact on motivation and test performance through internalized negative expectations and diminished self-concept (Anastasi & Urbina, 1997; Alston & McCowan, 1994).

Testing response styles may be strongly influenced by cultural factors. Hispanics may see the clinician as an authority figure, resulting in a tendency to acquiesce and to provide socially desirable responses (Smart & Smart, 1993). Social desirability may also be reflected in test responses of Asian Americans arising from a need not to lose face (Gainor, 2001). Some ethnic groups, especially Hispanics (Scheuneman & Oakland, 1998) and African Americans (Alston & McCowan, 1994), may be at a disadvantage on speeded tests because time is given less emphasis in these cultures than in European American culture. Having different orientations to time, these individuals may work at their own pace with a focus on quality rather than time constraints. This approach results in fewer correct items and thus a lower score, even though most items answered may be correct (Alston & McCowan, 1994). Individuals from diverse cultures are also more likely to omit items, rather than guessing (Scheuneman & Oakland, 1998). Since omitted items are considered incorrect in many cognitive tests, this response style means that results may not reflect their potential, especially for cognitive tests that have cut-off points after a certain number of incorrect answers. Clinicians can try to reduce these problems by observing clients' response styles during practice sections for tests or by providing additional practice, when feasible, and by ensuring that clients

understand the importance of working quickly and answering as many items as possible (Alston & McCowan, 1994).

ISSUES IN THE ASSESSMENT PROCESS FOR PERSONS WITH DISABILITIES

Test fairness and validity, appropriateness of norms, and provision of test accommodations are particular issues of concern in the assessment process of individuals with disabilities. Clinicians cannot assume equivalence of test content if a test requires certain skills that are affected by the disability (Geisinger, 1998). Legal requirements, beginning with Section 504 of the Rehabilitation Act of 1973, which stipulate that programs receiving federal assistance to provide accommodations to individuals with disabilities to ensure equality in access and program participation (Pitoniak & Royer, 2001), mandate consideration of test equivalence and fairness for persons with disabilities. These requirements were expanded to the private sector with the Americans with Disabilities Act (ADA) of 1990, which was applicable to employers with more than 15 employees. Provisions of the ADA mandate physical accessibility of assessment programs and test formats that allow persons with disabilities to demonstrate skills and knowledge related to job functions (Pullin, 2002). Assessors should, therefore, provide modifications of tests or test administration, such as time limits, unless these modifications invalidate measurement of the skill the test is designed to assess (Pratt & Moreland, 1998).

TEST FAIRNESS AND VALIDITY

Clinicians may need to change how a test is given to ensure test fairness, particularly with regard to test content and the skills needed to perform the test. Deviations from standardized administration, however, can adversely affect test reliability and validity (Pratt & Moreland, 1998). The key to appropriate accommodation is to provide enhanced access while preserving the validity of test results (Behuniak, 2002). A first step in this process is proper test selection; that is, clinicians should consider the skill requirements of the test, such as ability to read, turn pages, and manipulate objects (Pratt & Moreland, 1998). If a test requires abilities that the individual does not have, then the test is measuring disability, rather than the intended construct. Provision of appropriate test modifications requires clinicians to be knowledgeable about disabilities and the types of accommodations that are available. Smith (2002) provides a series of guidelines to assist clinicians in identifying testing accommodations. These include an identification of the client's receptive and

expressive skills (including motoric response), followed by an examination of the receptive and expressive skills required by the selected tests. If these skills do not match, then clinicians should determine what modifications are needed and if these modifications will compromise the validity of test results.

TEST ACCOMMODATIONS

The 1999 Standards for Educational and Psychological Testing (AERA, APA, & NCME) suggest the following strategies for test modifications:

- Presentation format (for example, Braille or large print for individuals with vision impairment and verbal instructions provided in manual communication for persons who are deaf);
- Response format (such as dictating answers to a scribe or into a tape recorder);
- Test timing, such as extended time limits;
- Test setting, such as individual administration instead of group administration for someone with attentional difficulties, and providing special lighting for an examinee with vision impairment;
- Using only portions of tests, for example, selected sections of a cognitive test battery;
- Using substitute tests, such as a test designed specifically for individuals with disabilities.

Extended time is the most frequently used accommodation (Pitoniak & Royer, 2001). Bradley-Johnson and Ekstrom (1998) advise clinicians not to use timed tests for individuals with vision impairment, as reading large print takes additional time, and Braille may take two and a half times longer, depending on the person's level of proficiency. Sirici and Geisinger (1998) suggest additional accommodations that may be appropriate for persons with learning disabilities as well as for individuals with psychiatric disabilities or metabolic disorders: providing more frequent breaks, presenting instructions or test questions aloud, and allowing use of a computer or calculator.

Due to a lack of research, the impact of test modifications on the assessment of persons with disabilities is largely unknown. One concern is to ensure that accommodated tests provide more accurate results than those that are not accommodated. Modifications may make a test easier or more difficult for the individual with a disability when compared to nondisabled examinees of comparable ability, thus affecting the ability of the test to predict future performance. For example, although extended time may be needed to ensure test fairness, it could also cause fatigue and thereby impair test performance

(Pratt & Moreland, 1998). Certain types of accommodations may hinder clinicians' ability to measure the intended construct of the test, such as reading questions aloud for tests designed to assess reading comprehension and removing or extending time limits for tests in which part of the construct being measured is speed (Sirici & Geisinger, 1998).

The 1999 Standards advise clinicians to "pilot test" modifications when possible, but in reality, this is seldom done. Studies of test accommodations for persons with disabilities are complicated due to (1) small sample sizes, especially for certain disabilities, resulting in a lack of quantitative data (Pullin, 2002), (2) group variability, and (3) accommodations variability (Pitoniak & Royer, 2001), which may include a combination of different types of accommodations, such as large print test format and extended time limits. Of the limited research that is available, most studies have examined results of accommodations on high stakes tests, such as the Scholastic Aptitude Test (SAT) or Graduate Record Examination (GRE). These studies were conducted during the 1980s and are described by Willingham, Ragosta, Bennett, Braun, Rock, and Powers (1988). According to Pullin (2002), since that time, there has been "little validity research on modifications to address disabilities" (p. 26).

Lusting and Saura (1996) suggest a potential solution to the validity issues raised by test modifications in that they outline a structured procedure for accommodations using criterion-referenced tests. This procedure could be applied in vocational assessment to predict work performance. It would allow the clinician to match test accommodations to the types of accommodations that could be provided in a work setting. With this criterion-based procedure, the client's test performance with accommodations can be compared to the knowledge and skill requirements of a job rather than through comparison to a norm group, which may be invalid, depending on the nature of the test modification.

Another assessment issue involves the debate about whether clinicians should use general or special norms when assessing individuals with disabilities. Comparison of an individual's test scores with a norm group that shares similar characteristics and for which predictive validity is available enables clinicians to make more accurate predictions about future behavior. Most tests, however, do not include persons with disabilities in the normative sample, or if they do, they are small in number (Pratt & Moreland, 1998). Practical issues may also make development of such norms unlikely, given the problems with sample size and the heterogeneity of individuals with disabilities. This issue becomes especially problematic for individuals with visual impairment, because they may require significant test modifications, and individuals with early-onset vision loss may have had different experiences

from sighted individuals on whom the norms are based, which could make the norms of ability and personality tests inapplicable for this population (Gallagher & Wiener, 2001). Very few tests provide standardized norms for persons with vision impairment, and those that are available usually are not new, as few have been published within the last 15 years (Bradley-Johnson & Ekstrom, 1998). One recent exception is the Cognitive Test for the Blind, which has shown promise as a useful instrument in assessing the intellectual capabilities of this population (Nelson, Dial, & Joyce, 2002).

SPECIAL NORMS

Parker (2001) suggests that a solution to the norms problem is to look at test scores as being descriptive, rather than predictive. If clinicians want to describe where a person stands in relation to a norm group, both general and special norms are acceptable. Normative scores become a problem when they are inappropriately used for predictive purposes, as prediction should be based on statistical data, such as regression equations. The purpose of testing will determine norms selection; for example, clinicians may need to compare an examinee's performance to norms of persons without disabilities when this is the context in which the person will be expected to perform, such as an educational or job setting (Pratt & Moreland, 1998). The 1999 Standards also indicate that regular norms may be used when comparison with the general population is needed. As already noted, test accommodations may substantially alter the test procedures upon which the test is standardized, which could make comparison to standardized competitive norms inappropriate. Competitive norms may underestimate the abilities of persons with disabilities (Berven, 1980). Some rehabilitation facilities have addressed this problem by developing local client norms, but Berven (1980) pointed out that this approach might lead to overestimation of abilities. He proposed a solution that could overcome the disadvantages of using either competitive or local norms: "If clients were followed-up after completing assessment, different client subpopulations could be defined on the basis of training or employment outcomes, and norms could be established for those various subgroups" (p. 61). Such norms would allow comparison to a norm group of similar individuals who experienced successful outcomes in various training programs, jobs, or other areas of concern. Development of these norms, however, would require a sufficiently large group of individuals.

6

CONCLUSION

We provided a general overview on psychological assessment. As noted, the process of psychological assessment is a multifaceted procedure. The added complexities of understanding an individual who is from a diverse background make psychological assessment a challenging task, especially given the impact of the results and recommendations for clinical and rehabilitation practice. Culturally sensitive rehabilitation professionals should be aware of the limitations of psychological assessment practices, from intakes to the use of standardized assessment instruments (Constantine, 1998; Helms, 2002; Ridley, Hill, & Li, 1998) and safeguard themselves from testing bias and misinterpretation of test results. In addition to knowing the "dos" and "don'ts," rehabilitation professionals should be aware of their own worldview and attitudes toward those who are different from them. As pointed out by Fiske (1998) there is a tendency, often unconscious, to exaggerate differences between groups and similarities within one group and favor one's in-group over the out-group. This becomes problematic when one group holds much more power than the other group. It is quite common for the in-group to form automatic biases and stereotypic attitudes about people in the out-group.

The American Psychological Association (1990) warns that automatic biases and attitudes may lead to miscommunication, since normative behavior in one context may not be necessarily understood or valued in another. Rehabilitation professionals should realize that the responsibility of selecting, administering, and interpreting test results in a culturally sensitive manner remains with themselves. It is our hope that issues and considerations discussed in this chapter would heighten rehabilitation professionals' multicultural awareness and sensitivity and assist them in performing psychological assessments in a culturally sensitive manner.

REFERENCES

Alston, R. J. & McCowan, C. J. (1994). Aptitude assessment and African American clients: The interplay between culture and psychometrics in rehabilitation. *Journal of Rehabilitation, 60* (1), 41-46.

American Educational Research Association, American Psychological Association, & National Council on Measurement in Education (1999). *Standards for educational and psychological testing* (2nd ed.). Washington, DC: American Educational Research Association.

American Psychiatric Association. (1994). *Diagnostic and statistical manual of mental disorders* (4th ed.). Washington D.C.: Author.

American Psychological Association. (1990). Guidelines for providers of psychological services to ethnic, linguistic, and culturally diverse populations. Retrieved March 1, 2003 from http://www.apa.org/pi/oema/guide.html

American Psychological Association. (1992). Ethical principles of psychologists and code of conduct. Washington, DC: Author.

Anastasi, A. (1992). What counselors should know about the use and interpretation of psychological tests. *Journal of Counseling & Development, 70*, 610-615.

Anastasi, A., & Urbina, S. (1997). *Psychological testing* (7th ed.). Upper Saddle River, NJ: Prentice Hall.

Arnold, B. R., & Matus, Y. E. (2000). Test translation and cultural equivalence methodologies for use with diverse populations. In I. Cuellar & F. A. Paniagua (Eds.), *Handbook of multicultural mental health* (pp.121-136). San Diego, CA: Academic Press.

Behuniak, P. (2002). Types of commonly requested accommodations. In R. B. Ekstrom & D. K. Smith (Eds.), *Assessing individuals with disabilities in educational, employment, and counseling settings* (pp. 45-58). Washington, DC: American Psychological Association.

Berven, N. L. (1980). Psychometric assessment in rehabilitation. In B. Bolton & D. W. Cook (Eds.), *Rehabilitation client assessment* (pp. 46-64). Baltimore: University Park Press.

Berven, N. L. (2001). Assessment interviewing. In B. F. Bolton (Ed.), *Handbook of measurement and evaluation in rehabilitation* (3rd ed., pp. 197-213). Gaithersburg, MD: Aspen.

Bradley-Johnson, S., & Ekstrom, R. (1998). Visual impairments. In J. Sandoval, C. L. Frisby, K. F. Geisinger, J. D. Scheuneman, & J. R. Grenier (Eds.), *Test interpretation and diversity: Achieving equity in assessment* (pp.271-295). Washington, DC: American Psychological Association.

Brauer, B. A. (1992). The signer effect on MMPI performance of deaf respondents. *Journal of Personality Assessment, 58*(2), 380-388.

Brauer, B. A., Braden, J. P., Pollard, R. Q., & Hardy-Braz, S. T. (1998). Deaf and hard of hearing people. In J. Sandoval, C. L. Frisby, K. F. Geisinger, J.D. Scheuneman, & J. R. Grenier (Eds.), *Test interpretation and diversity: Achieving equity in assessment* (pp.297-315). Washington, DC: American Psychological Association.

Chan, F., Lam, C. S., Wong, D., Leung, P., & Fang, X. (1988). Counseling Chinese Americans with disabilities. *Journal of Applied Rehabilitation Counseling 19*(4), 21-25.

Cole, N. S. (1981). Bias in testing. *American Psychologist, 36*, 1067-1077.

Comas-Diaz, L., & Grenier, J. R. (1998). Migration and acculturation. In J. Sandoval, C. L. Frisby, K. F. Geisinger, J.D. Scheuneman, & J. R. Grenier (Eds.), *Test interpretation and diversity: Achieving equity in assessment* (pp.231-239). Washington, DC: American Psychological Association.

Constantine, M. (1998). Developing competence in multicultural assessment: Implications for counseling psychology training and practice. *The Counseling Psychologist, 6,* 922-929.

Cuellar, I. (2000). Acculturation as a moderator of personality and psychological assessment. In R.H. Dana (Ed.), *Handbook of cross-cultural and multicultural personality assessment* (pp. 113-1129). Mahwah, NJ: Lawrence Erlbaum Associates.

Cuellar, I., Arnold, B., & Maldonado, R. (1995). Acculturation Rating Scale for Mexican Americans -II: A revision of the original ARSMA scale. *Hispanic Journal of Behavioral Sciences, 17,* 275-304.

Dana, R. H. (2000). Culture and methodology in personality assessment. In I. Cuellar & F.A.

Paniagua (Eds.), *Handbook of multicultural mental health* (pp. 97-120). San Diego, CA: Academic Press.

Dana, R. H. (2001a). Multicultural issues in assessment. In B. F. Bolton (Ed.), *Handbook of measurement and evaluation in rehabilitation* (pp. 449-469). Gaithersburg, MD: Aspen.

Dana, R. H. (2001b). Clinical diagnosis of multicultural populations in the United States. In L.A. Suzuki, J. G. Ponterotto, & P. J. Meller (Eds.), *Handbook of multicultural assessment* (2nd ed., pp. 101-131). San Francisco: Jossey-Bass.

Day, S. X & Rounds, J. (1998). Universality of vocational interest structure among racial and ethnic minorities. *American Psychologist, 53*(7), 728-736.

Eby, L. T., & Russell, J. E. A. (1998). A psychometric review of career assessment tools for use with diverse individuals. *Journal of Career Assessment, 6*(3), 269-310.

Elliott, T. R., & Umlauf, R. L. (1995). Measurement of personality and psychopathology following acquired physical disability. In L.A. Cushman & M. J. Scherer (Eds.), *Psychological assessment in medical rehabilitation* (pp. 325-358). Washington, DC: American Psychological Association.

Feist-Price, S., Harley, D. A., & Alston, R. J. (1996). A cross-cultural perspective for vocational evaluation and assessment. *Vocational Evaluation and Work Adjustment Association Bulletin, 29* (2), 48-54.

Fiske, S. T. (1998). Stereotyping, prejudice, and discrimination. In D. T. Gilbert & S. T. Fiske (Eds.), *The handbook of social psychology, Vol. 2* (4th ed., pp.357-411). New York: McGraw-Hill.

Fouad, N. A. (1993). Cross-cultural vocational assessment. *Career Development Quarterly, 42,* 4-13.

Fouad, N. A. (2002). Cross-cultural differences in vocational interests: Between-groups differences on the Strong Interest Inventory. *Journal of Counseling Psychology, 49*(3), 283-289.

Frisby, C. L. (1998a). Culture and cultural differences. In J. Sandoval, C. L. Frisby, K. F. Geisinger, J. D. Scheuneman, & J. R. Grenier (Eds.), *Test interpretation and diversity: Achieving equity in assessment* (pp.51-73). Washington, DC: American Psychological Association.

Frisby, C. L. (1998b). Poverty and socioeconomic status. In J. Sandoval, C. L. Frisby, K. F. Geisinger, J. D. Scheuneman, & J. R. Grenier (Eds.), *Test interpretation and diversity: Achieving equity in assessment* (pp.241-270). Washington, DC: American Psychological Association.

Gainor, K. A. (2001). Vocational assessment with culturally diverse populations. In L. A. Suzuki, J. G. Ponterotto, & P. J. Meller (Eds.), *Handbook of multicultural assessment* (2nd ed., pp. 169-189). San Francisco: Jossey-Bass.

Gallagher, J. T. & Wiener, W. R. (2001). Assessment of individuals with visual impairment. In B. F. Bolton (Ed.), *Handbook of measurement and evaluation in rehabilitation* (pp. 365-384). Gaithersburg, MD: Aspen.

Geisinger, K. F. (1998). Psychometric issues in test interpretation. In J. Sandoval, C. L. Frisby, K. F. Geisinger, J. D. Scheuneman, & J. R. Grenier (Eds.), *Test interpretation and diversity: Achieving equity in assessment* (pp.17-30). Washington, DC: American Psychological Association.

Gray-Little, B. & Kaplan, D. A. (1998). Interpretation of psychological tests in clinical and forensic evaluations. In J. Sandoval, C. L. Frisby, K. F. Geisinger, J. D. Scheuneman, & J. R. Grenier (Eds.), *Test interpretation and diversity: Achieving equity in assessment* (pp.141-178). Washington, DC: American Psychological Association.

Greene, R. L. (1991). *MMPI-2/MMPI: An interpretive manual.* Needham Heights, MA: Allyn & Bacon.

Greenfield, P. M. (1997). You can't take it with you: Why ability assessments don't cross cultures. *American Psychologist, 52*(10), 1115-1124.

Hale, R. L. (1991). Intellectual assessment. In M. Hersen, A. E. Kazdin, & A. S. Bellack (Eds.), *The Clinical Psychology Handbook* (2nd ed., pp. 374-405). Elmsford, NY: Pergamon Press.

Hall, G. C. N., & Phung, A. H. (2001). Minnesota Multiphasic Personality Inventory and Millon Clinical Multiaxial Inventory. In L.A. Suzuki, J. G. Ponterotto, & P. J. Meller (Eds.), *Handbook of multicultural assessment* (2nd ed., pp. 307-330). San Francisco: Jossey-Bass.

Handel, R. W., & Ben-Porath, Y. S. (2000). Multicultural assessment with the MMPI-2: Issues for research and practice. In R. H. Dana (Ed.), *Handbook of cross-cultural and multicultural personality assessment* (pp. 229-245). Mahwah, NJ: Lawrence Erlbaum Associates.

Harrington, R. G., & McDermott, D. (1993). A model for the interpretation of personality assessments of individuals with visual impairments. *Journal of Rehabilitation, 59*(4), 24-29.

Hays, P. A. (2001). *Addressing cultural complexities in practice: A framework for clinicians and counselors.* Washington, DC: American Psychological Association.

Helms, J. E. (2002). A remedy for the Black-White test-score disparity. *American Psychologist, 57,* 303-304.

Janda, L. H. (1998). *Psychological testing: Theory and applications.* Needham Heights, MA: Allyn & Bacon.

Jenkins, J. O., & Ramsey, G. A. (1991). Minorities. In M. Hersen, A. E. Kazdin, & A. S. Bellack (Eds.), *The Clinical Psychology Handbook* (2nd ed., pp. 724-740). Elmsford, NY: Pergamon Press.

Katz, I. (1968). Factors influencing Negro performance in the desegregated school. In M. Deutsch, I. Katz, & A. Jensen (Eds.), *Social class, race, and psychological developments* (pp. 254-289). New York: Holt, Rinehart & Winston.

Leung, P. & Sakata, R. (1988). Asian Americans and rehabilitation: Some important variables. *Journal of Applied Rehabilitation Counseling 19*(4), 16-19.

Lonner, W. J. (1985). Issues in testing and assessment in cross-cultural counseling. *The Counseling Psychologist, 13*(4), 599-614.

Lusting, D. C. & Saura, K. M. (1996). Use of criterion-based comparisons in determining the appropriateness of vocational evaluation test modifications for criterion referenced tests. *Vocational Evaluation and Work Adjustment Association Bulletin, 29* (1), 15-18.

Marsella, A. J. & Yamada, A. (2000). Culture and mental health: An introduction and overview of foundations, concepts, and issues. In I.

Cuellar & F. A. Paniagua (Eds.), *Handbook of multicultural mental health* (pp.3-24). San Diego, CA: Academic Press.

Meyer, G. J., Finn, S. E., Eyde, L. D., Kay, G. G., Moreland, K. L., Dies, R. R., et al. (2001). Psychological testing and psychological assessment: A review of evidence and issues. *American Psychologist, 56*(2), 128-165.

Morris, E. F. (2000a). An Africentric perspective for clinical research and practice. In R.H. Dana (Ed.), *Handbook of cross-cultural and multicultural personality assessment* (pp.17-41). Mahwah, NJ: Lawrence Erlbaum Associates.

Morris, E. F. (2000b). Assessment practices with African Americans: Combining standard assessment measures within an Africentric orientation. In R.H. Dana (Ed.), *Handbook of cross-cultural and multicultural personality assessment* (pp.573-603). Mahwah, NJ: Lawrence Erlbaum Associates.

Myers, H. F., & Rodriguez, N. (2003). Acculturation and physical health in racial and ethnic minorities. In K.M. Chun, P.B. Organista, & G. Marin (Eds.), *Acculturation: Advances in theory, measurement, and applied research* (pp. 163-185). Washington, DC: American Psychological Association.

Nelson, P. A., Dial, J. G., & Joyce, A. (2002). Validation of the Cognitive Test for the Blind as an assessment of intellectual functioning. *Rehabilitation Psychology, 47*(2), 184-193.

Olkin, R. (1999). *What psychotherapists should know about disability.* New York: Guilford Press.

Padilla, A. M. (2001). Issues in culturally appropriate assessment. In L. A. Suzuki, J. G. Ponterotto, & P. J. Meller (Eds.), *Handbook of multicultural assessment* (2nd ed., pp. 5-27). San Francisco: Jossey-Bass.

Paniagua, F. A. (1998). *Assessing and treating culturally diverse clients.* Thousand Oaks, CA: Sage.

Paniagua, F. A. (2000). Culture-bound syndromes, cultural variations, and psychopathology. In I. Cuellar & F. A. Paniagua (Eds.), *Handbook of multicultural mental health* (pp.139-169). San Diego, CA: Academic Press.

Parker, R. M. (2001). Aptitude testing. In B. F. Bolton (Ed.), *Handbook of measurement and evaluation in rehabilitation* (pp. 103-123). Gaithersburg, MD: Aspen.

Pitoniak, M. J., & Royer, J. M. (2001). Testing accommodations for examinees with disabilities: A review of psychometric, legal, and social policy issues. *Review of Educational Research*, 71(1), 53-104.

Power, P. W. (2000). *A guide to vocational assessment.* (3rd ed.). Austin, TX: Pro-Ed.

Pratt, S. I., & Moreland, K. L. (1998). Individuals with other characteristics. In J. Sandoval, C. L. Frisby, K. F. Geisinger, J. D. Scheuneman, & J. R. Grenier (Eds.), *Test interpretation and diversity: Achieving equity in assessment* (pp.349-3371). Washington, DC: American Psychological Association.

Puente, A. E., & Perez-Garcia, M. (2000). Psychological assessment of ethnic minorities. In G. Goldstein & M. Hersen (Eds.), *Handbook of psychological assessent* (3rd ed., pp. 527-551). Oxford: Elsevier Science.

Pullin, D. (2002). Testing individuals with disabilities: Reconciling social science and social policy. In R. B. Ekstrom & D. K. Smith (Eds.), *Assessing individuals with disabilities in educational, employment, and counseling settings* (pp. 11-31). Washington, DC: American Psychological Association.

Ridley, C., Hill, C., & Li, L. (1998). Revisiting and refining the multicultural assessment procedure. *Counseling Psychologist, 6,* 939-947.

Rodevich, M. A., & Wanlass, R. L. (1995). The moderating effect of spinal cord injury on MMPI-2 Profiles: A clinically derived T score correction procedure. *Rehabilitation Psychology, 40*(3), 181-190.

Rohe, D. E., & Athelstan, G. T. (1982). Vocational interests of persons with spinal cord injury. *Journal of Counseling Psychology, 29*(3), 283-291.

Samuda, R. J. (1998). *Psychological testing of American minorities: Issues and consequences* (2nd ed.). Thousand Oaks, CA: Sage.

Scheuneman, J. D. & Oakland, T. (1998). High-stakes testing in education. In Sandoval, J., Frisby, C. L., Geisinger, K. F., Scheuneman, J. D., & Grenier, J. R. (Eds.), *Test interpretation and diversity: Achieving equity in assessment.* Washington, DC: American Psychological Association.

Sireci, S. G. & Geisinger, K. F. (1998). Equity issues in employment testing. In J. Sandoval, C. L. Frisby, K. F. Geisinger, J. D. Scheuneman, & J. R. Grenier (Eds.), *Test interpretation and diversity: Achieving equity in assessment (pp.105-140).* Washington, DC: American Psychological Association.

Smart, J. F. & Smart, D. W. (1993). Vocational evaluation of Hispanics with disabilities: Issues and implications. *Vocational Evaluation and Work Adjustment Association Bulletin, 26* (3), 111-122.

Smith, D.K. (2002). The decision-making process for developing testing accommodations. In R. B. Ekstrom & D. K. Smith (Eds.), *Assessing individuals with disabilities in educational, employment, and counseling settings* (pp. 71-86). Washington, DC: American Psychological Association.

Sternberg, R. J., &: Grigorenko, E. L. (2001). Ability testing across cultures. In L. A. Suzuki, J. G. Ponterotto, & P.J. Meller (Eds.), *Handbook of multicultural assessment* (2nd ed., pp. 335-357). San Francisco: Jossey-Bass.

Suzuki, L. A., & Valencia, R. R. (1997). Race-ethnicity and measured intelligence: Educational implications. *American Psychologist, 52*(10), 1103-1114.

Suzuki, L. A., Short, E. L., Pieterse, A., & Kugler, J. (2001). Multicultural issues and the assessment of aptitude. In L. A. Suzuki, J. G. Ponterotto, & P. J. Meller (Eds.), *Handbook of multicultural assessment* (2nd ed., pp. 359-382). San Francisco: Jossey-Bass.

U.S. Bureau of the Census. (1996). *Poverty in the United States: 1995.* Washington, DC: U.S. Government Printing Office.

Van de Vijver (2000). The nature of bias. In R. H. Dana (Ed.), *Handbook of cross-cultural and multicultural personality assessment* (pp. 87-106). Mahwah, NJ: Lawrence Erlbaum Associates.

Velasquez, R. J., & Callahan, W. J. (1992). Psychological testing of Hispanic Americans in clinical settings: Overview and issues. In K. F. Geisinger (Ed.), *Psychological testing of Hispanics* (pp. 253-265). Washington, DC: American Psychological Association.

Velasquez, R. J., Ayala, G. X., Mendoza, S., Nezami, E., Castillo-Canez, I., Pace, T., et al. (2000). Culturally competent use of the Minnesota Multiphasic Personality Inventory-2. In I. Cuellar & F. A. Paniagua (Eds.), *Handbook of multicultural mental health* (pp. 389-417). San Diego, CA: Academic Press.

Vernon, M. (2001). Assessment of individuals who are deaf or hard of hearing. In B. F. Bolton (Ed.), *Handbook of measurement and evaluation in rehabilitation* (3rd ed., pp. 385-397). Gaithersburg, MD: Aspen.

Westermeyer, J. (1987). Cultural factors in clinical assessment. *Journal of Consulting and Clinical Psychology, 55*(4), 471-478.

Willingham, W.W., Ragosta, M., Bennett, R.E., Braun, H., Rock, D.A., and Powers, D.E. (1988). *Testing handicapped people.* Needham Heights, MA: Allyn and Bacon. Zane, N., & Mak, W. (2003). Major approaches to the measurement of acculturation among ethnic minority populations: A content analysis and an alternative empirical strategy. In K. M. Chun, P. B. Organista, & G. Marin (Eds.), *Acculturation: Advances in theory, measurement, and applied research* (pp. 39-60). Washington, DC: American Psychological Association.

CHAPTER 7

PSYCHOSOCIAL ADJUSTMENT TO DISABILITY: A MULTI-ETHNIC APPROACH

ALO DUTTA

MADAN M. KUNDU

Chapter Highlights

➡ Guiding models of allied health

➡ Multiculturalism from an American perspective

➡ Effects of social movement

➡ Stages of adjustment and adaptation to chronic illness and disability

➡ Disability in the context of Maslow's hierarchy of needs

➡ Conclusion

7

*Only through diversity of opinion is there, in the existing state
of human intellect, a chance of fair play to all sides of the truth.*
John Stuart Mill

Since time immemorial, human beings have been overly concerned about their outward appearances, and have held the belief that, somehow, the characteristics of the physique were reflections of the inner self. The philosophy of mind and body being two interconnected parts of the human unity may have inadvertently generated the notion of intimate interdependence of physique and personality. Even today, disability is considered a challenge. It is perceived as a misfortune that results in a very long and arduous journey through life unique to those with disabilities. Spread is defined as the ability of a single characteristic to evoke inferences about the person as a whole. The effects of spread continue to devalue and dehumanize the individual to an object of intervention. A person with a disability may be perceived as unhappy, eager to please, frustrated, child-like, and incompetent. Though society has made progress in becoming sensitive to the needs of this population, significant levels of prejudice, ignorance, and stereotypes continue to impact the quality of lives of people with disabilities (Dembo, Leviton, & Wright, 1956; Marinelli & Dell Orto, 1999; Wright, 1983).

In an effort to identify and explain the psychosocial effects of a disability, this chapter will focus on (1) an overview of selected models of conceptualizing disability in general and from a cultural perspective, (2) the effects of civil and women's rights on the disability rights movement, (3) conceptualization of multiculturalism from an American perspective and its effects on disability in general, (4) stages of adjustment to a disability as a function of one's environment, and (5) the role of culture and ethnicity in the acceptance of a disability. We are aware that a certain type of physical and mental health condition may cause specific coping, adjustment, and psychosocial issues for a person with a disability. It is beyond the purview of this chapter, however, to delve into specific implications of each type of disability. The focus is on the effects of disability in general, and as a function of a person's contextual factors.

GUIDING MODELS OF ALLIED HEALTH

Chronic health conditions and disability due to congenital anomalies or accidents or illnesses, are a natural part of life. Rapid medical and technological advancements have resulted in enhanced longevity, higher survival rates for people with life threatening illnesses, and an increase in the population of those with disabilities. More than 54 million Americans report some form of disability that interferes with one or more activities of daily living (ADL), and almost 50% of that population has a severe disability. There is a differential distribution of disability by age, gender, and ethnicity. Prevalence of disability is (1) higher in females than in males and among ethnic minorities than in the Caucasian population; (2) inversely proportional to educational level; and (3) directly proportional to poverty (National Institute on Disability and Rehabilitation Research [NIDRR], 2005). The hindrances imposed by functional limitations, prolonged treatment, subsequent social stereotypes, and an uncertain future can have significant physical, emotional, vocational, social, and economic affects on the person and significant others (Eisenberg, Gleuckauf, & Zaretsky, 1993; Shapiro, 1994). In order to address the unique socio-environmental challenges of those with disabilities, it is necessary to comprehend the principal dimensions of a few selected conceptual models.

MEDICAL MODEL AND SOCIAL MODEL

The following table presents a comparative discussion of two philosophically opposing models of disability (Hahn, 1988; NIDRR, 1999; World Health Organization [WHO], 2002).

Medical Model	Social Model
1. Disability is a personal, biological, and physical problem, directly caused by trauma or other health condition. It is one of the oldest models linking western science to human body functions.	1. Disability is a socially created problem. It is a collection of interactive conditions, many of which are created by the social environment.
2. Disease, impairment, disabilities, handicaps, disadvantage for an individual, limits or prevents the fulfillment of a role for that individual.	2. Disability is not an attribute of an individual; rather it is a function of the external surroundings.
3. Disability requires medical care provided in the form of individual treatment by professionals. Therefore, the person, sum of his or her body parts, is an object of intervention.	3. The hindrances imposed by disability can be addressed by promoting full integration, equity, universal design, wellness, and health.

4. Management of disability is aimed at cure or elimination of disability or disease. In other words, it advocates for the individual's adjustment and behavior change.

4. Management of disability requires consumer-driven social action.

5. At the political level, the primary mode of response is the change of healthcare policy. Due to its person-centered, reductionist, and body-mind-environment separationist foci, the model is challenged by disability activists.

5. It is the collective responsibility of society to make the environmental modifications necessary to promote full participation in all areas of social life. Therefore, it is an attitudinal or ideological issue that requires social change. At the political level, it is a human rights issue.

The medical model promotes the elimination and prevention of disease and disability. For example, with reasonable effort, a condition like smallpox will be completely eradicated. It is just a matter of time. However, in parts of society where the nearest physician is 100 miles away, the next meal is several days away, and/or the effect of the color of the skin superimposes all other desirable human characteristics, the word disability can only mean invalidity and the need for charity. In communities where participation of all members is a dire necessity for survival, the medical model premised on the concept of "normal" people, but applying only to those with disabilities, can promote wholesale rejection of individuals with disabilities. Because a large proportion of the socially disadvantaged population (including non-mainstreamed Americans and minorities) lives in environments as described above, policy making and service delivery based on the medical model will only enhance dependence on public assistance and reduce the potential for successful community integration (WHO, 2002).

The social model, on the other hand, challenges the age-old concept of natural linear progression from normality through disease to disability and social exclusion. Since incarceration under despicable conditions, living in a segregated society, and destitution are not inevitable consequences of disease, there is a need to address contextual factors that affect the perception of disability. High prevalence of disability among those living in poverty and those experiencing lack of access to proper health care can be attributed to their exposure to new etiologies as a direct function of the high-risk life style and work environment. People of ethnically and linguistically diverse origins are more likely to live in poverty, be less educated, have lower access to medical care, experience malnutrition, give birth to babies with low birth weight, and be exposed to violence in their day-to-day lives. The differential distribution of disability according to age, gender, ethnicity, education, socioeconomic status, and geographic location warrants emphasis on dynamic interactions of the person and the environment. This shift in conceptualizing the phenomenon of disability encourages the development of innovative methods of helping people with various disabilities, including ethnic minorities, to achieve their fullest potential (NIDRR, 2005; WHO, 2002).

ENERGY MODEL

The concept of the energy model is that health and wellness are influenced by the body, mind, emotions, and the soul. This paradigm, generated by oriental philosophy and medicine some 500 years ago, re-establishes the innate connection between humanity and nature. Energy is omnipotent, omnipresent, omniscient, and the mother of all living and non-living beings. There exists a natural equilibrium among all types of matter that, in turn, produces peace, happiness, and health. Therefore, human health is linked to environmental health, which, in turn, is connected to the health of the universe. The concept of energy, the foundation for quantum physics, is the universal operating force. Humans owe most of their advancement to the discovery of energy in form of electricity. Therefore, the model focuses on the interdependence of all systems and all aspects of life (Trieschmann, 1995; Trieschmann, 2001).

The consequence of any change in the equilibrium of energy affects the entire system. Emotional disturbance, one of the principal causes of disharmony in human, often results in unnecessary drainage of energy that needs to be replenished. Continued emotional reactions to external events of day-to-day life, such as social stereotypes to disability, cause the body to remain out of balance for a prolonged period of time. This extended state of imbalance eventually leads to underlying and chronic physical disorders, e.g., pain, headache, cancer, ulcers, and cardiovascular diseases. It is essential, therefore, for people with disabilities to achieve energy balance by effectively managing emotional reactions to stressors and maintaining a healthy level of composure.

Medical diagnosis only considers the physiological cause of the disorder without looking at the patterns of human energy. One way to replenish the depleted supply of energy is to engage in meditation through tai chi, Shen Qi, and Yoga. Lifestyle and behavior change is often necessary to reduce emotional disturbance by avoiding stressful situations (Trieschmann, 1995; Trieschmann,

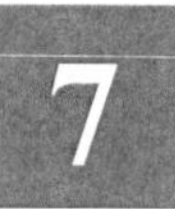

2001). Happiness, a precursor to psychological and physical well-being, can be achieved by finding an optimal functional environment and gaining control over one's mind (Csikszentmihalyi, 1993). As rehabilitation revolves around the concept of the whole person from womb to tomb, this relatively eastern paradigm provides the field with a credible theoretical and philosophical basis.

MULTICULTURALISM FROM AN AMERICAN PERSPECTIVE

The principal component of multiculturalism is diversity of opinion. It entails being uncritical, understanding, and respectful of values that are different from our own. If there is an opinion and an insight, it is worth being heard, not necessarily being agreed upon. Such consideration often helps dispel ignorance of other people and cultures, i.e., the causative agent of ethnocentrisms and racial intolerance. By choosing to remain ignorant, we fail to realize the innumerable similarities of human kind and the potential of our competitors who can become our future partners in the continued prosperity of planet earth. In this era of globalization of resources that causes millions of people to live and work in cultures different from their own, myopic knowledge of human capital will fast become counterproductive. In other words, the survival of the Western civilization will increasingly depend on a global understanding of that part of the world where a major segment of the population lives, i.e., the developing countries (Blum, 1991).

Development of multicultural sensitivity and competence is a means to increasing one's power, energy, and decision-making abilities by adjusting to the effects of different perceptions of the same situation. It is a person-specific process characterized by the following stages of gaining: (1) awareness of the common beliefs about the differences and similarities; (2) knowledge and insight of culturally learned assumptions; and (3) skills to effectively interact with people of different cultures (Pedersen, 1988). Among this diversity of values, cultures, morals, and lifestyles, the overarching question remains, what determines appropriateness or inappropriateness of a specific action?

Since multicultural awareness is a personal responsibility that is to be fulfilled in a social context, a comparative discussion of western and non-western perspectives is in order. Western belief is centered around mastery and control of nature, aggressive and highly competitive quest for individualism, a perfect body image, a time driven and action oriented lifestyle, and the concept of people being products of their environment. However, the concepts of time, social relationship, meaning of existence, and human worth vary widely between cultures and religions. The following table presents a brief, incomplete,

160

comparison of beliefs, traditions, and life styles of five different cultures (Blum, 1991; Sue & Sue, 1990).

African	American Indian	Asian	Hispanic	Islamic
1. A person is a function of the entire community.	1. A deep-seated respect for and commitment to the tribe.	1. Non-violence and pacifism is the way to end suffering and promote well-being.	1. Family traditions and family unity are important aspects of life.	1. Lifestyle must be congruent with the specificat-ions of the Koran.
2. Due to high poverty, economic needs are more important than civil rights.	2. Existence in harmony with nature and mother earth.	2. A philosophy of non-attachment and not non-commitment. Attachment gives rise to greed and conflict.	2. A strong belief that sacrifices in this world will promote salvation.	2. Religious rules are stricter for women than for men.
3. Importance is on non-verbal behavior.	3. The spirit is immortal and is a part of all humans, plants, and animals.	3. Silence, lack of eye contact, and restraint of feelings are signs of respect.	3. Present is more important than past and future.	
4. It is important to learn from history and tradition.	4. People have an innate ability to grow positively.	4. People are by nature good.	4. Humans must accommodate nature and not try to change it.	

Cultural differences encountered by a person with or without a disability are functions of one's country of origin, unique social background, and experiences with inequality.

There are three components geared to minimize the affects of perceived diversity among people. First, anti-racism promotes the belief that all humans are

161

equal. One aspect of anti-racism is learning to perceive intended or unintended patterns of racism, and when it is occurring. Second, multiculturalism entails becoming aware of one's own cultural identity, respecting and learning about other cultures, and valuing the richness and worth of diverse religious or cultural groups. Third, sense of community embraces both ethnic and cultural differences (Blum, 1991). As of 2002, about 11.5% of the American population was foreign-born, 17% is ethnic minority, and the prevalence of disability is quite high in this population (Stone, 2005). Coming to terms with the myriad of differences in the American pluralistic community is the only way to promote a sense of belongingness and shared humanity among its stakeholders (Bellah, 1985). The field of rehabilitation is no exception.

EFFECTS OF SOCIAL MOVEMENT

Rights are the basic tenets of moral and social ethics. Existence of rights, both human and civil, enables a person to engage in behaviors or make claims against another individual, or society as a whole. Rights are anti-majoritarian in nature and de-emphasize the salience of collective good. People have human rights solely because they are human. The major components of human rights are thought to be globally applicable. Civil rights encompass the basic rights of a person as a member of society, e.g., rights to vote, assemble, and speak. The United Nations' Universal Declaration of Human Rights was unanimously accepted in 1948 as a proof of its worldwide applicability. However, more than five decades after its ratification, the question of its universality, or lack thereof, still looms large over humanity (May, Collins-Chobanina, & Wong, 1998).

In spite of the existence of this U.N. Declaration and the Constitution of the U.S., structured inequality on the bases of ethnicity, gender, health status, and socio-economic level continues to prevail in all spheres of American society. Assimilation theory, the most common mode of studying social relations, attributes the perceived deficiencies of immigrants of color to their biological and cultural identity. As a result, victim blaming became the principal criterion in explaining racial discrimination. One reason for such an erroneous finding was the focus of assimilation studies on European immigrants rather than American Indians and Hispanics who have settled in the American mainland long before the arrival of the Mayflower (Aguirre & Baker, 2000). The investigation of the historical roots of institutional racism has repeatedly established inappropriateness of subjugation of a particular group of people in the U.S. The inequitable treatment and segregation of African Americans, Asians, American Indians, Hispanics, women, and people with disabilities prompt many to enquire, are human rights universal in scope or do they vary according to gender or ethnicity (May, Collins-Chobanina, & Wong, 1998)?

CIVIL RIGHTS OF AFRICAN AMERICANS AND WOMEN

Public awareness of and interest in ethnic populations began to escalate in the 1950s and gained momentum in the 1960s. The movement that was initiated in Montgomery, Alabama by the bus boycott in 1955 culminated in the Civil Rights Act of 1964. The African American "Black" power movement acted as a catalyst to generate sensitivity towards the unique needs of people who were disadvantaged, powerless, and disenfranchised, including racial minorities, women, people with disabilities, the elderly, gays, and lesbians. Due to heavy immigration, high birth rate among immigrants, and changing ethnographic composition of the country, an increasing need to respect the human rights of the people of diverse cultural origins was felt. The American public was forced to recognize the inequities of the "separate but equal" policies (Faragher, Buhle, Czitrom, & Armitage, 2003). This realization prompted the advent of international activism geared to liberate another segment of the "oppressed class," the women.

"Gender is what culture makes out of the raw material of biological sex" (Unger & Crawford, 1996, p. 18). Since it is impossible for men and women to function in an environment with no expectation for gender-related behavior, a system of power relations between the two genders is the center of all human interactions. As a direct consequence of the largely male driven social norms and expectations, the status of women is often relegated to that of minorities. Discriminations encountered by women and people of ethnic origin, therefore, show striking similarities (Enns, 2000).

Although non-African American women did not experience slavery like the African Americans, women in general did not have the right to vote until the 20th century and lacked many of the legal protections enjoyed by Caucasian men. Therefore, strategies enacted to reduce the inequality between the mainstream and minority populations were also applicable to women (Hinman, 2000). In the 1970s, the change in the social status of minorities evoked a strong belief in the government's power to initiate legal actions for addressing social inadequacies. Several pieces of legislation were passed to dismantle workforce barriers for women. The women's liberation movement acted as a catalyst to the implementation of affirmative action programs, state equal opportunity laws, and the establishment of women's studies programs and research centers (Bunch, 1998).

RIGHTS OF PERSONS WITH DISABILITIES

People with disabilities are the largest group of minorities in the U.S. The attitudes of the mainstream population toward minorities often predict their impressions of people with disabilities. Although historically these two groups have shared common problems, there are a few significant differences between minorities and people with disabilities. First, there is a lack of group endorsement of behavior typical to a particular disability. Since there is no fixed social norm indicative of the type of disability, most people with disabilities are expected to imitate a "normal" state as closely as possible. There is some resistance from both people with and without disability to behaviors that unnecessarily draw attention to the disability. Contrary to this largely American mainstreamed expectation, certain ethnic groups, such as American Indians, take pride in their unique characteristics (Wright, 1980).

Second, the difference of a person with a disability is not usually shared by other members of his/her family. Racial characteristics are genetic and, therefore, inherited by virtue of being born in that family. On the contrary, a person with a disability may often be the only member of a family to have the specific condition. As a result, children are often unaware of the existence of others with a similar condition and do not affiliate with any particular minority group. The psychological make-up of minorities is quite different from those with disabilities. In spite of the above dissimilarities, any changes in the social and economic condition of groups disadvantaged by virtue of race, religion, gender, and ethnicity were generally accompanied by parallel transformation in the status of people with disabilities (Wright, 1980). For example, the civil rights movement in the early 1960s was followed by the independent living movement in the mid 1960s and incorporation of Sections 501-504 of the Rehabilitation Act in 1973.

CONTEXTUAL AND MULTICULTURAL ISSUES IN ACCEPTANCE OF LOSS

The existence of disability often causes a person to feel devalued, incomplete, and almost ashamed of one-self. The onset of a sudden traumatic event or insidious condition produces an emergency for the person and the family. The following section presents a brief account of how disability is treated in different cultures. In the Hindu culture, the existence of a disability is believed to be the cause of wrong doing in a previous life. As a result, there is little sympathy for those with disabilities. The attribution of the responsibility for disability is an important factor in determining people's attitude (Hanks & Hanks, 1948). In Nordic mythology, Gods have disabilities. Some believe that suffering is a test for high-level future pursuits. Suffering provides deep insight into life and is a means of self-sacrifice to achieve higher purposes (Wright, 1983). It is a fact that the prevalence of disability is high among the elderly. However, with age comes wisdom. American Indians, therefore, revere the elderly as the most knowledgeable and often having a connection between life and the afterlife (Marshall, 2001).

The drastic change in body image, functional capabilities, social role, and individual autonomy produced by disability often trigger a sense of tremendous loss and self-pity. The person and the family feel the absence of something valuable and experience a sense of misfortune. In an effort to keep the issue of disability from becoming a social reality, the person tries to conceal the effects of disability as much as possible. If concealment is not possible, the person makes himself or herself believe that the effects of the disability are not significantly limiting, i.e., as if nothing has happened. This "as if" behavior, feeling of inferiority, and effort to "idolize the normal standards," confirm one's belief that disability is, in fact, a punishment. These reactions to disability are often the first steps toward the striving to comprehend the importance of accepting one's disability and adjusting to a new body image. Ethnic minority groups that are often devalued by the American mainstream experience a heightened sense of loss and anger following the onset of a functional limitation. As disability is an inextricable part of one's identity, denial of its existence may only mean that there is a need to restructure the basis of a person's entire value system (Livneh & Antonak, 1997; Wright, 1983).

The issues of acceptance and denial of disability are considered two mutually exclusive responses to a chronic condition resulting in functional limitations. Denial, characterized by a failure to accept one's disability, is often a precursor to poor psychosocial adjustment (Stewart, 1999) and compromised mental health status (Matthews & Harrington, 2000). Although the above perspective is quite prevalent, but not universal, it is important to briefly discuss the various stages of adjustment to a disability. The following paragraphs will provide a brief summary of the theories of adjustment to disability in general, and modes of facilitating community integration of people with disabilities.

STAGES OF ADJUSTMENT AND ADAPTATION TO CHRONIC ILLNESS AND DISABILITY

Humans have a powerful need to feel connected through meaningful, regular, and positive interactions. According to Daneshpaur (1998), Neumark-Sztainer, Story, French, and Resnick (1997), Newcomb (1990), and Rosen (1999), the concept of connectedness includes a self-in-relation-to-others component. Some refer to the connectedness as relationships with other individuals and systems. In other words, it is an enduring experience of self in relation to the world. When this fundamental human need is not addressed, a person may experience negative impact on health, adjustment, and well-being. Psychological distress, social isolation, and dearth of purpose in life are other significant consequences of lack of connectedness with others for an extended period of time (Townsend & McWhieter, 2005). The impact of connectedness to self, others, and a purpose of life can be significant in the life of a person with a disability. In this regard, a brief discussion of cultural differences in connectedness is in order.

As per Tamura and Lau (1999), many cultures demonstrate significantly more preference for greater connectedness. The perception and practice of individualism and collectivism vary as a function of culture. For example, Rude and Burham (1995) state that many non-western, minority, and non-European American societies are more community-oriented and are thought to be more connected as individuals and group members than the U.S. mainstream. According to Wong (1997), a strong feeling of connectedness to one's ethnic group is often related to educational expectations, resiliency, and perceived positive peer characteristics. It is apparent that social and cultural connectedness is an important determinant of psychosocial adjustment for people with and without disabilities (Townsend, 2003). The various stages of adaptation to disability, therefore, must be considered in light of the above-mentioned concept.

Adaptation to any form of life altering loss such as injury, illness, disability, and death, is often characterized by the phases of shock, realization, denial, depression, anger, hostility, acknowledgment, and adjustment. These stages are not sequential and can be revisited several times in no particular order on the way to adjustment to a disability (Antonak & Livenh, 1995; Bray, 1978; Russell, 1981; Shontz, 1965).

Shock is the initial phase of heightened emotional reaction to the onset of a disability or diagnosis of a life-threatening condition. It may be characterized by overwhelming depersonalization, a sense of loss, and psychological numbness. Realization of the magnitude of the disability often produces anxiety, panic, confusion in thinking, fear of death, uncertainty about the future, and purposeless over-activity. Denial or defensive retreat is a significant but problematic form of coping strategy against painful realization of the long-term effects of a disability or a disease. A person in denial often experiences wishful and unrealistic expectation of recovery, i.e., I am going to recover fully and walk out of this hospital. Depression may accompany an initial accurate understanding of the nature of the disability or loss. This is especially noted among persons experiencing a sudden onset of disease or disability. It is a natural grief reaction to loss associated with feelings of distress, helplessness, and hopelessness.

Anger, characterized by feelings of guilt, may be perpetrated by self-directed resentment and self-blame. Mostly reported by people with adventitious chronic disability, anger often results in self-destructive behaviors and suicidal ideation. Hostility, often directed toward other people and the environment believed to be responsible for the condition, is an effort to retaliate against functional limitations. Obstruction of treatment, verbal aggressiveness and criticism, and feelings of antagonism are some of the external manifestations of this phase. Acknowledgment and adjustment is the final phase of adaptation. This acceptance phase is characterized by an individual's emotional readiness to be realistic about the functional limitations, to realize one's self-worth as a person with a disability, and to start making use of his or her newly discovered potentials for a productive life. The order, duration, and repetition of these stages largely depend on an individual's feeling of physical and psychological well-being in connection to self and the environment.

DISABILITY IN THE CONTEXT OF MASLOW'S HIERARCHY OF NEEDS

In western society, it is traditionally believed that a person's self-worth and self-esteem can be developed from a sense of personal achievement. In other words, a good way to enhance one's self-esteem is to offer plenty of opportunities to experience success. At par with this belief, standards of performance are often changed to allow completion of a task (with or without accommodation) by persons with disabilities, and thereby foster trust in their abilities. Contrary to the general anticipation, such practices not only diminish society's expectation of persons with disabilities but also help them learn that their worth as individuals is contingent upon being able to fit into the prescribed norms (Villa, Thousand, Stainback, & Stainback, 1992). Therefore, it is essential for people in general to be able to live and be accepted in the context of a community.

Maslow (1968 and 1970) expounds on the importance of satisfying personal needs for physiological (food, water, shelter, and warmth), safety (security, freedom from fear, and stability), and love (friendship, family, and belongingness) before attempting to self-actualize. For the first time, the need for community as a function of connectedness, relatedness, and interdependence is emphasized as a pre-requisite for self-sufficiency. It professes that the need for self-actualization implies that a person has the required abilities to become proficient to a certain level. However, according to Villa, Thousand, Stainback, and Stainback (1992), society has a unique way of identifying the "gifted" and the "mediocre," and providing the "gifted" with the opportunity to develop the areas in which they naturally excel. People with disabilities, with their apparent or unapparent limitations, often do not appear to possess the need to self-actualize as per society's pre-existing standards. In addition, people with disabilities from non-mainstreamed ethnic backgrounds experience further lack of social expectation and support as a direct consequence of their cultural affiliation and value differences with the mainstream. This conflict between American core values and the reality of life for citizens across the nation continues to undermine the potential of minorities with disabilities.

As the central tenet of the western society, uniformity becomes the criterion for belongingness and diversity the criterion for exclusion. The general consensus is one must earn the right to belong through physical (appearance), academic, professional, and social achievements. This leaves people with disabilities with two options, both with significant negative effects for the target population. First, they can decide that the standards are too difficult for them to accomplish, and resign themselves to feelings of inadequacy. Second, exert considerable effort, at the cost of one's overall quality of life, to gain acceptance through achievement (Villa, Thousand, Stainback, & Stainback, 1992). It is imperative, therefore, that inclusion and belongingness be adopted by the stakeholders in rehabilitation as cornerstones for facilitating a person's adjustment to and minimizing the effects of a disability.

VALUE CHANGES IN ACCEPTANCE OF DISABILITY

According to Dembo, Leviton, and Wright (1956) and Wright (1980), adjustment to and acceptance of disability are characterized by changes in the value system that helps one perceive the loss as non-devaluating. The following are the components of value change.

First, enlargement of the scope of value. During the period of adjustment, a person is overwhelmed by the need to address the physical and psychological effects of disability. As a part of the shock reaction, disability becomes the center of one's entire existence. At this time, the person must learn to genuinely appreciate other existing values in addition to the one(s) lost. This renews interest in satisfactions that are accessible and assists in acceptance of the loss.

Second, subordination of the importance of physique relative to other aspects of the person. Although a person is convinced that life is worth living, he or she may still harbor deep-rooted feelings about perceived consequences of the loss. This may either be attributed to overemphasis on physical normalcy or to insufficient weight placed on other values. In other words, the potency of physique far out weighs the satisfactions derived from the accessible values in life. The value of outward appearance is directly proportional to the effect of physique as a prime mover.

Third, containment of the effects of disability so as not to overshadow other aspects of a person. Spread often results in false perceptions about the effects of disability in many facets of life. Since all aspects of life are not affected by disability and people's perceptions of its effects are largely misconstrued, it is necessary to conceptualize disability as a possession, and not as a personal characteristic. Separation of disability from the holistic person reduces its devaluing effects. For example, if physical abilities were viewed as tools used to perform actions, one could substitute for an impaired tool, i.e., doing it another way. Crutches, wheelchairs, leg braces may be considered substitutes for walking.

Fourth, transformation of comparative-status values to asset values. The characteristics of a person, such as the person's looks, may carry status implications for persons who are evaluating themselves. Status judgments are often made by comparing a person against a standard of presumed average. The concept of physique as an asset value promotes the importance of the residual capabilities rather than the functional limitations.

ROLE OF SPIRITUALITY IN ADAPTATION TO DISABILITY

Disability poses several challenges to the achievement of goals and desires. A logical consequence of such hindrance and frustration is anger. Anger is a part and parcel of the (1) overwhelming grief cycle, (2) social stigma and stereotypes, (3) experiences of pain and vulnerability, (4) loss of control, autonomy, equality, and power, (5) lack of self-confidence resulting from the knowledge of functional limitations, and (6) reduced self-worth and image that often follow the advent of a disabling condition. Anger is an attempt to retrieve choice, respect, freedom, and self-importance (Thompson, 1985). Expression of anger is considered an important step toward spiritual and psychological growth and subsequent adjustment to a disabling condition.

Anger, the inner energy, and one of the significant facts of life, can promote justice, enhance health, and facilitate positive lifestyle changes. When repressed or denied, anger can only cause ill health, self-destructive behaviors, hopelessness, and generalized devastation in life. Failure to express anger often causes depression, guilt, self-blaming attitudes, withdrawal from outside contacts, and prolonged frustration. In addition, suffering is caused by fatigue as a result of (1) living with a disability, (2) needing to struggle for one's rights and equal opportunity, (3) educating people in one's surrounding, and (4) always being under the effects of the disability (Campbell, 1986; McClosky, 1986). The most common form of coping response is to be angry with God, and to try to find meaning in the problem of suffering. One way of addressing this issue is to fearlessly challenge God with the question of why. In order to heal, the pain of suffering must be honestly presented before God. Repressing this anger will only cause one's relationship with God to weaken. Confronting God and forming a dialectic relationship with him or her will re-establish one's faith in God. One can both confront and obey God. "Both are spiritual acts; discovering when each is appropriate in the life of faith requires discernment" (McCarthy, 1995, p. 104).

From time immemorial, humans were at the mercy of Mother Nature. Religion was often considered a foundation of life and a spiritual consciousness of God. Even currently, the sense of God's presence often contributes to one's sense of security, and hope or optimism. As per Dr. Paul Pedersen, issues of spirituality and culture always go together. As most religious behaviors and spiritual states are culturally learned, it is important to understand them in terms of where the behavior was learned and displayed (Cartwright & D'Andrea, 2005). It is important to fully understand the individualized perception of God in the process of rehabilitation.

Both spirituality and rehabilitation are journeys of discovery, i.e. paths to experiencing the readiness for a new awareness, defining the self, and settings goals for the future (Nosek, 1995). When operationalized, the above concepts strive to invigorate the person as a whole. There exists a direct link between holistic thinking and medical concerns. The words holy and holistic have originated from the Greek word "holos" meaning whole. Holos, on the other hand, is closely related to the Greek words for heal and health. Religion has traditionally played a significant role in treating medical conditions and addressing health care issues (McCarthy, 1995). Indigenous healers and local religious leaders, such as gurus in Indian culture and medicine men in African countries, continue to be the main source of health care for millions who value the importance of being one with nature, and the role of a formless higher power in their lives. The World Health Organization recognizes indigenous healing or traditional medicine as the "knowledge and practices, whether explicable or not, used in diagnosis, prevention and elimination of physical, mental or social disequilibrium and relying exclusively on practical experience and observation handed down from generation to generation, verbally or in writing" (WHO, 1978, p. 3). On a futuristic note, it can be stated that psychoneuro-immunologists have empirically established the influences of metaphysical practices and inner energy on a number of physical phenomena such as mental states and functions of the immune system (McCarthy, 1995). It is imperative, therefore, that the immense power of this natural human energy be utilized to promote acceptance of disability and loss.

CONCLUSION

The dynamic process of adaptation is characterized by a series of highly individualized steps determined by the interaction of (1) psychodynamic and disability-triggered phases of adaptation, i.e., short- or long-term psychosocial reactions to disability, and (2) a group of intrapersonal (biopsychological), interpersonal (sociocultural), and extrapersonal (environmental) factors, i.e., contextual issues (Livneh, 2001). Although several theories have been proposed, adjustment to disability should essentially be viewed as an evolutionary, changing, highly individualized, and temporarily ordered hierarchical process. The sequential nature of the process is dependent on factors such as the type of disability, nature of onset, pre-disability personality, cultural identity, social environment, and perception of the residual functional abilities. In other words, the process is characterized by (1) learning the techniques to live with a disability, (2) making the most of one's residual abilities, and (3) striving to have a productive and satisfying life (Antonak & Livneh, 1991; Carpenter & Strauss, 1977; Sue & Sue, 1990; Trieschmann, 1988).

The literal meaning of rehabilitation is return to something. This something holds different meaning for different people and changes its meaning with transforming life situations. For those with congenital disability, rehabilitation is a misnomer because they have not known any other way of living. Instead of returning, they should grow and enhance their capabilities in the dimensions accessible to them. Adaptation to a disability or a chronic condition is a life-long process of successfully coping with the loss of health, transformed social standing, environmental restrictions, and reduced vocational roles (Livneh, 2001; Nosek, 1995). Rehabilitation is the process of defining or re-defining oneself and reveling in the fact that one's spiritual essence is eternal and unchanging.

REFERENCES

Aguirre, Jr., A. & Baker, D. V. (2000). *Structured inequality in the United States - Discussions on the continuing significance of race, ethnicity, and gender.* Upper Saddle River, NJ: Prentice Hall.

Antonak, R. F., & Livneh, H. (1991). A hierarchy of reactions to disability. *International Journal of Rehabilitation Research, 14*, 13-24.

Antonak, R. F., & Livneh, H. (1995). Adaptation to disability and its investigation among persons with multiple sclerosis. *Social Sciences and Medicine, 40*, 1099-1108.

Bellah, R. N. (1985). *Habits of the heart: Individualism and commitment in American life.* Berkeley, CA: University of California Press.

Blum, L. A. (1991). *Antiracism, multiculturalisn, and interracial community: Three educational values for a multicultural society.* Boston: University of Massachusetts.

Bray, G. P. (1978). Rehabilitation of spinal cord injured: A family approach. *Journal of Applied Rehabilitation Counseling, 9,* 70-78.

Bunch, C. (1998). Women's rights as human rights: Toward a re-vision of human rights. In L. May, S. Collins-Chobanina, and K. Wong, K. (Eds.). *Applied ethics – A multicultural approach* (pp. 61-71). Upper Saddle River, NJ: Prentice Hall.

Campbell, A. V. (1986). *The gospel of anger.* London: SPCK.

Carpenter, W. T., & Strauss, J. S. (1977). Methodological issues in the study of outcome. In J.S. Strauss, H. M. Babigian, & M. Roff (Eds.). *The origin and course of psychopathology* (pp. 345-367). New York: Plenum Press.

Cartwright, B. Y., & D'Andrea, M. (2005). A personal journey toward culture-centered counseling: An interview with Paul Pedersen. *Journal of Counseling and Development, 83*(2), 214-221.

Csikszentmihalyi, M. (1993). *The evolving self: A psychology for the third millennium.* New York: Harper perennial.

Daneshpaur, M. (1998). Muslim families and family therapy. *Journal of Marriage and Family Counseling, 24,* 355-368.

Dembo, T., Leviton, G. L., & Wright, B. A. (1956). Adjustment to misfortune: A problem of social-psychological rehabilitation. *Artificial Limbs, 3*(2), 4-62.

Eisenberg, M. G., Gleuckauf, R. L., & Zaretsky, H. H. (Eds.). (1993). *Medical aspects of disability: A handbook for rehabilitation professional.* New York: Springer.

Enns, C. Z. (2000). Gender issues in counseling. In S. D. Brown & R. W. Lent (Eds.). *Handbook of counseling psychology* (3rd ed.) (pp. 601-638). New York: John Wiley & sons.

Faragher, J. M., Buhle, M. J., Czitrom, D., & Armitage, S. H. (2003). *Out of many: A history of American people* (3rd ed.). Upper Saddle River, Prentice Hall.

Hahn, H. (1988). The politics of physical differences: Disability and discrimination. *Journal of Social Issues, 44*(1), 39-48.

Hanks, J. R., & Hanks, L. M., Jr. (1948). The physically handicapped in certain non-occidental societies. *Journal of Social issues, 4*(4), 11-20.

Hinman, L. M. (2000). *Contemporary moral issues: Diversity and consensus* (2nd ed.). Saddle River, NJ: Prentice Hall.

Livneh, H., & Antonak, R. (1997). *Psychosocial adaptation to chronic illness and disability.* Frederick, MD: Aspen.

Livneh, H. (2001). Psychosocial adaptation to chronic illness and disability: A conceptual framework. *Rehabilitation Counseling Bulletin, 44*(3), 151-160.

Marinelli, R. P., & Dell Orto, A. E. (1999). *The psychological and social impact of disability* (4th ed.). New York: Springer Publishing Company.

Marshall, C. (Ed.). (2001). *Rehabilitation and American Indians with disabilities: A handbook for administrators, practitioners, and researchers.*

Maslow, A. H. (1968). *Toward a psychology of being* (2nd ed.). New York: D. Van Nostrand Company.

Maslow. A. H. (1970). *Motivation and personality.* New York: Harper & Row.

Matthews, C. K., & Harrington, N. G. (2000). Invisible disability. In D. O. Braithwaite, T. L. Thompson, et al. (eds). *Handbook of communication and people with disabilities: Research and application* (pp. 405-421). Mahwah, NJ: Lawrence Erlbaum.

May, L., Collins-Chobanina, S., & Wong, K. (1998). *Applied ethics - A multicultural approach* (2nd ed.). Upper Saddle River, NJ: Prentice Hall.

McCarthy, H. (1995). Integrating spirituality into rehabilitation in a technocratic society. *Rehabilitation Education, 9*(2&3), 87-96.

McClosky, P. (1986). *When you are angry with God.* New York: Paulist Press.

National Institute on Disability and Rehabilitation Research. (2005). *Long-range plan: 2005-2009.* Washington, D.C.: Author.

Neumark-Sztainer, D., Story, M., French, S. A., & Resnick, M. D. (1997). Psychosocial correlates of health compromising behavior among adolescents. *Health Education Research, 12,* 37-52.

Newcomb, M. D. (1990). Social support by many other names: Toward a unified conceptualization. *Journal of Social and Personal Relationships, 7,* 479-494.

Nosek, M, (1995). The defining light of Vedanta: Personal reflections on spirituality and disability. *Rehabilitation Education, 9*(2&3), 171-182.

Pedersen, P. (1988). *A handbook for developing multicultural awareness.* Alexandria, VA: American Association for Counseling and Development.

Rosen, W. B. (1999). Moments of truth: Notes from a lesbian therapist. *Smith College Students in social Work, 69,* 293-308.

Rude, S. S., & Burham, B. L. (1995). Connectedness and neediness: Factors of DEQ and SAS dependency scales. *Cognitive Therapy and Research, 19,* 323-340.

Russell, R. A. (1981). Concepts of adjustment to disability: An overview. *Rehabilitation Literature, 42,* 330-338.

Shapiro, J. P. (1994). *People with disabilities forging a new civil rights movement - No pity.* New York: Times books.

Shontz, F. C. (1965). Reactions to crisis. *Volta Review, 67,* 364-370.

Stewart, J. R. (1999). Applying Beck's cognitive therapy to Livneh's model of adaptation. In R. P. Marinelli and A. E. DellOrto (Eds.). *Psychological and social impact of disability* (pp. 303-315), New York: Springer.

Stone, J. H. (2005). (Ed.) *Culture and disability*. Thousand Oaks, CA: Sage Publications, Inc.

Sue, D. W., & Sue, D. (1990). *Counseling the culturally different: Theory and practice* (2nd ed.). New York: John Wiley & Sons.

Tamura, T., & Lau, A. (1999). Connectedness versus separateness: Applicability of family therapy to Japanese families. In K. S. Ng (Ed.), *Counseling Asian families from a systems perspective. The family psychology and counseling series* (pp. 95-125). Alexandria, VA: American Counseling Association.

Thompson, R. D. (1985). *Anger: The misunderstood emotion*. New York: Simon and Schuster.

Townsend, K. C. (2003). Late adolescent psychological adjustment: Roles of individuation, sex, social connectedness, and ambivalence over emotional expression (Doctoral dissertation, University of Oregon, 2003). *Dissertation Abstracts International, 64*, 4115.

Townsend, K. C., & McWhieter, B. T. (2005). Connectedness: A review of the literature with implications for counseling, assessment, and research. *Journal of Counseling and Development, 83*(2), 191-201.

Trieschmann, R. B. (Ed.). (1988). *Spinal cord injuries: Psychological, social, and vocational rehabilitation* (2nd ed.). New York: Demos.

Trieschmann, R. B. (1995). The energy model: A new approach to rehabilitation. *Rehabilitation Education, 9*(2&3), 217-228.

Trieschmann, R. B. (2001). Spirituality and Energy Medicine. *The Journal of Rehabilitation, 67*(1), 26-32.

Unger, R., & Crawford, M. (1996). *Women and gender: A feminist psychology* (2nd ed.). New York: McGraw-Hill.

Villa, R., Thousand, J., Stainback, W. & Stainback, S. (1992). *Restructuring for caring and effective education: An administrative guide to creating homogeneous schools*. Baltimore, MD: Paul H. Brooks.

Wong, C. A. (1997). The risks and protective factors of the content of racial stigma on African-American and early adolescents' development (Doctoral dissertation, University of Michigan, 1997). *Dissertation Abstracts International, 58*, 5675.

World Health Organization. (1978). *The promotion and development of traditional medicine*. Technical reports services, 666. Geneva, Switzerland: Author.

World Health Organization. (2002). *International classification of functioning, disability and health*. Geneva, Switzerland: Author.

Wright, G. N. (1980). *Total rehabilitation*. Boston: Little Brown and Company.

Wright, B. A. (1983). *Physical disability - A psychosocial approach* (2nd ed.). New York:

CHAPTER 8

Addressing the Independent Living Needs of Ethnic/Racial Minority Groups

Joan Looby

Chapter Highlights

➡ Perceptions of people with disabilities

➡ The historical roots of the independent living movement

➡ Independent living and significant social movements of the 1960's and 1970's

➡ Ethnic/racial minority group and independent living

➡ Issues impacting ethnic/racial minority group participation in independent living

➡ Incorporating ethnic/racial minority groups into independent living

➡ Conclusion

8

$\mathcal{T}$he independent living movement originated in the late 1960's and is often described as a social or civil rights movement involving persons with disabilities, who not only demanded their rights to inclusion in mainstream United States (U.S.) culture and more humane service delivery, but also control for determining the services they require (DeJong, 1979; Mackleprang & Salsgiver, 1999; Shreve, 1982; Wilson, 1998). Title VII of the Rehabilitation Act Amendments of 1978 authorized the addition of, and funding for, independent living rehabilitation programs. This funding was made available through the federal-state rehabilitation programs (Rubin & Roessler, 2001). The independent living movement has had tremendous impact on redefining traditional notions of disability (the sick/impaired role) and has influenced the development of new service paradigms among disability professionals, researchers, and policy makers. However, more than a quarter century after the Berkeley model had been established by Ed Roberts, independent living services still continue to elude many persons with disabilities and, in particular, persons from ethnic/racial minority groups.

This chapter focuses on independent living. It begins with a brief review of societal perceptions of individuals with disabilities, and legislation that helped to remove critical barriers to their successful integration into mainstream U.S. culture. A historical overview of the independent living movement, the other movements with which it dovetailed, and the legal mandates that gave rise to its inception, are presented. Ethnic/racial minority group participation is discussed, specifically in the context of the four largest minority groups in the United States (Hispanics, African Americans, Asians, and Native Americans). Following this is a comprehensive discussion of issues impacting ethnic/racial minority group participation in independent living. The chapter concludes with suggestions for how independent living can better incorporate racial/ethnic minority groups into its paradigm of services.

PERCEPTIONS OF PEOPLE WITH DISABILITIES

Society has always viewed persons with disabilities as anomalies of nature, evil, God's punishment for a sin, or incapable of making any significant contribution to mankind (Olkin, 1999; Pren, 1976; Rubin & Roessler, 2001; Smart, 2001; Stein, 1979). Such negative perceptions are steeped in history. The Nomads considered people with disabilities useless; the Greeks and Romans specialized in infanticide, murder, and exposure to the elements for children who were disabled. Early Christians pitied people with disabilities and sought to exorcize their conditions through intense ritual and prayer. During the

Middle Ages, persons with disabilities were considered evil and often tortured and persecuted. While people with disabilities were institutionalized during the Renaissance, they were subject to horrific treatment and living conditions (Garrett, 1969; Mackelprang & Salsgiver, 1999; Preen, 1976; Rubin & Roessler, 2001; Shapiro, 1993; Shreve, 1982).

In America, colonists enacted laws restricting people with disabilities from entering the country. Those born with or who acquired disabilities were sent "away" for treatment, education, or to live elsewhere. For the mentally ill, if one's family was rich, the person was kept at home, but locked in dungeons, cells, attics, and other places, to be kept away from society and others. Those of more tenuous financial circumstances were subjected to inhumane treatment such as whippings, hangings, incarceration, and other cruel, harsh punishment (Deutsch, 1949, as cited in Rubin & Roessler, 2001; Shreve, 1982).

Near the end of the Nineteenth century, the eugenic movement led to the passage of laws prohibiting persons with disabilities from immigrating to the U.S., marrying, or having children. Eugenics also promoted forced sterilization of people with disabilities, a practice that continued well into the Twentieth century. The rise of the Social Gospel Movement and the American Charity Movement in the 19th century advocated compassion and assistance to persons with disabilities; however, the moral superiority of the helpers, and the moral inferiority of people with disabilities were always underscored (Conyers, 2002; Harber, 1963; Judge, 1976; Pfeiffer, 1994; Rubin & Roessler, 2001; Smart, 2001).

Landmark political, social, and legislative initiatives since the early 1990's, culminating in The Rehabilitation Act of 1973 and its subsequent amendments, and the Americans with Disabilities Act of 1990, have given a voice to persons with disabilities, have helped to remove some critical environmental barriers to their success, and have emphasized their right to self-determination, independence, and choice (Conyers, 2002; Mackelprang & Salsgiver, 1999; Olkin, 1999; Rubin & Roessler, 2001). As significant as these developments have been, in the 21st century, attitudinal barriers still exclude people with disabilities from equal opportunity and access to society's mainstream.

The independent living movement represented a breaking away from the shackles of confinement imposed by the traditional rehabilitation paradigm, to the participation of persons with disabilities in all decisions impacting their lives. However, there has been and continue to be tensions between both philosophies. Mainstream U.S. culture still limits the rights of persons with disabilities, controls their choices, enables their dependency, and continues to embrace the medical model of service delivery as the only model of rehabilitation (Conyers, 2002; Rubin & Roessler, 2001).

THE HISTORICAL ROOTS OF THE INDEPENDENT LIVING MOVEMENT

The independent living movement did not suddenly rise out of the ashes like a Phoenix. It was influenced heavily by the turbulent, socio-cultural milieu of the 1960s and 70s (DeJong, 1979; Flowers, Edwards, & Pusch, 1996; Mackelprang & Salsgiver, 1999; McDonald & Oxford, 2003; Shreve, 1982).

This was the era of the Vietnam War, where anti-war protests, demonstrations, and marches, particularly by university students, occurred almost daily. This was the time of the Hippie generation who rejected traditional values and advocated sexual freedom, drugs, and rock and roll. This was the time of Black militancy, challenging society and advocating equality. This was the time of the passage of The Civil Rights Act in 1964. This was also the time of the rise of the Women's Movement. This was the time of the founding of Disabled in Action by Judith Heumann in 1970, and the Physically Disabled Students Program at the University of California Berkeley in 1970, by Ed Roberts and others. The message reinforced by all these events was that turmoil and challenge would produce change (DeJong, 1979).

Frustrated by their second class citizenry, poor service delivery, and lack of opportunity for self-determination, and encouraged by the successes of the civil rights and other movements, persons with disabilities joined together to demand their full participation in the mainstream 70s (Conyers, 2002;DeJong, 1979; Mackelprang & Salsgiver, 1999; McDonald & Oxford, 2003; Shapiro, 1993; Shreve, 1982). They too felt that they were being denied access to similar services accorded to persons without disabilities. It was in this context that the independent living movement was born. The movement blossomed at a time when several other complementary movements developed, such as the civil rights movement, consumerism, self-help, demedicalization, and deinstitutionalization (DeJong, 1979; Flowers, Edwards, & Pusch 1996; McDonald & Oxford, 2003; Shapiro, 1993; Shreve, 1982).

INDEPENDENT LIVING AND SIGNIFICANT SOCIAL MOVEMENTS OF THE 1960'S AND 1970'S

THE CIVIL RIGHTS MOVEMENT

The Civil Rights Act of 1964 did not include people with disabilities as a
protected class, but made vulnerable groups such as persons with disabilities
cognizant of their rights to equal societal participation (DeJong, 1979;
McDonald & Oxford, 2003; Shreve, 1982). The civil rights movement stressed
entitlement (vote, trial by a jury of peers, hold political office) and benefits
rights (Medicare, attendant care, income assistance), as well as alternative
techniques of social protest (DeJong, 1979). The independent living
movement's battle for entitlement is manifested in Section 504 of the
Rehabilitation Act of 1973 that prohibits various forms of discrimination, and
in the provisions of the Americans with Disabilities Act of 1990 (Mackelprang
& Salsgiver, 1999; Rubin & Roessler, 2001). The movement's fight for benefits
is reflected in the Social Security Disability Amendments of 1980, and
subsequent revisions in 1986, 1987, and 1990 (Mackelprang & Salsgiver, 1999;
Rubin & Roessler, 2001). Demonstrations and sit-ins, practices inherent in the
civil rights movement, were used effectively by members of the independent
living movement to secure their rights (DeJong, 1979).

One of the tenets of the civil rights movement is that racism and prejudice
are endemic to American society. Although legislation eliminated many
barriers to the equal participation of African Americans in mainstream U. S.
culture, it did not change the negative societal perceptions of these individuals.
This tenet applies equally well to persons with disabilities. They continue to
realize all too frequently that prejudice against disability will continue to thrive
in this culture because it glorifies beauty, youth, and able-bodied people, and
belittles differences or anomalies (DeJong, 1979; Shreve, 1982).

CONSUMERISM

Another movement that influenced independent living was consumerism
(McDonald & Oxford, 2003; Shreve, 1982). Its outspoken leader, Ralph
Nader, preached consumer sovereignty, that consumers have ultimate control of
the choice of goods and services available to them. The independent living
movement promoted similar ideology—that persons with disabilities should
determine which of their own services they required not professionals. This
concept was incorporated into one of the mandates in the Rehabilitation Act of
1973, which stipulated consumer involvement throughout the rehabilitation
process, especially in crafting the components of the Individual Written
Rehabilitation Plan (Mackelprang & Salsgiver, 1999). If the consumer is
deemed ineligible for services, the professional had to stipulate the reasons for
such a decision, and the consumer has the right to appeal the ruling (Rubin &
Roessler, 2001). The independent living movement also helped to create a

number of advocacy centers offering consumer protection to various groups uneducated about, or who have been denied, their legal rights and benefits (Shreve, 1982).

THE SELF-HELP MOVEMENT

The self-help movement gained momentum in the 1970's with the profusion of self-help literature, and the proliferation of support groups for every conceivable problem imagined (McDonald & Oxford, 2003; Shreve, 1982). Many were modeled after Alcoholics Anonymous whose premise was that sharing with similar others promotes solidarity, support, understanding, and healing (Shreve, 1982). Self- help and group support are hallmarks of the independent living philosophy that places emphasis on people with disabilities assisting each other by virtue of their similar circumstances. Independent living centers, like self-help groups, provide services which may be lacking in traditional helping systems, and allow members to control their own choices.

DEMEDICALIZATION

The voices of many in the independent living movement resonated with support for a shift in paradigm from the traditional medical model of disability as illness and dependency, to individual empowerment and responsibility for ones own health (McDonald & Oxford, 2003; Shreve, 1982). The movement took issue with various aspects of the medical model, such as a continued medical presence despite stability of the disability; emphasis on the sick and dependent roles; acute/restorative care well beyond what is needed; prescribing unnecessary surgery, drugs, and medical care; the physician as the only decision maker; and repeated diagnostics, certification, or treatment services although the person is familiar enough with his or her condition to monitor it effectively (DeJong, 1979).This overarching medical presence in the lives of persons with disabilities runs counter to the independent movement's concept of self-determination.

DEINSTITUTIONALIZATION

Another societal movement that impacted independent living was deinstitutionalization, an attempt to move people out of institutions and back to their communities (McDonald & Oxford, 2003; Shreve, 1982). It was felt that with the right support services, these individuals could live normal, fulfilled lives. This philosophy closely parallels that of the independent living movement that stresses providing community based services that will ultimately enable people with disabilities to be mainstreamed into everyday life.

181

8

MOVERS AND SHAKERS

The philosophy of the independent movement is rooted in self-determination, choice, and consumer control (Nosek, 1992; Nosek, & Howland, 1992; Rubin & Roessler, 2001). Self-determination includes choice, goal setting, optimal control, and responsibility for decision-making while, control implies freedom from coercion, independence, and manipulation of the environment to enable participation in all aspects of the mainstream (Giordano& D'Alonzo, 1994; Smith & Smith, 1994; Wilson, 1998).

Berkeley is generally recognized as the birthplace of the independent living movement; however, in 1962, the University of Illinois at Urbana-Champaign pioneered community living for persons with severe disabilities by transferring four disabled students from the campus's nursing facility to a modified home nearby (DeJong, 1979). Its disabled students program has placed the university as one of the most architecturally accessible institutions of its kind (DeJong, 1979).

The first independent living center was incorporated in 1972 by the efforts of Ed Roberts and a group of severely disabled students who were enrolled at the University of California at Berkeley (Conyers, 2002; DeJong, 1979; Mackelprang & Salsgiver, 1999; Nosek, 2002; Oklin, 1999). Roberts, a polio survivor, a quadriplegic, and on a respirator, along with other students with severe disabilities, was housed in the campus hospital because of lack of accessible housing (Olkin, 1999; Zukas, 1975). Roberts and his peers organized into a group called the "Rolling Quads", and saw their mission as advocating full community integration for people with disabilities by providing necessary support services to enhance the quality of their lives (Conyers, 2002; Nosek, 1992; Olkin, 1999).

The group opened a program office to provide needed support services unavailable elsewhere, and within a year were deluged with so many requests, particularly from the surrounding communities, that they established a Center for Independent Living (CIL) for the community at large (DeJong, 1979; Olkin, 1999; Rubin & Roessler, 2001; Zukas, 1975). Its basic tenets were that persons with disabilities know the needs of their peers best; service delivery is best provided by people with disabilities; full community integration; services should enhance independence and self-determination; self-determination, independence, and choice (Matthews, 1990; Nosek, 1992; Nosek, Zhu, & Howard, 1992; Olkin, 1999; Smith & Smith, 1994; Wilson, 1998; Zukas, 1975).

Following the successful efforts at Berkeley, CILs were established in Boston, Houston, Columbus, Ann Arbor, and other parts of the country (Conyers, 2002; DeJong, 1979; Mackelprang & Salsgiver, 1999; Smith & Smith, 1994), and today over 400 independent living centers operate in the United States (Mackelprang & Salsgiver, 1999; Pelka, 1994). Title VII of the Rehabilitation Act Amendments of 1988 stipulate that independent living centers must provide multiple services to persons with a wide array of disabilities; that at least 51% of the policymaking board and the majority of its staff must be persons with disabilities; that consumers with disabilities must be intimately involved in service delivery, program and center design, planning, and training activities, and facilitating consumer and community needs, and that every CIL funded through the Rehabilitation Act must provide information and referral services, advocacy, independent living skills training, and peer counseling (Frieden, 1983; Potter, 1996; Rubin & Roessler, 2001; Wilson, 1998).

ETHNIC/ RACIAL MINORITY GROUPS AND INDEPENDENT LIVING

DeJong (1979) claimed that at its beginning, the independent living movement garnered its constituency from severely disabled, older adolescents and younger working age adults including those with spinal cord injury, muscular dystrophy, cerebral palsy, multiple sclerosis, and post polio disablement. DeJong believed that this narrow age range was a function of disabling conditions that are more likely to occur during the late teen or early adulthood years. In addition, the movement took root in academic communities. Severely disabled older individuals and ethnic/racial minorities were missing from the group. This is ironic because African Americans as well as other ethnic/racial minority groups including Hispanics and Native Americans have more severe and higher rates of disabling conditions than Caucasians (Capella, 2002; Clay, 1992; McNeil, 1993; Smart & Smart, 1992; Walker, 1987; Wilson, Turner, Liu, Harley & Alston, 2002) and the independent living movement drew its impetus from the gains made by African Americans during the civil rights movement (National Center for the Dissemination of Disability Research (NCDDR),1996).

Since its inception, the constituency of the independent living movement has been Caucasian consumers with disabilities and not ethic/racial minority consumers with disabilities (DeJong, 1979). Although some ethnic/racial minority consumers may have benefited from its outcomes, the numbers pale in comparison to the service delivery benefits of Caucasian consumers. For

example, in a national study of independent living centers, Nosek, Zhu, &
Howland (1992) found that almost 80% were white consumers and 20%
ethnic/racial minority consumers. In a regional study of 32 centers for
independent living, Flowers, Edwards, & Pusch (1996) reported that, of the
8,000 persons served, almost 90 % were white. To address this problem, a
committee established by the National Center for Independent Living
recommended that more independent living centers be established in areas with
large ethnic/racial minority populations (Parkin & Nosek, 2001). However,
there is not overwhelming evidence that ethnic/racial minority individuals with
disabilities are accessing independent living services. The obvious question is,
Why not? Answers to this question are provided in the discussion below.

ISSUES IMPACTING ETHNIC/ RACIAL MINORITY GROUP PARTICIPATION IN INDEPENDENT LIVING

Title VII of the Rehabilitation Act Amendments of 1988 stipulate that every
center for independent living funded through the Rehabilitation Act must
provide the following: (a) information and referral services; (b) advocacy; (c)
independent living skills training; and (d) peer counseling (Frieden, 1983;
Parkin & Nosek, 2001; Potter, 1996; Rubin & Roessler, 2001; Wilson, 1998).

According to Rubin & Roessler (2001) *information and referral services*
may encompass housing, attendant, adaptive equipment, transportation,
community, employment, support group, interpreter and reader, recreational,
medical, civil rights, benefits, and other supplementary resource information.
Independent living skills and training may include instruction in services such
as daily survival skills, self- management, social interaction, self- advocacy,
community training, utilization of public transportation, pre-vocational training
and other tools necessary for successful independent living. Persons with
disabilities serve as role models and mentors by providing *peer counseling* and
serving as credible resources for helping persons with disabilities develop
autonomy, improve their coping skills, and effectively navigate their place in
the community. *Advocacy* services involve individual and community systems;
they empower people with disabilities to develop the skills required to achieve
their independent living goals, and promotes the elimination of barriers and
other disincentives that limit full mainstream participation of all persons with
disabilities.

The National Center for the Dissemination of Disability Research (1999)
points out that the key components of the independent living philosophy,

184

however, were ultimately shaped by the norms, beliefs, and values of mainstream U.S. culture articulated through educated Caucasian men with disabilities. Little attempt was made to include other perspectives such as those of ethnic/racial minority groups. Services were often provided in a manner that was inconsistent with their cultural beliefs and values. Therefore, ethnic/racial minority individuals with disabilities did not, and still do not access independent living services as readily as consumers from the mainstream U.S. culture. Another major concern has been the even wider cultural and value differentials between ethnic/racial minorities with disabilities and service delivery personnel. This concern continues to be echoed in the work of rehabilitation researchers and others concerned with diversity in the helping professions such as Alston & Bell, 1996; Alston & Mngadi, 1992; Atkinson, 2004; Conyers, 2002; Herbert & Cheatham, 1988; Leal-Idrogo, 1993; Parkin & Nosek, 1991; Peterson, 1996; Sue & Sue, 2003; Walker, et al., 1986; Wilson, 1997; Wilson, Jackson, & Doughty, 1999; Wright, 1988. Utilization of independent living services by ethnic/racial minority groups is also hampered by a number of barriers specifically related to cultural values and the independent living philosophical orientation. Some of these barriers are articulated below.

DIFFERING WORLDVIEWS

Central to understanding the clash of cultural values that exists between mainstream U. S. culture and ethnic/racial minority groups is the concept of worldview. Sue and Sue (2003) define worldview as one's perceptions of his/her relationship to the world via nature, institutions, other people, and things. In other words, it is the lens through which the person discerns and responds to the environment or the person's belief system about how the world works. There is a striking disconnect between the worldview of the four largest ethnic/racial minority groups and mainstream U.S. culture. Individuals from these groups generally tend to be more collectivist in nature and focus on the group, while individuals from mainstream U. S. culture hold worldviews that are more individualistic in nature (McLaughlin & Braun, 1998; Nosek & Howland, 1992; Nosek & Hughes, 2004; Sue & Sue, 2003; Triandis, 1994; Westbrook & Legge, 1993). Differences between the worldviews of ethnic/racial minority groups and the mainstream U.S. culture, especially in regards to accessing mental health and other health related services, have been cited frequently in the literature (Atkinson, 2004; Atkinson & Hackett, 2004; Looby& Webb, 2002; Parkin & Nosek, 2001; Smart & Smart, 1993; Sue & Sue, 2003; Wilson, 2002; Wright, Martinez & Dixon, 1999). Many of these

differences directly impact ethnic/racial minority group utilization of
independent living services.

INDIVIDUALISM

It is imperative in this discussion to address the concept of "individualism"
itself and what it means to individuals from ethnic/racial minority groups.
Individualism is one of the most dominant values shaping mainstream U. S.
culture, and has directly influenced and shaped rehabilitation service delivery,
procedures, rules, and independent living philosophy (NCDDR, 1999). As
Parkin & Nosek (2001) reiterate, individualism stresses achievement of
personal goals, self- determination, autonomy, and choice. The notion of
individualism fits like a glove in the context of independent living where the
individual controls his life, makes decisions, has choices, manages resources,
and is an active participant in the independent living community (Nosek,
Fuhrer, & Howland, 1992; Parkin & Nosek, 2001). Independent living also
means having the resources to achieve the aforementioned goals.

The notion of individualism in the context of the cultural values of
ethnic/racial minorities runs counter to their group orientation, interdependence,
collectivity, shared decision making, and strong community focus (NCDDR,
1999; Parkin & Nosek, 2001; Sue & Sue, 2003). For example, many
ethnic/racial minority groups define themselves in the context of their family,
and view family as a referent point for social economic, emotional, financial,
and psychological support (Looby & Webb, 2002; Sue & Sue, 2003). The
philosophy of independent living, which stresses empowerment, advocacy,
personal choice, and independence from others, may negate the importance of
family choice and involvement. Family choice and involvement may run
counter to the aims of independent living. Therefore, ethnic/racial minority
individuals with disabilities may devalue the notion of independence, refuse to
access independent living services, and, instead, choose the security of the
family.

FAMILY AS REFERENT POINT

The cohesiveness, and security found in ethnic/racial minority families and the
sense of collective responsibility for each other may encourage over-
protectiveness, paternalism, protection from and distrust of outsiders, and
strong sanctions against airing family problems to strangers (Looby & Webb,
2002). In ethnic/racial minority families, family relationships are held sacred,
and the family takes precedence over all other matters (Hines & Boyd-Franklin,
1996; Falicov, 1996; Herring, 1999; Uba, 1994). Hence, individuals with

disabilities may be sheltered from outsiders and are taken care of by family members, or help may be sought from the priest or other significant individuals in the community (NCDDR, 1999; Smart & Smart, 1993). There is an inherent distrust of outsiders, counselors, and also social service agencies; therefore, if help is sought, it may be done as a last resort (Falicov, 1996; Garcia-Preto, 1996; Garrett & Garrett, 1994; Hines & Boyd-Franklin, 1996; Ho, 1987; Uba, 1994). In Asian families, the preservation of family honor is very important; an individual with a disability may be viewed as bringing shame to the family or perceived as weak and lacking will (NCDDR, 1999; Sue & Sue, 2003). Asian families may be less comfortable accessing independent living services because this may cause the family to lose face.

RELIGIOUS AND SPIRITUAL PRACTICES
Individuals from ethnic/racial minority groups are firmly grounded in religious and spiritual practices that emphasize some of the following ideas: suffering as a natural consequence of life; that the greater the sacrifice, suffering, and pain one endures, the greater the salvation; that faith in God/a spiritual power is the best medicine for dealing with crisis, turmoil, and illness; that having a disability or illness is God's will, a punishment from God/an offended spirit, something caused by supernatural forces, or as the sins of the parents handed down to their children; that illness results from the failure to live in harmony with nature and the dictates of the culture (Looby & Webb, 2002; McLaughlin & Braun, 1998; Smart & Smart, 1991; Sue & Sue, 2003; Yamamoto & Acosta, 1982). What logically follows is that these groups believe that having a disability is God's will, and altering or seeking services cannot change the path that God has laid out (Looby & Webb, 2002; Sue & Sue, 2003; Yamamota & Acosta, 1982).

CAUSES OF DISABILITY
Having a different understanding of the causes of disability may lead individuals with disabilities from ethnic/racial minority groups to seek help through sources other than independent living services. Such systems may include informal and familiar indigenous healing and helping networks (NCDDR, 1999). Consequently, accessing independent living services may not be viewed as beneficial.

DEFINITIONS OF DISABILITY
Attitudes about the causes and treatment of disability within mainstream U.S. culture are influenced by the philosophy of individuality, and are rooted in the scientific or medical model which views disability as a disease emanating from

the individual, and treats it in isolation from other aspects of the person
(NCDDR, 1999). Individuals from ethnic/racial minority groups may define
disability differently.

African Americans, for example, view disabilities in a spiritual context, as
God's will, hold more varied perceptions of what constitutes "developmental
normalcy," and rely heavily on a number of environmental resources for
treatment of individuals with disabilities (NCDDR, 1999). Hispanics view
many disabling conditions as individual differences rather than disabilities, and
consider it their duty to care for those family members with disabilities (Smart
& Smart, 1993). Although Asians may view disabling conditions as a sign of
weakness or bringing shame to one's family, they honor their obligation to care
for that person and consider it personal and family shame and dishonor if they
are unable to take care of family members (McLaughlin & Braun, 1998).
Native Americans have no word for disability in their language, treat each
person with respect and dignity, and their belief in the interconnectedness of
body and spirit and all things within the universe (Clay, 1992; NCDDR, 1999)
is in direct contrast to the medical model of rehabilitation delivery services.

Consequently, if a service agency advertises itself as serving people with
disabilities, it may not reach the consumers it wants to reach because of the
differing minority perspectives of what constitutes a disability (Clay, 1992).
These beliefs may help to explain why individuals with disabilities from
ethnic/racial minority groups may not access independent living services, and
the failure of independent living centers to provide culturally appropriate
services to these groups.

INFORMATION AND REFERRAL SERVICES

Information and referral services and independent living skills and training are
two mandated domains of independent living centers service delivery.
However, there is not overwhelming evidence that individuals with disabilities
from ethnic/racial minority populations are accessing these important services.
Wright, Martinez, & Dixon (1999) conducted a pilot investigation of minority
consumers of independent living services via focus groups to determine (a)
existing barriers to independent living and their impact on transportation,
housing, vocational skills, and health services; and (b) provide
recommendations for alleviating said barriers. Participants presented with 17
different disabilities, and included African Americans, Hispanic Americans,
Asian Americans, American Indians, and Anglo Americans of varying age
ranges.

The researchers reported that specific concerns related to transportation included unreliability, insensitive personnel, little or no attempts to inform consumers about services provided, and inaccessibility in rural areas. Suggestions, such as consumer education and information dissemination, sensitivity training for drivers, and developing a more consumer friendly transit system, were articulated.

Inaccessible and unaffordable housing, limited or no attempts to make accommodations for consumers with disabilities, long waiting lists, and financial constraints were mentioned by the researchers as the major obstacles to obtaining suitable housing. Government sponsored initiatives, tax incentives for developers who build accessible housing, ongoing education and training of landlords about disability, reasonable accommodations, cultural sensitivity, and creating an advertising program focusing on available housing for persons with disabilities, were some proposed solutions.

According to the researchers, participants were also openly critical of the medical community. Frequent complaints included lack of sensitivity and cultural knowledge among providers; negative bedside manner and inadequate medical treatment; limited accessibility to and unaffordable services; and poor medical insurance coverage. Recommendations included major health care changes, employment of culturally competent and sensitive providers, the development of an adequate health network system to address the needs of persons with disabilities, and effective information dissemination systems.

The researchers also indicated that vocational training issues included unsystematic eligibility determination criteria; exclusion from the rehabilitation process; frequent counselor turnover; questionable evaluation methods; prolonged waiting periods for and limited access to services; inadequate testing, training and placement methods; and a lack of cultural sensitivity among providers. More reliable and efficient testing and training techniques, adherence to the Americans with Disabilities Act (ADA), sensitivity training, and community outreach programs on persons with disabilities were some suggested corrective measures.

The researchers claimed that the most significant responses addressed the inadequacy of independent living services. Participants were not only uninformed, but also unable to access information about available services. Other concerns mentioned which directly impacted independent living included little consumer empowerment, inaccessible communities, lack of transportation, restricted opportunities for social relationships and activities, safety concerns, and the inability to access essential survival needs. The authors concluded that ethnic/racial minority consumers with disabilities continue to face many obstacles in their attempts to navigate independent living services.

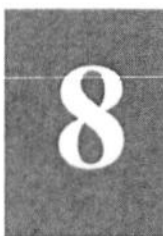

PEER COUNSELING

One of the services of centers for independent living is to provide peer
counseling with individuals with disabilities acting as role models and
informational resources, helping consumers develop self sufficiency and
autonomy, providing support, and modeling self sufficiency (Rubin & Roessler,
2001).

For ethnic/racial minority individuals with disabilities, their support comes
from family members who may not have the experience or knowledge of
working with disability issues, and may or may not define the family member's
problem as a disability (Clay, 1992; NCDRR, 1999). Family, not outside
agencies or individuals, is the referent point for information, teaching coping
skills, providing emotional, psychological, economic, and physical support, and
the one positive constant in the lives of ethnic/racial minority individuals
(Smart, 1991; Smart & Smart, 1992, 1993; Sue & Sue, 2003; Looby &Webb,
2002).

Equally important, asking an individual with a disability from an
ethnic/racial minority group to develop autonomy and personal independence
may be asking that person to reject cultural and family dictates that emphasize
cohesiveness and the importance of the collective over the individual (Sue &
Sue, 2003). This may be interpreted as asking the individual to reject important
family values and traditions. Because the family prefers to take care of its own,
opportunities to interact with other individuals with disabilities may not be
frequent because these individuals may not access the system.

ADVOCACY

Self and community advocacy is another core service of independent living
centers. This involves learning about and exercising ones right to equal access,
to non-discrimination, to appropriate services, and to develop the skills required
to achieve independent living goals (Clay, 1992; Rubin & Roessler, 2001).
Self-advocacy involves the individual taking charge of his/her own life and
acting in his/her own best interest. This requires having appropriate
information, understanding how social agencies function, having the ability to
communicate with others, and persistence in the face of denial (Clay, 1992).

Individuals from ethnic/racial minority groups typically suppress individual
interests to the good of the collective or family (Looby & Webb, 2002; Parkin
& Nosek, 2001; Sue & Sue, 2003). Further, families and other significant
persons view their role as supporters and advocates for the needs of the member
with a disability (Clay, 1992). Advocating for one's needs places emphasis on

190

the individual. This may be viewed as being boastful, focusing on self, and disrespecting family rules and dictates, since the needs of the group are priority. Self-advocacy requires persistence with bureaucracy, communicating effectively, and withstanding rejection (Clay, 1992). Individuals from ethnic/racial minority groups may not choose to subject themselves to this discomfort, especially if it involves violating family values and beliefs.

Looby & Webb (2002) claim that individuals from some ethnic/racial minority groups may be introverted and reserved (e.g., Asian); others may not have the language facility to articulate their needs (e.g., Hispanics, Asian Americans); others may honor and value maintaining harmony and acceptance of a particular outcome (e.g. Asians, Native Americans); and others may value respecting authority (e.g. Asians, Native Americans, Hispanics). Therefore, individuals from ethnic/racial minority groups who honor these values may see little benefit in advocacy and may not understand it. When they apply for services and are denied, they may not complain or advocate for their rights because of cultural imperatives which promote maintaining harmony and balance in one's life and with others (Clay, 1992; Sue & Sue, 2003).

CONSUMER CONTROL AND INVOLVEMENT

Consumer control and involvement is another core mandate of independent living centers. The mandate stipulates that the consumer controls and directs the services received and makes major decisions regarding the management of the independent living center (Clay, 1992). Flowers, Edwards, & Pusch, (1996) conducted a regional survey of cultural diversity within 53 centers for independent living in RSA Region V (Illinois, Indiana, Michigan, Minnesota, Ohio, and Wisconsin). The major focus was on staff diversity and outreach to underserved ethnic minorities.

Responses from 32 of the 53 centers indicated that almost 19% of the directors and 15% of the management staff were racial or ethnic minorities and that they served over 8, 000 persons. Caucasians comprised 89.3% and African Americans 7.02% (9.05 % of the general population in that area was African American) of the consumers utilizing independent living services. Administrators were queried about outreach efforts to increase diversity. Fifty eight percent had no plan; sixty six percent of the centers with plans were unsure of their effectiveness; thirty seven percent had staffing plans in place; twenty five percent felt that their plans were effective; and 19 % did not know if such a plan existed.

The researchers also asked the centers to indicate their specific outreach activities. Activities included direct mailings to organizations, personal visits and presentations to groups, participation in cultural diversity programs and events, and distribution of agency information at sites where persons from ethnic/racial minority groups are served.

The results of the above study seem to indicate that Caucasian consumers with disabilities have more accessibility to independent living centers and services than do individuals with disabilities from ethnic/racial minority groups. Equity of independent living services for persons from ethnic/racial minority groups is mixed. Obviously, without minority consumers, there can be no minority consumer involvement, which is one of the core mandates of independent living.

Research continues to document long-standing problems among ethnic/racial minority groups with disabilities that may or may not be aware of independent living services. These problems include transportation difficulties, limited outreach efforts by social service agencies and rehabilitation service providers, lack of information about services, inaccessibility to rural areas, no community outreach programs, little consumer empowerment, poor finances, limited community resources, and culturally insensitive service delivery (McLaughlin & Braun, 1998; Nosek, 1992; Nosek & Howland, 1992; Parkin & Nosek, 2001; Wright, Martinez, & Dixon, 1999).

It is obvious that centers for independent living must engage in a more concerted and comprehensive effort to involve ethnic/racial minority groups in independent living. There are several ways that this may be accomplished.

INCORPORATING ETHNIC/RACIAL MINORITY GROUPS INTO INDEPENDENT LIVING

The following is a list of general recommendations to improve participation of ethnic/racial minority groups in independent living. This list is by no means exhaustive:

- Include family members and/or significant support entities (individual and community) in consultations with ethnic/ racial minority consumers. Individuals from ethnic/racial minority groups value the importance of family relationships and may not participate in the rehabilitation process without family involvement. Disrespect of the family hierarchy may be interpreted as disrespect for the consumer also, thereby precluding participation in services.
- Current independent living services and policies reflect the values of mainstream U.S. culture to the exclusion of values of ethnic/racial minority consumers. For example,

consideration must be given to critical issues such as the importance of family, communication styles, independence versus the good of the group, definitions of disability, definitions of independence, self sufficiency and dependence, and the significance of guilt and shame in Asian cultures. These concepts serve as guiding principles in the lives of ethnic/racial minority consumers. In order for these individuals to fully participate in independent living, there should be a redefinition of the independent living philosophy to incorporate these and other important cultural values of ethnic/racial minority groups. Perhaps then, ethnic/racial minority consumers may access independent living services.

- The inability of service providers to network and build alliances with resources existing in ethnic/racial minority communities may prevent minority group participation in independent living. Grass roots, credible, respected individuals from the four ethnic/racial minority groups identified in this chapter can serve as spokespersons to adapt, explain, educate, and even illustrate application of varied components of the independent living mandates in ethnic/racial minority communities. These individuals can be excellent resources for educating service providers and rehabilitation administrators about how to effectively mesh the independent living philosophy with the varied cultural values, practices, and beliefs of ethnic/racial minority groups.

- Recruit and hire ethnic/racial minority service providers with disabilities, and who are bilingual-if possible, and place them in management/decision making roles at the independent living center and on the Board of Directors. These individuals may be better able to articulate the needs of the targeted ethnic/racial minority consumers, serve as role models with whom the consumers can identify, and communicate with them in their native language. These service providers could provide added voices to the concerns of ethnic/racial minority consumers. They could also have an impact on the shaping and development of programs and policies that take into account issues which affect ethnic/racial minority consumer utilization of independent living services.

- Make a more concerted effort to outreach to ethnic/racial minority consumers, especially since research has indicated that they know very little about independent living centers and even less about the services provided (Parkin & Nosek, 2001; Wright, Martinez, & Dixon, 1999). Outreach efforts should be active, high profile, conducted in ethnic/racial minority communities, and involve all community members, not just those individuals with disabilities. Flowers, Edwards & Pusch (1996) feel that outreach efforts should be approached systematically. They suggest that prior to initiating, it is important that independent living centers identify their target group, assess previous efforts, review current policies and procedures, especially recruitment strategies, and then implement their plan/program.

- Given the mistrust that ethnic/racial minority groups may have of strangers and individuals from the "bureaucracy," it is imperative that independent living center staff build personal relationships with members of the ethnic/racial minority group(s) and the community(ies) they wish to serve. Developing relationships with significant community personnel who have been successful in reaching ethnic/racial minority individuals with disabilities can help in a number of ways: making referrals; introduction to other community members and agencies; facilitating entry or outreach to targeted ethnic/racial minority consumers; having an influential and supportive ally; having a respected individual explaining the significance of independent living services to ethnic/racial minority consumers; and adding credibility and trust to the service provider. All of these efforts may serve a critical role in encouraging ethnic/racial minority consumers to access independent living services.

- One of the major findings of the study done by Wright, Martinez, & Dixon (1999), and reported by ethnic/racial minority consumers, was a lack of awareness of services provided by independent living centers. To address this problem, multiple methods of communicating and disseminating information should be utilized. For example, word of mouth, providing interpreters, phone calls, mailings, brochures and forms written in the appropriate language of the consumer; pamphlets; flyers; email; newspaper and radio advertisement; mailing lists; setting up booths and displays at

8

events in ethnic/racial minority communities; speaking at churches and other community venues; placing information in local social services, mental health, and other agencies; going from door to door; and placing information in areas populated by ethnic/racial minority consumers with disabilities are some avenues which may be utilized.

- Diversity training as well as training in the Americans with Disabilities Act (ADA) is imperative for effective outreach to ethnic/racial minority populations with disabilities so that they may access independent living services. Staff that are culturally sensitive and educated about rehabilitation mandates, including ADA and independent living, will be able to provide services that are more effective to ethnic/racial minority consumers who want to access independent living services.

- Help to decrease additional existing barriers to independent living for ethnic/racial minority consumers as cited in the Wright, Martinez, & Dixon (1999) study. These include, but may not be limited to, transportation, inaccessibility to rural areas, suitable housing, medical treatment, vocational training issues, eligibility determination criteria, dealing with the rehabilitation bureaucracy, advocacy, restricted opportunities for social relationships and activities, safety issues, and accessing basic survival needs.

CONCLUSION

The independent living movement revolutionized rehabilitation and presented a new paradigm within which to view persons with disabilities. This paradigm resulted in considerable social and political changes for persons with disabilities from mainstream U.S. culture. They asserted themselves, demanded access to, and were allowed to participate in mainstream society, became active and capable consumers, and took control of their own lives.

However, the independent living philosophy, though well intentioned, did not take into account the different cultural values and perspectives of individuals with disabilities from ethnic/racial minority groups. As the literature has indicated, today, more than 30 years after the establishment of the first independent living center in Berkeley, California, ethnic/racial minority individuals with disabilities continue to be underserved by independent living centers. As articulated previously, the reasons are varied, but suffice it to say that a major theme has been the differing value systems of individuals from the mainstream U.S. culture and those from ethnic/racial minority groups. This gap can and must be remedied if independent living is to fulfill its mandate for all people with disabilities—full participation in mainstream U. S. society.

REFERENCES

Alston, R. J., & Bell, T. J. (1996). Cultural mistrust and the rehabilitation enigma for African Americans. *The Journal of Rehabilitation, 10*(4), 73-82.

Alston, R. J., & Mngadi, S. (1992). The interaction between disability status and the African American experience: Implications for rehabilitation counseling. *Journal of Applied Rehabilitation Counseling,* 12-15.

Atkinson, D. R. (2004). Counseling *American minorities* (6th ed.). Boston, MA: McGraw-Hill.

Atkinson, D. R., & Hackett, G. (2004). Counseling *diverse populations*. New York, NY: McGraw-Hill (172-187).

Capella, M. E. (2002). Inequities in the VR system: Do they still exist? *Rehabilitation Counseling Bulletin, 45*(3), 143-153.

Clay, J.A. (1992). Native American independent living. *Rural Special Education Quarterly, 11(1),* 41-50.

Conyers, L. M. (2002). Disability: An emerging topic in multicultural counseling. In J. Trusty, E. J. Looby, & D. Sandhu (Eds.), *Multicultural counseling: Context,theory and practice, and competence,* pp. 173-201. New York: Nova Science Publishers.

De Jong, G. (1979). The *movement for independent living: Origins, ideology, and implications for disability research.* East Lansing: University Center for International Rehabilitation, Michigan State University.

Deutsch, A. (1949). The *mentally ill in America* (2nd ed.). New York: Columbia University Press.

Falicov, C. J. (1996). Mexican families. . In M. McGoldrick, J. Pearce, & J. Giordano (Eds.) *Ethnicity and family therapy (*2nd ed.), pp 169-182. New York: Guilford Press.

Flowers, C. R., Edwards, D., & Pusch, B. (1996). Rehabilitation cultural diversity Initiative: A regional survey of cultural diversity within CILs. *Journal of Rehabilitation, 62*(3), 22-28.

Frieden, L. (1983). Understanding alternative program models. In N. M. Crewe and I. K. Zola (Eds.), *Independent living for physically disabled people,* pp. 62-72. San Francisco: Jossey-Bass Publishers.

Frieden, A. (1990). Substance abuse and disability: The role of independent living centers. *Journal of Applied Rehabilitation Counseling, 21*(3), 33-36.

Garcia-Preto, N. (1996). Puerto Rican families. . In M. McGoldrick, J.Pearce, & J. Giordano (Eds.), *Ethnicity and family therapy (*2nd ed.), pp. 183-199. New York: Guilford Press.

Garrett, J. F. (1969). Historical background. In D. Malikin & H. Rusalem (Eds.), *Vocational rehabilitation of the disabled,* pp. 29-38. New York: New York University Press.

Garrett, J.T., & Garrett, M.W. (1994). The path of good medicine. Understanding and counseling Native American Indians. *Journal of Multicultural Counseling and Development, 22,* 134-144.

Giordano, G., & D'Alonzo, B. J. (1994). The link between transition and independent living. *American Rehabilitation, 20*(1), 2-7.

Harber, M. H. (1963). Eugenics*: Hereditarian attitudes in American thought.* New Brunswick, NJ: Rutgers University Press.

Herbert, J. T., & Cheatham, H. E. (1988). Africentricity and the Black disability experience: A theoretical orientation for rehabilitation counselors. *Journal of Applied Rehabilitation Counseling, 19*(4), 50-54.

Herring, R. (1996). Counseling indigenous American youth. In C.C. Lee (Ed.), *Multicultural issues in counseling: New approaches to diversity* (2nd ed.), pp.53-70. Alexandria, VA: American Counseling Association.

Hines, P., & Boyd-Franklin, N. (1996). African American families. In M. McGoldrick, J.Pearce & J. Giordano (Eds.), *Ethnicity and family therapy (*2nd ed.), pp. 66-84. New York: Guilford Press.

Ho, M.K. (1987). *Family therapy with ethnic minorities.* California: Sage.

Judge, M. (1976). A brief history of social services, part I. *Social and Rehabilitation Records, 3*(5), 2-8.

Leal-Idrogo, A. (1993). Vocational rehabilitation of people of Hispanic origin. *Journal of Vocational Rehabilitation, 3*(1), 27-37.

Looby, E.J., & Webb, T. (2002). Counseling ethnically diverse families.). In J. Trusty, E. J. Looby, & D. Sandhu (Eds.), *Multicultural counseling: Context, theory and practice, and competence,* pp. 144-171. New York: Nova Science Publishers.

Mackelprang, R.., & Salsgiver, R. (1999). Disability*: A diversity model approach in human service practice.* California: Brooks/Cole.

Mathews, R. M. (1990). Independent living as a lifelong community service. *Journal of Head Trauma Rehabilitation, 5*(1), 23-30.

McDonald, G., & Oxford, M. (2003). History of independent living. Article retrieved May 20, 2003, from www.acils.com.

McLaughlin, L., & Braun, K. (1996). Asian and Pacific Islander cultural values: Considerations for health care decision making. *Health & Social Work, 23* (2), 116-126.

McNeil, J. M. (1993). Americans *with disabilities: 1991-92.* U. S. Bureau of the Census Current Population Reports, p. 70-133. Washington, DC: U. S. Government Printing Office.

National Center for the Dissemination of Disability Research. (1999). A review of literature on topics related to increasing the utilization of rehabilitation research outcomes among diverse consumer groups. Article retrieved, April 20, 2004, from www.ncddr.org/du/products/DisabilityDiversity.pdf

Nosek, M. A. (1992). Independent living. In R. M. Parker (Ed.), *Rehabilitation counseling: Basics and beyond* (2nd ed.), pp. 103-133. Austin, TX: Pro-Ed.

Nosek, M. A., Fuhrer, M. J., & Howland, C. A. (1992). Independence among people with disabilities: II. The personal independence profile. *Rehabilitation Counseling Bulletin, 36,* 21-36.

Nosek, M.A., & Howland, C. A. (1992). The role of independent living centers in delivering rehabilitation services to rural communities. *American Rehabilitation, 18*(1), 2-6.

Nosek, M. A., Hughes, R. B. (2004). Navigating the road to independent living. (pp. 172-192). In D. Atkinson, & G. Hackett (Eds.), *Counseling diverse populations,* pp.172-192. New York NY: McGraw-Hill.

Nosek, A. N., Zhu, Y., & Howard, C. A. (1992). The evolution of independent living programs. *Rehabilitation Counseling Bulletin, 35*(3), 175-189.

Swedlund, N., Taylor, H. B., & Swank, P. (in press). Self- esteem and women with disabilities. *Social Science and Medicine.*

Olkin, R. (1999). What *psychotherapists should know about disability.* New York: The Guilford Press.

Parkin, E. K., & Nosek, M. A. (2001). Collectivism versus independence: Perceptions of independent living and independent living services by Hispanic Americans and Asian Americans with disabilities. *Rehabilitation Education, 15*(4), 375-394.

Pelka, F. (1993). Fire in the belly: Just how independent is the independent living movement. *Mainstream, 4,* 35-38.

Peterson, G. E. (1996). An analysis of participation, progress, and outcome of individuals with diverse racial and ethnic backgrounds in the public vocational rehabilitation program in Nevada. *Dissertation Abstracts International, 57*(4A), Abstract retrieved December 19, 2000, from Dissertation Abstracts Online: First Search.

Pfeiffer, D. (1994). Eugenics and disability discrimination. *Disability and Society, 9, 481-499.*

Potter, C. G. (1996). After independent living, what next? A primer on independence for people with disabilities, their families, and service providers. *Journal of Applied Rehabilitation Counseling, 27*(2), 36-39.

Preen, B. (1976). Schooling *for the mentally retarded: A historical perspective.* New York: St. Martin's Press.

Rubin, S. E., & Roessler, R. T. (2001). Foundations of the vocational rehabilitation process. (5th ed.). Austin, TX: Pro-Ed.

Shapiro, J. P. (1993). No *pity.* New York: Times Books.

Shreve, M. (1982). The movement for independent living: A brief history. Written under federal grant for an ILC Training Module. Article retrieved May 20, 2003, from www.ilusa.com.

Smart, J. (2001). Disability, *society, and the individual.* Gaithersburg, MD: Aspen Publishers, Inc.

Smart, J., & Smart, D. (1992). Curriculum changes in multicultural rehabilitation. *Rehabilitation Education, 6,* 105-122.

Smart, J. F., & Smart, D. W. (1993). The rehabilitation of Hispanics with disabilities: Sociocultural constraints. *Rehabilitation Education, 7,* 167-184.

Smith, L. W., & Smith, Q. W. (1994). Independent living centers: Moving into the 21st century. *American Rehabilitation, 20*(1), 14-22.

Stein, H. F. (1979). Rehabilitation and chronic illness in American culture: The cultural psychodynamics of a medical and social problem. *Journal of Psychological Anthropology, 2*(2), 153-176.

Sue, D. W., & Sue, D. (2003). Counseling *the culturally diverse: Theory and practice.* New York: Wiley & Sons.

Triandis, H.C. (1994). *Culture and social behavior.* New York: McGraw-Hill.

Trusty, J., Looby, E.J. & Sandhu, D. (Eds.) (2002). *Multicultural counseling: Context, theory and practice, and competence.* New York: Nova Science Publishers.

Uba. L. (1992). Cultural barriers to health care for southeast Asian refugees. *Public Health Reports, 107,* 544-548.

Walker, S., Akpati, E., Roberts, V., Palmer, R., & Newsome, M. (Eds.). (1986). Frequency and distribution of disabilities among blacks: Preliminary findings. In S. Walker et al (Eds.), *Equal to the challenge: Perspectives, problems, and strategies in the rehabilitation of non-white disabled.* Proceedings of the national conference of the Howard University model to improve rehabilitation services to minority populations with handicapping conditions. (ERIC Education Reproduction Service No. ED 276 198).

Westbrook, M., & Legge, V. (1993). Health practitioners' perceptions of family attitudes toward children with disabilities. A comparison of six communities in a multicultural society. *Rehabilitation Psychology, 38,* 177-185.

Wilson, K. B. (1997). The *relationship between consumer race and vocational rehabilitation services and outcomes.* Unpublished doctoral dissertation, The Ohio State University.

Wilson, K. B. (2002). The exploration of vocational rehabilitation acceptance and ethnicity: A national investigation. *Rehabilitation Counseling Bulletin, 45,* 168-176.

Wilson, K. B., Jackson, R., & Doughty, J. (1999). What a difference a race makes: Reasons for unsuccessful closures within the vocational rehabilitation system. *American Rehabilitation, 25,* 16-24.

Wilson, K. B., Turner, T., Liu, J., Harley, D. A., & Alston, R. J. (2002). Perceived vocational rehabilitation service efficacy by race/ethnicity: Results of a national customer survey. *Journal of Applied Rehabilitation Counseling, 33*(3), 26-34.

Wilson, K. E. (1998). Centers for independent living in support of transition. *Focus on Autism and Other Developmental Disabilities, 13*(4), 246-252.

Wright, T. J. (1988). Enhancing the professional preparation of rehabilitation counselors for improved services to ethnic minorities with disabilities. *Journal of Applied Rehabilitation Counseling, 19*(4), 4-10.

Wright, T. J., Martinez, Y. G., & Dixon, C. G. (1999). Minority consumers of independent living services: A pilot investigation. *Journal of Rehabilitation, 65*(2), 20-25.

Yamamoto, J., & Acosta, F.X. (1982). Treatment of Asian Americans and Hispanic Americans: Similarities and differences. *American Academy of Psychoanalysis, 10,* 585-607.

Zukas, H. (1975). CIL history. Report of the state of the art conference, center for independent living (RSA Grant 45-P-45484/9-01). Berkeley, CA: Center for Independent Living.

CHAPTER 9

HUMAN RESOURCES DEVELOPMENT AND ISSUES IN REHABILITATION

MICHELLE P. POINTER

Chapter Highlights

➡ Introduction

➡ Human resources management and development

➡ Diversity and disability in human resources management

➡ Human resources management and development in rehabilitation

➡ Training needs in rehabilitation

➡ Programs and resources designed to address human resources needs

➡ Issues for rehabilitation in human resources management and development

➡ Conclusion

9

INTRODUCTION

$\mathcal{R}$esources are crucial to the successful operation of an organization, agency, or business. Although there are different types of resources, it is human resources that are most crucial to organizations. The heart of a business is the group of organized individuals that operate the business. State Vocational Rehabilitation Services Programs provide services to individuals with disabilities. Agencies assess, plan, develop, and provide services "consistent with their strengths, resources, priorities, concerns, abilities, capabilities, interests, and informed choice" (Rehabilitation Act, 1998, Sec. 100(a) (2)). People are important to the provision of services, and people must be prepared to be effective. These human resources come with varied training and competencies, and from diverse cultures and backgrounds. It is through recruitment, retention, and promotion that human resources development occurs. For purposes of this discussion, human resources development is defined as recognizing and realizing the possibilities and potential for human growth within an agency that make it better, and providing avenues for such development/growth.

As diversity has become integral in American society and disability is inherent in life, vocational rehabilitation counselors must be qualified to serve all individuals with disabilities (Szymanski, Leahy, & Linkowski, 1993). It is, therefore, imperative that professional counseling be founded on an understanding and appreciation of diversity (Lee, 1997). Diversity and disability in the workplace, reflective of the vast human resources available today, lends itself to a carefully woven approach to personnel development and is significant during three distinct human resources development phases: recruitment, retention, and promotion. As personnel retention and promotion are considered, issues such as the relationship between knowledge, education, and rehabilitation leadership must be addressed (Pointer, 2002).

In this chapter, human resources development will be examined in the context of multiculturalism and diversity as it is manifested during personnel recruitment, employee retention and development, and promotion. This context is significant as the culture in the 21st century has become increasingly diverse, and pluralism has become the way of society (2000 US Census, Lee, 1997). Lee states, "people who represent diverse cultural backgrounds characteristic of this pluralism will be attempting to develop their abilities and interests within this new social order" (Lee, 1997, p 10). A brief, yet comprehensive discussion of training and development of rehabilitation personnel, reflective of diversity and inclusive of rehabilitation administration and leadership, will also be conducted. Issues that impact the current trends and future direction of rehabilitation will be identified.

As a result of reading this chapter, graduate students are expected to have a more comprehensive understanding of rehabilitation human resources development. Students will also be able to delineate from a multicultural perspective, the complex components of human resource development pertinent to the rehabilitation profession.

A literature review was conducted primarily from a framework of four disciplines: human resources; rehabilitation; diversity and disability; and leadership, which enlarged the pool of available research studies. This chapter will unravel literature and group the information into distinct areas: (1) human resources development and management literature; (2) diversity and disability as it impacts human resources; and (3) human resources in the rehabilitation profession, including both public and private settings. The specific focus of the review will be on diversity, disability, and human resources development, along with related current issues. Implications of the literature review will be drawn.

HUMAN RESOURCES MANAGEMENT AND DEVELOPMENT

Human resources are a valuable commodity, the development of which enhances the continuation of the agency or organization. This development is future-focused, and training and educationally based. It involves planning, managing, and motivating people for the purposes of performance enhancement (Goss, D., 1994). Developing employees to carry on the business extends beyond traditional on-the-job-training, focusing more on preparing people for additional responsibilities. Conceptually, human resources development provides for employees' personal growth (DeCenzo & Robbins, 1999).

The people who work in the agency are the means to the accomplishment of the agency's purpose and goals, and their competency, growth, and development are necessary. Successful agencies invest in their employees in order to ensure employee growth and agency success. As it relates to human resources management (structural component) and human resources development (growth component), the literature contains various approaches, research findings, and issues. There is, however, agreement on three essential processes that occur: recruitment, retention, and promotion.

Management is the organizational component responsible for acquiring and providing for the employee's growth. It is a mechanism motivated by thought, which seeks, prepares, provides for, and deliberately integrates agency/organizational personnel into its purposeful, goal-directed, and functional operations. Whether it is handled informally or formally, human resources management guides recruitment, retention, and the promotional processes.

Rehabilitation agencies or commissions have separate, dedicated personnel or human resources departments that may be located within the agency or a host organization. For instance, human resources management for VR may be in Education, Labor, Labor and Industry, Family and Social Services, Public Health and Human Services, or Employment and Training. Private and other rehabilitation agencies also have dedicated personnel or HR departments. Employee development begins with recruitment and leads to retention, and in many cases, promotion.

RECRUITMENT

Practices in recruitment are surprisingly similar cross-nationally (Huo, et al., 2002) as human resource managers are concerned about three general areas: (a) ability/potential to do the job; (b) interpersonal/interorganizational skills; and (c) longevity or return on investment. Employers consider whether a person encompasses the skills, knowledge, and abilities required for the job when reviewing candidates (DeCenzo, & Robins, 1999; Rehabilitation Services Administration). Recruitment initiates the process of human resources development by seeking out and developing a pool of job appropriate applicants. Recruitment has long been a concern of rehabilitation (Parker, & Szymanski, 1992). In a study specific to individuals with disabilities, Keys and Balcazar (2000) reviewed 37 research studies, and concluded that even with generally positive employer attitudes and willingness to hire, negative attitudes persisted when specifics (e.g., promotability, accommodation costs) were involved. In another study, Gilbride, Stensrud, Ehlers, Evans, and Peterson (2000) found employers satisfied with the individuals whom they hired, but concerned about hiring individuals with specific types of disabilities.

Recruitment efforts vary according to agency and policies. For example, recruitment efforts in VR are guided by federal legislation that requires state rehabilitation agencies to develop a Comprehensive System of Personnel Development (CSPD), and specify its components in the State Plan. One component of the CSPD is the statement of what shall constitute a "qualified" rehabilitation professional in that agency.

Competition among organizations for the most qualified employee is tighter when unemployment rates are lower, and some researchers have suggested using persuasion during interviewing, as well as promoting the agency reputation as a mechanism for obtaining competitive advantage (Ferris, Berkson, & Harris, 2002). The outside perception of the agency can be enhanced through the organizational management of diversity. Cross (2000), for example, suggests the use of a social-justice approach where executives explore less oppressive hierarchical and money driven work environments. Thus, the work of executives in more culturally sensitive work settings will impact other areas of employees' lives and will enhance the agency's reputation.

LEARNING STYLES

Recognition of ways individuals work and subsequent utilization of this information in advertising, can positively impact recruitment. Tobias (1999) suggested learning style differences are more the cause of employee conflict than culture. Consequently, marketing approaches utilizing the four Gregoric learning styles would most likely appeal to individuals in accordance with their dominant style of learning. In other words, the question to answer when promoting the agency would vary for individuals:

- Concrete Sequential Dominant learner—What will we accomplish?
- Abstract Sequential Dominant Learner—What will we learn?
- Abstract Random Dominant Learner—What difference will we make?
- Concrete Random Dominant Learner—What makes us unique?

Recruitment can be accomplished internally as well as externally. Internal searches have many benefits. For example, internal searches are good for public relations and organizational reputation, organizational morale, individual ambition, good selection probability, and training mechanisms. They are also less costly. Work on task forces and committees provide experience, training, and promotional exposure for likely candidates. Properly used personnel files may be sources for internal recruitment. Internal advertisement and subsequent interviews may yield appropriate candidates.

When external searches are utilized, the choice of local, statewide, regional, national, or international advertisement will depend on the scope of the job and the specific knowledge and skills required of the candidates. The modes of communicating vacancies could involve any combination of the following: newspapers; newsletters; Internet postings; web pages; job hotlines; departmental kiosks; employment office listings; job banks; and personnel offices. Announcements may be posted, mailed, emailed, or delivered to schools, colleges and universities, disability and minority organizations, professional organizations, chambers of commerce, churches, civic groups, and other local establishments. Referral sources are many and varied, ranging from employee referrals to placement referral agencies and executive personnel companies.

Diversity is a major concern with recruitment and, in fact, has become a major priority within the Federal government. Specifically, the law states

> Recruitment efforts within vocational rehabilitation at the level of pre-service training, continuing education, and in-service training must focus on bringing larger numbers of minorities into the profession in order to provide appropriate practitioner knowledge, role models, and sufficient manpower to address the clearly changing demography of vocational rehabilitation.

Section 21(a)(4), Rehabilitation Act

Goss (1994) explained recruitment as the place where principles of assessment involving judging attributes and abilities, operate. There are three distinct functions: (1) recruitment (e.g., creating a selection pool, evaluating performance needs); (2) selection (e.g., performance potential and succession planning); and (3) appraisal (e.g., reward, performance, career and development planning, and training needs). These three functions directly impact the employee's commitment to the organization.

In order for an organization to continue profitably, employees must invest in it. Whether it is a private or public human services program, its survival, and effectiveness is contingent upon accountability in management (Harley, 2002). People make investments where there is a commitment to fulfilling their needs. The question in today's multicultural society becomes, how does human resources management recognize, respect and capitalize on their employees' similarities and differences, and encourage organizational commitment?

RETENTION AND EMPLOYEE DEVELOPMENT

Retention precedes employee development. Employees tend to remain with an agency or organization if the rewards are sufficient. However, rewards are not always monetary. The individual and agency fit is also significant. Both intrinsic (e.g., self-fulfillment, opportunities for growth, job satisfaction) and extrinsic (salary, benefits, work environment) rewards play a role in employee commitment and, ultimately, tenure with the agency (Goss, 1994; DeCenzo & Robbins, 1999).

Tenure is impacted by appraisal, although appraisals can be uncomfortable and training may not ease the discomfort. Blankenship and Crimando (2003) found no significant correlation between appraisal training and increasing

206

comfort in a study of the effectiveness of performance appraisal among three Illinois community rehabilitation agencies. In another study with community rehabilitation organizations, Mallik and Lemarie (2003) examined perceptions of departing community-based rehabilitation program employees as a means to reduce staff turnover. Among other things, they found that employees with a high school, associate, and/or bachelors degrees reported being in the right job, unlike those with less than a high school diploma and those with a doctoral degree. Overall, employees reported being properly trained.

BURNOUT

Exhaustion from the work arising from long-term stress and specifically identified as *burnout* is real, and has often been explored. Gomez and Michaels (1995) observed low to moderate levels of burnout among public and private human service workers. Caseload size was, surprisingly, not significant. It was found that traditional coping strategies were employed. The researchers concluded that increased direct contact with the individuals being served and less paperwork provided more of a sense of personal accomplishment to the human service works.

Stress is especially significant for individuals from minority groups. According to a study by Clark, Anderson, Clark, and Williams (1999). A stressor for African-Americans is racism; and racism is still very much prevalent today (Embrick, 2005). For example, "Black people have had to re-narrate themselves and re-negotiate their identities as workers..." (Yancy, 2004, p 352), thus giving an outward appearance of accommodation.

Whether individuals stay, remain in entry positions, become stagnant, grow, and develop, or progress promotionally is influenced by many factors, among which is motivation. Human resources has looked to other disciplines for a theoretical base in the absences of a distinctly human resources theory. Motivational theory is one way to explain human behavior. At this point, a brief discussion of selected theories explaining motivation is warranted.

MOTIVATIONAL THEORY AND HUMAN RESOURCES DEVELOPMENT

Abraham Maslow, Douglas McGregor, Frederick Hertzberg, David McCelland, Stacey Adams, and Victor Vroom are major contributors of motivational theories. Maslow is known for identifying five hierarchical order needs (physiological, safety, belonging, esteem, and self-actualization). McGregor proposed Theory X - Theory Y, which postulated that supervisors viewed human motivation as either negative (Theory X) or positive (Theory Y). On the other hand, Hertzberg proposed motivation hygiene suggesting that motivation was connected to intrinsic and extrinsic factors. Another theorist, McClelland, suggested achievement, affiliation, and power motives were connected to human motivation, and that these were tied directly to situations specific to the work environment (i.e., achievement, affiliation, power). A higher achievement need, for example, is related to higher performance. Adams is recognized for Equity Theory as he examined equity and the impact of perceived inequity in the work place. Finally, Vroom examined value of effort and reward (Decenzo & Robbins (1999).

REHABILITATION ACT OF 1973 AS AMENDED

Federal legislation impacting rehabilitation human resources development includes the Comprehensive System of Personnel Development (CSPD) delineated in the Rehabilitation Act. This is a legal requirement for VR agencies and directs an examination of the personnel needs and plan for adequate rehabilitation personnel. In their research on 1996 CSPD state documents, Froehlich, Garcia, and Linkowski (1998) examined hiring requirements. Recognizing an increase in hiring qualified counselors, they also identified inconsistencies between minimum education requirements and federal law.

The CSPD is specific in requirements and purposes to increase qualified personnel. Guidelines include the following directives: (a) describe procedures and activities that ensure an adequate supply of qualified State rehabilitation professionals and paraprofessionals; (b) specify the number and type of personnel currently needed, and projected to be needed in *five* years; and, (c) delineate a system for the continuing education of professionals and paraprofessionals within VR, especially for the retraining or hiring of personnel consistent with the State's professional requirements. As a result of CSPD, agencies have developed specific plans (incorporated in State Plans) to increase qualified personnel. Collaboration with local colleges and universities has yielded partnerships that lead to paid and unpaid internships, and in some instances, direct hires for rehabilitation students from minority and other groups.

A replication study on the Rehabilitation Cultural Diversity Initiative (RCDI) with Region V Centers for Independent Living was conducted by Flowers, Forbes, Crimando, & Riggar (2005). Their conclusion was that "the way to initiate cultural diversity is to retrain current rehabilitation professionals and to train future professionals in racial/demography of disability" (p 20) using an experiential knowledge approach.

In 1998, the RSA Commissioner reinforced the need to "ensure the quality of personnel who provide VR services and assist individuals with disabilities to achieve employment outcomes through the VR program (Schroeder, 1998). RSA has also dedicated funds to enhance the development of Rehabilitation personnel.

AMERICANS WITH DISABILITIES ACT

In 1990, the Americans with Disabilities Act (ADA) made it illegal to discriminate against individuals with disabilities (United States Equal Employment Opportunity Commission, 1991). The ADA is divided into five titles: Title I, Employment; Title II, Public Services; Title III, Public Accommodations; Title IV, Telecommunications; and, Title V, Miscellaneous. The legislation is especially important to human resources development, as Title I prohibits discrimination by employers in hiring, promotion, and dismissal. The United States Equal Employment Commission (US EEOC) enforces job discrimination, and any discrimination in state and local government programs and activities is enforced by the Department of Justice (DOJ). Work place accommodations are required by employers with 15 or more employees, according to the Americans with Disabilities Act of 1990. In fact, the ADA specifically prohibits employment discrimination and provides for the hiring of qualified employees who can perform the essential functions of the job with or without reasonable accommodation.

In an effort to examine the conditions that influence accommodations, Geyer and Schroedel (1999) conducted a study involving employees who were deaf or hard of hearing. Using a sample of 232 employees, the researchers sought to determine if accommodations were provided more frequently to individuals with higher education, and in more professional and managerial positions. The findings were consistent with their hypotheses. For employees at higher levels, their is greater investment and the employer may "...more readily conclude that these employees perform the types of essential job functions for which an accommodation can be justified" (p. 48).

It is also important to consider coworker attitudes regarding individuals with disabilities. Hagner (2003) reviewed the literature and made recommendations for specific strategies for employers. Suggestions included having a more supportive culture in the work place, plans for career advancement beyond entry level, and assisting employees' social inclusion and mentoring.

9

DIVERSITY AND DISABILITY IN
HUMAN RESOURCES MANAGEMENT

Culture is significant to the work environment, and subsequently to employee commitment and agency retention. Understanding culture is a significant part of HRD and HRM (Cross, 2000; Huo, Hang, and Napier, 2002; Jackson, 2002; Budwar & Sparrow, 2002). Recall that people learn differently and consider that they also work differently. In their investigation from a feminist framework of hundreds of papers on HRD, Bierema, and Cseh (2002) determined that analysis of race, ethnicity, and gender were severely limited in the literature (Tobias, 1995). The fact that people come from diverse racial, ethnic, gender, disability, and cultural backgrounds is significant in understanding human resources development. Individual values, possibly influenced by national culture, influence organizational commitment (Glazer, Daniel, Short, 2004).

In their study with white counseling students, Evans and Foster (2000) concluded that simple multicultural training, although helpful with information processing, might not lead to the complex thinking necessary for moral development. Cross (2000) stated "cross-cultural management training has mushroomed, and now includes approaches that take into account patterns of racism, sexism, classism, and anti-immigrant sentiment" (p 161). It can be concluded that managing diversity is multifaceted, and involves addressing the ways employees are different and providing fundamental change in the life of the corporation. "Changing the root culture is at the heart of the managing diversity approach" (Thomas, 1991, p 26).

The significance of culture in human resource management and development is reflected in the literature. In their examination of international hiring practices, Huo, Huang, and Napier (2002) determined that as cultures remain different in various countries and regions, and therefore human resources practices vary, there tends to be more divergence of practices as it relates to international recruitment. It is likely that there will be some convergence. Nevertheless, the "...best international human resources management practices ought to be the ones best adapted to cultural and national differences" (p. 42).

In another organizational study examining the differences in valuing people across cultures, Jackson (2002) identified differences in seven nations regarding the locus of human value, and concluded that the West sees people as a means to an end. In a related study on culture, Budwar, and Sparrow (2002) saw the need to develop an integrated framework in order to study human resources

9

policies across nations, noting distinctive differences among variables, strategies, and polices.

Minority recruitment is enhanced legislatively through Section 21(a)(4), Rehabilitation Act, 1998). Section 21 findings indicate a disproportionately high rate of disabilities among ethnic and racial minorities and support recruitment equity. If minority recruitment is to succeed, however, diversity in the work place must be a reality. The approach to the management of diversity is more of an attitudinal concept that directs a comprehensive process of creating an atmosphere of inclusion. Organizations committed to managing and facilitating diversity must provide resources and set policies to support and embrace diversity.

There are multiple strategies for rehabilitation human resources to consider to obtain diversity, and may include the following initiatives: (1) mentoring programs; (2) diverse focus groups; (3) policy revision sessions inclusive of individuals from minority and disability groups; (4) cultural workshops; (5) shadow days; (6) formal recognition programs; (7) accountability measures; and (8) rewarding creative diversity actions. The American Psychological Association (Smith, 2000) provided awards to three universities for their initiatives with recruitment and retention of ethnic minorities.

HUMAN RESOURCES MANAGEMENT AND DEVELOPMENT IN REHABILITATION

Rehabilitation has grown from an occupation into a profession (Parker, & Szymanski (1992). In support of this, the concept of a career development tool for educators has been introduced (Koch, Schultz, and Cusick, 1998). Specifically, this involves the creation of a portfolio for rehabilitation counselors that serve three purposes: (1) educational planning; (2) employment; and (3) career advancement. The rehabilitation profession has historically been synonymous with the State-Federal agency. This is no longer the case (Jenkins, Patterson, Szymanski, 1992) as the field has grown tremendously, and includes private (for profit and not for-profit) agencies.

All rehabilitation agencies, in order to continue effectively, realize that investing in personnel from all backgrounds has become essential. Strategic planning, goal setting, human resources, and personnel needs assessments similar to American businesses, must be done in the rehabilitation profession to shape its future (Wright, 1986). Current practices among public rehabilitation agencies reflect acceptable human resources strategies. Vision and mission statements are incorporated in policy and widely distributed. Agencies also

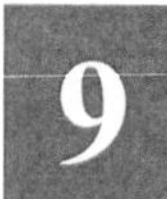

recognize and reward performance. Additionally, federal money has been provided for rehabilitation staff training.

ACCEPTING DIVERSITY

Recognizing differences among agency personnel is an important ingredient in agency functioning. For example, Andrew and Robertson (2001) found consistency between private sector and public rehabilitation agencies as it relates to expecting computer skills in prospective candidates. However, retention is linked to development that extends beyond initial skills. Equally important is the process of developing diverse individuals within the agency. This requires an understanding of the social structure of the agency as well as how the agency functions, leading to insight into how learning and the acquisition of new skills occurs.

Understanding personal beliefs and attitudes regarding others who are different is a start to "helping people master the intrapersonal and interpersonal awareness needed to apply principles of group dynamics and adult learning to race, gender, and other forms of visible difference" (Cross, 2000, p. 144). Sensitivity to diversity is crucial to human resources development in the 21st century. Although some individuals simply embrace the richness that emanates from diversity, diversity is a reality and goes beyond choice (Thomas, 1991). The United States Census Projections for 1999 - 2010 indicate a major increase in minority populations in the United States. This increase in population will impact legislation and become a major component of human resources development.

ACCEPTING DISABILITY

Individuals with disabilities are an integral part of the fabric of society; therefore, a significant factor in the human resources development equation. Stigmas still exist, and confidence and success is directly related to how this is addressed in the work place. Smart (2001) suggests that individuals with disabilities learn to recognize and manage stigmas, acknowledging that although judgments and actions of others may hurt, they do not have to become a part of the individuals' self-concept. Nevertheless, employers have responsibilities.

Employer responsibilities include attention to workplace quality, which impacts employee retention and subsequent organizational commitment. Issues include staff competency, growth, and development. Differences in education, training, abilities, experience, skills, and performance dictate training needs.

212

9

TRAINING NEEDS IN REHABILITATION

This section will examine training and preparation using two categories: (1) Rehabilitation specialists; and (2) Rehabilitation administrators and leaders.

REHABILITATION SPECIALISTS

The concept of rehabilitation specialists is inclusive of such professional areas as counseling, vocational evaluation, and job placement. Specific knowledge and skills as well as specific training areas have interested researchers. Over ten years ago, Linkowski, Thoreson, Diamond, Leahy, Szymanski, and Witty (1993) designed an instrument to validate rehabilitation knowledge standards used in counselor certification. The 57-item instrument included several subscales: (1) Vocational Services; (2) Case Management and Services; (3) Group and Family Issues; (4) Medical and psychological aspects; (5) Foundations of Rehabilitation; (6) Workers Compensation, Employer Services and Technology; (7) Social, Cultural, and Environmental Issues; (8) Research; (9) Individual Counseling and Development; and, (10) Assessment. Subsequently, Szymanski, Linkowski, Leahy, Diamond, and Thoereson (1993), examined human resources development needs of rehabilitation professionals. Counselor knowledge areas, as well as importance, were examined for validation purposes relative to the practice of rehabilitation counseling (Leahy, Szymanski, Linkowski, 1993).

Rehabilitation counselor and specialist knowledge and responsibilities has been of interest for some time, and efforts to measure these factors has resulted in the development of instruments and inventories (Beardsley & Rubin, 1988; Szymanski, et al., 1993). The training and preparation of rehabilitation professionals is essential and impacts effectiveness. For example, training and experience with HIV/AIDS significantly impacts counselor knowledge and skills when working with people with the disease (Glenn, Garcia, Li, Moore, 1998).

Research has clearly demonstrated a direct relationship between the level and type of educational degree and competency (Shapson, Wright, and Leahy, 1987) relative to successful closure (Cook & Bolton, 1992) and this actually varies according to employment settings (Leahy, Shapson, & Wright, 1987). One thing that remains consistent is that multicultural competencies are increasingly in demand (Middleton, Rollins, Sanderson, Leung, Harley, Ebeener, Leal-Idrogo, 2000).

Remaining current is the challenge for the rehabilitation profession, as changes occur rapidly. In fact, several years ago, while counselor education programs tried to keep up with swift legislative shifts, the professional identity and independence of the profession was actually hampered (Hershenson, 1988). That is no longer the case and the profession is firmly established and growing with the support of professional organizations.

PROFESSIONAL BODIES AND ORGANIZATIONS

Today there are four major national professional bodies: (1) Commission on Rehabilitation Counselor Certification; (2) American Rehabilitation Counseling Association; (3) Alliance for Rehabilitation; and (4) National Rehabilitation Counseling Association. The rehabilitation code of ethics, which was established in the 1980s, has remained current and alive through revisions.

The Foundation for Rehabilitation Education and Research (2000) has identified professional credentialing options as indicated in Table I.

Table I

ORGANIZATIONS OFFERING CREDENTIALS RELATED TO REHABILITATION

National Credentials	
CCMC	Certified Case Manager (CCM)
CDMSC	Certified Disability Management Specialist CDMS)
CRCC	Certified Rehabilitation Counselor (CRC);
	Canadian Certified Rehabilitation Counselor (CCRC)
NAADAC	National Certified Addiction Counselor I (NCAC I)
	National Certified Addiction Counselor II (NCAC II)
NBCC	National Certified Counselor (NCC)
	Certified Career Counselor (CCC)
	Certified Clinical Mental Health Counselor (CCMHC)
CCWAVES	Certified Vocational Evaluator (CVE)
State Credentials	
(CADAC)	Certified Alcohol and Drug Abuse Counselor
	Licensed Professional Counselor (LPC)

Other professional organizations include the National Association of Multicultural Rehabilitation Concerns (NAMRC) and the Council of State Administrators of Vocational Rehabilitation (CSAVR), in which every State Director of Public Vocational Rehabilitation usually maintains membership.

9

REHABILITATION ADMINISTRATORS AND LEADERS

Leadership is evolutionary and has generally been studied extensively over the years (Stodgill, 1974, Burns 1978, Bennis, 1989, Bass, 1990). Some will argue that skillful movement of disciplined, decisive, and responsible risk-takers is how leadership talent enters the pipeline (Kesler, 2002). Others declare a connection between relationships and members of groups, and thereby agree with what Stodgill (1948) said:

> Leadership appears to be a working relationship among members of a group, in which the leader acquires status through active participation and demonstration of his [her] capacity for carrying cooperative tasks through to completion.

p. 66

With the recent focus on transformational leadership and extensive research (Yammarino & Bass, 1990; Yammarino & Dubinsky, 1994; Kuhnert & Lewis, 1987, Lowe, Kroeck, & Sivasubramaniam, 1996; Fuller, Morrison, Jones, Bridger, & Brown 1999; Carless, 1998; Sashkin, 1999) many define leadership as transformational. Transformational leaders "use transactional, managerial roles not simply to define, assign, and accomplish tasks and achieve goals, but also to educate, empower, and ultimately transform followers" (Sashkin, 1993, p.20). This is common in public administration. In fact, in a recent study, 97.4% of State VR Directors were found to be transformational leaders (Pointer, 2001).

Public rehabilitation administrators and leaders often develop within the agency and move through internal promotional opportunities. Executive leaders can be appointed, however, and vary substantially in experience and training. Pointer (2001), for example, found 42.3% of respondents to have training fields unrelated to rehabilitation, and State VR Directors were almost equally divided between bachelor and doctoral degrees.

Administrators and leaders have training needs (Matkin, Sawyer, Lorenz, & Rubin, 1989) and require training and preparation in management and competencies (Atkinson, 1997; Corriagan, Garman, Canar, & Lam, 1999; Ford, 1998). As leaders must have the ability to influence, energize, (Glenn, Hawley, & Mann, 2000), lead change, (Crimando, Riggar, & Bordieri, 1988) and provide vision (McFarlane & Griswold, 1992), training and development is also necessary. Due to the nature of rehabilitation, some argue for leader credentialing (Jewkes, 1998), as is the case with rehabilitation specialists.

Leadership occurs through preparation and planning and, conversely, succession planning should be considered more as an assessment and human resources development rather than planning for replacement (Kessler, 2002). Nevertheless, diversity remains an area to consider. In her survey of State

Directors of VR, Pointer (2004) found similar demographic characteristics among state leaders, as was found in a study twenty years ago. The leadership in public rehabilitation continues to be predominately white males who have certain dynamics. On the other hand, in instances when the boss is from a minority group (e.g., African American, Latina), other dynamics are inevitable.

In an unrelated agency, research conducted by Embrick (2005) with males in lower level management positions revealed that racial prejudice is alive and there is a bond between white males. Women, especially minority women, in leadership positions are at a disadvantage. Some benefit has been identified with social capital/mentors (Palgi & Moore, 2004). In another study, Vianello (2004) concluded that although women need more conditions of advantages, once they achieve top positions in public life "they are equal to men in feeling that they exercise power to the same extent as men without the need to be backed by more favorable conditions."

PROGRAMS AND RESOURCES DESIGNED TO ADDRESS HUMAN RESOURCES NEEDS

LONG-TERM AND SHORT-TERM TRAINING PROGRAMS

There are a variety of programs and resources designed to address rehabilitation human resources needs. Colleges and universities with programs accredited by the National Council on Rehabilitation Education (NCRE) exist throughout the nation. Many colleges offer scholarships through federal long-term training grants. Regional Continuing Education Programs and Community Continuing Rehabilitation Programs exist. In addition, there are regional and national rehabilitation leadership programs, all of which can be located via the Internet.

RESOURCES

Selected resources available to rehabilitation are included in this section.

RSA	Rehabilitation Services Administration	Federal agency that administers the Rehabilitation Act
NCRE	National Council on Rehabilitation Education	The association of rehabilitation educators
NIDRR	National Institute on Disability and Rehabilitation Research	Federal agency that funds disability related research
IRI	Institute on Rehabilitation Issues	Federal program that develops training materials on rehabilitation

NARIC	National Rehabilitation Information Clearinghouse	A clearing house of rehabilitation research and training materials
IARP	International Association of Rehabilitation Professionals	Professional organization focusing on consulting, case management, and expert testimony
CSAVR	Council of State Administrators of Vocational Rehabilitation	Has a standing committee on human resource development

ISSUES FOR REHABILITATION IN HUMAN RESOURCES MANAGEMENT AND DEVELOPMENT

Several issues confront the human services nature of rehabilitation, and they are presented briefly for consideration and professional discussion: (1) *Leadership and qualified rehabilitation specialists pools* are impacted as the massive exit (retirement) of rehabilitation professionals continues; (2) *Funding for training and preparedness* is of concern due to the 2003 reauthorization of the Rehabilitation Act which relaxes legislative control of funds; (3) *Tailored training* as globalization leads to subsequent changes in the nature of work (Ryan, 2000), consumer expectancies of community-based rehabilitation programs (Thomas, Menz, Rosenthal, 2001) and other agencies, and continuous advances in assistive technology (Riemer-Reiss, 2003; (4) *Spirituality and subsequent counselor education* (Green, Behshoff, Harris-Forbes, 2003); (5) *Diversity* (6) *Performance appraisals*; (7) *Job functions and guidelines* in workforce investment centers; and, (8) *Education on-line*, as a mechanism to reach diverse and distributed rehabilitation personnel (Glenn, M., Danczyk-Hawkey, C., & Mann, D, 2000).

CONCLUSION

This chapter has examined human resources development and issues in rehabilitation from a review of the literature. Delineation between management and development of personnel was made. Human resources have been examined within the context of theory and legislation, using an approach of diversity (which includes disability) as the underlying theme within the profession of rehabilitation. Personnel training needs, leadership and succession, and related issues have been explored, and programs and resources identified.

SIGNIFICANCE AND IMPLICATIONS FOR TRAINING, PRACTICE, AND RESEARCH

Guided by the ADA, the Rehabilitation Act, and the CSPD, equity in recruitment, retention, training and development, and promotion is strengthened. Training needs exist at every level of personnel (Pointer, 2001; Froelich, et al., 1998; Linkowski, et, al., 1993), and in specific areas (Glenn, et al., 1998). Issues such as succession planning, credentialing, leadership, diversity, funding, on-line education (Glenn, et al., 2000), and spirituality will continue to surface and move to the forefront.

Higher education will be especially challenged as a result of this literature review, as it is significant and has implications for training, practice, performance, and future research. First, there is urgency in training. Recruitment and retention of qualified personnel will be guided by societal, technological, and economic changes, and the applicant pool will reflect increased diversity and disability. Appropriate, continuous upgrading of skills in a cost effective and refined timeframe is necessary. Funding sources for training may become scarce with the 2003 reauthorization changes in the Rehabilitation Act. Consequently, more creative ways to include a larger and more diversified personnel pool will be critical. Finally, transformational leadership will be essential in a global and increasingly diverse environment.

Areas for future research include rehabilitation human resources development, agency leadership, support personnel needs, agency effectiveness, personnel needs in a workforce environment, and differences in human resources development practices.

REFERENCES

Americans with Disabilities Act (1990).

Andrew, J., & Robertson, J. (2001. Private-sector computer skills expectations for rehabilitation counselor job applicants. *Rehabilitation Education, 15*(3), 295-299.

Atkins, D. (1997). Rehabilitation management and leadership competencies. *Journal of Rehabilitation Administration, 21*(4), 249-261.

Beardsley, M., & Rubin, S., (1988). Rehabilitation service providers: An investigation of generic job tasks and knowledge. *Rehabilitation Counseling Bulletin 32*, 122-135.

Bierema, L., & Cseh, M. (2003). Evaluating AHRD research using a feminist research framework. *Human Resource Development Quarterly, 14*(1), 5-21.

Blankenship, C., & Crimando, W. (2003). Effectiveness of a performance appraisal training program in increasing knowledge and decreasing discomfort among   rehabilitation supervisors. *Journal of Rehabilitation Administration, 27*(1), 11-22.

Budwar, P., & Sparrow, P. (2002). An integrative framework for understanding cross-national human resource management practices. *Human Resource Management Review, 12*(2002), 377-403.

Clark, R., Anderson, N. B., Clark, V., & Williams, D. R. (1999). Racism as a stressor for African Americans: A biopsychosocial model. *American Psychologist, 54,* 805-816.

Cook, D., & Bolton, G. (1992). Rehabilitation counselor education and case performance: An independent replication. *Rehabilitation Counseling Bulletin, 36*(1), 37-43.

Crimando, W., Riggar, R., Bordieri, J.(1988). Proactive change management in rehabilitation: An idea whose time has been. *Journal of Rehabilitation Administration*, February 1988, 20-22.

Cross, E. (2000). *Managing Diversity: The Courage to Lead*. Connecticut: Quorum Books.

DeCenzo, D. & Robbins, S. (1999). *Human Resource Management. 6th ed.* New York: John Wiley & Sons.

Embrick, D. G. (2005). Race-talk within the workplace: Exploring ingroup/outgroup and public/private dimensions. *The Journal of Intergroup Relations, 32*(51), 3-17.

Evans, K. M. & Foster, V. A. (2000). Relationships among multicultlural training, moral development, and racial identity development of white counseling students. *Counseling and Values, 45*(1), 39-48.

Ferris, G., Berkson, H., Harris, M (2002). The recruitment interview process: Persuasion and organization reputation promotion in competitive labor markets. *Human Resource Management Review, 12*(2002), 359-375.

Flowers, C. R., Forbes, W. S., Crimando, W., Riggar, T. F. (2005). A regional survey of rehabilitation cultural diversity within CILs: A ten-year follow-up. *Journal of Rehabilitation 71*(2), 14-21.

Ford, L. H. (1998). Measuring rehabilitation management and leadership competencies. *Journal of Rehabilitation Administration, 21*(4), 263-272.

Foundation for Rehabilitation Education and Research (2000). *Rehabilitation Counseling: The Profession and Standards of Practice*, Illinois.

Froehlich, Garcia, & Linkowski (1998). Minimum hiring requirements for rehabilitation counselors in states: A comparison across federal regions. *Rehabilitation Education 12*(3), 193-203.

Geyer, P., & Schroedel, J. (1999). Conditions influencing the availability of accommodations for workers who are deaf or hard-of-hearing. *Journal of Rehabilitation 65*(2), 42-50.

Glazer, S. Daniel, S.C., Short, K. M. (2004). A study of the relationship between organizational commitment and human values in four countries. *Human Relations 57*(3), 323-345.

Glenn M., Danczyk-Hawley, C., & Mann, D. (2000). Rehabilitation leadership on line. *Journal of Rehabilitation 24*(1), 25-35.

Glenn, M., Garcia, J., Li. L., & Moore, D. (1998). Preparation of rehabilitation counselors to serve people living with HIV/AIDS. *Rehabilitation Counseling Bulletin, 41(3)*, 190-199.

Gomez, J., & Michaelis, R., (1995). As assessment of burnout in human service providers. *Journal of Rehabilitation*, January/February/March, 23-26.

Goss, D. (1994). *Principles of Human Resource Management*. Routledge: New York.

Green, R. L., Benshoff, J.J., & Harris-Forbes, J., A. (2003). Spirituality in rehabilitation counselor education: A pilot survey. *Journal of Rehabilitation, 67*(3), 55-60.

Hager D. (2003). What we know about preventing and managing coworker resentment or rejection. *Journal of Applied Rehabilitation Counseling 34*(1).

Harley, D. (2002). Book review of management of human service programs. *Journal of Rehabilitation Administration, 26*(3), 193-195.

Hernandez, B., Balcazar. F. (2000). Employer attitudes toward workers with disabilities and their ADA employment rights: A literature review. *Journal or Rehabilitation, 66*(4), 4-16.

Hershenson, D. B. (1988). Along for the ride: The evolution of rehabilitation counselor education. *Rehabilitation Counseling Bulletin, 31*, 204-217.

Huo, P., Huang, H., & Napier, N. (2002). Divergence or convergence: A cross-national comparison of personnel selection practices. *Human Resource Management, 41*(1), 31-44.

Jackson, T. (2002) The management of people across cultures: valuing people differently. *Human Resource Management, 41*(4), 455-475

Jenkins, W. J., Patterson, J. B., & Symanski, E. M. (1992). Philosophical, historical, and legislative aspects of the rehabilitating counseling profession. In R. M. Parker & E. M. Szymanski (Eds.) *Rehabilitation Counseling* (2nd ed.) Texas: Pro-ed.

Jewkes, L. F. (1988). Professional rehabilitation comments and challenges in *Journal of Rehabilitation Administration*, November 1988.

Kesler, G. (2002). Why leadership bench never gets deeper: Ten insights about executive talent development. *Human Resource Planning, 25*(3), 32-44.

Lee, Courtland. (1997). The promise and pitfalls of multicultural counseling. In C. C. Lee (Ed.). *Multicultural Issues in Counseling* (2nd ed.). Virginia: American Counseling Association.

Leahy, M. J., Shapson, P., & Wright, G. (1987). Rehabilitation practitioner competencies by role and setting. *Rehabilitation Counselor Bulletin*, December 1987, 119-130.

Leahy, M., Szymanski, E., & Linkowski, D. L. (1993). Knowledge importance in rehabilitation counseling. *Rehabilitation Counseling Bulletin*, 37(2), 130-145.

Linkowski, D. L., Thoreson, R. W., Diamond, E., E., Leahy, M., J., Szymanski, E. M., & Witty, T., (1993). Instrument to validate rehabilitation counseling accreditation and certification knowledge areas. *Rehabilitation Counseling Bulletin, 37*(2), 123-129.

Mallik, K. & Lemaire, G. (2003). Assessing departing employee's perceptions may lead to organizational change to reduce staff turnover. *Journal of Rehabilitation Administration, 27*(1), 23-32.

Matkin, R. E., Sawyer, H. W., Lorenz, J. R., & Rubin, S. E.(1982). Rehabilitation Administrators and supervisors: Their work assignments, training needs, and suggestions for preparation. *Journal or Rehabilitation Administration*, 170-187.

Middleton, R., Rollins, C., Sanderson, P., Leung, P., Harley, D., Ebener, D., & Leal-Idrogo, A. (2000) Endorsement of professional multicultural rehabilitation competencies and standards: A call to action. *Rehabilitation Counseling Bulletin, 43*(4), 219-240.

Palgi, M. More, G. (2004). Social Capital: Mentors and contracts. *Current Sociology, 52*(3), 459-480.

Parker, R., & Szymanski, E. (1992). *Rehabilitation Counseling: Basics and Beyond (*2nd ed.) Texas: Pro-ed.

Pederson, P. (1994). *A Handbook for Developing Multicultural Awareness*, 2nd ed. Virginia: ACA.

Pointer, M. P., (2004). Characteristics and leadership styles of state administrators of vocational rehabilitation. *Journal of Rehabilitation Administration, 27*(3 & 4), 83-93.

Pointer, M. P. (2002). The relationship between transformational leadership, self-reported knowledge, education, educational relevancy, and experience among state vocational rehabilitation directors and rehabilitation rate. *Dissertation Abstracts International*, (UMI No. 3029590).

Powell, G. & Butterfield, D. (2002). Exploring the influence of decision makers race and gender on actual promotions to top management. *Personnel Psychology, Inc., 55*, 397-428.

Rehabilitation Services Administration United States Department of Education, (1998). *Rehabilitation Act of 1973 As Amended*, Washington, DC.

Riemer-Reiss, M. Rehabilitation professionals' perceived competencies in assistive technology selection and referral: A preliminary analysis (2003). *Journal of Applied rehabilitation Counseling, 34*(2), 33-36.

Rosenbach, W. E., & Taylor. R. L., (1994). *Contemporary Issues in Leadership 4th ed*. Westview Press.

Ryan, C., (1995). Work isn't what it used to be: Implications, recommendations, and strategies for vocational rehabilitation. *Journal of Rehabilitation* October/November/December, 8-15.

Schroeder, F. (1998). Commissioner's memorandum cm-98-12. *Rehabilitation Services Administration*, Washington, DC.

Shapeson, P., Wright, G., & Leahy, M. (1987). Education and attainment of rehabilitation competencies. *Rehabilitation Counseling Bulletin*, December 1987, 131-145.

Smith, D. (2000). Psychology departments recognized for ethnic-minority recruitment, retention. *Monitor on Psychology, 31*(11), 14.

Souza, G. (2002). A study of the influence of promotions on promotion satisfaction and expectations of future promotions among managers. *Human Resource Development Quarterly, 13*(3), 325-340.

Stodgill, R. (1948). Personal factors associated with leadership: A survey of the literature. *Journal of Psychology, 25*, 35-71

Szymanski, E., Leahy, M., & Linkowski, D.(1993). Reported preparedness of certified counselors in rehabilitation counseling knowledge areas. *Rehabilitation Counseling Bulletin, 37*(2), 146-161.

Szymanski, E., Linkowski, D., Leahy, M., Diamond, E., & Thoreson, R. (1993). Human resource development: An examination of perceived training needs of certified   rehabilitation counselors. *Rehabilitation Counseling Bulletin, 37*(2), 163-181.

Szymanski, E. Linkowski, D., Leahy, M., Diamond, E., & Thoreson, R. (1993). Validation of rehabilitation counseling accreditation and certification knowledge areas: Methodology and initial results. *Rehabilitation Counseling Bulletin, 37*(2), 13-121.

Thomas, R. R. (1991). *Beyond Race and Gender*. New York: AMACOM.

Tobias, C. U. (1995). *The Way We Work: What you Know About Working Styles Can Increase Your Efficiency, Productivity, and Job Satisfaction.* Tennessee: Broadman and Holman.

Wolf, A. W. Wright, G. (1986). Professional perspectives and planning. In T. F. Riggar, D.T. Maki, & A. W. Wolf (Eds.), *Applied Rehabilitation Counseling,* 12-20. New York: Springer.

Valle, M. (1999). Crisis, culture and charisma: The new leader's work in public organizations. *Public Personnel Management, 28*(2) 245-257.

Vianello, M. (2004). Gender differences and power. *Current Sociology, 52*(3), 507-517.

Yancy, G. (2004). Historical varieties of African American labor: Sites of agency and resistance. *Western Journal of Black Studies, 28*(2), 337-353.

CHAPTER 10

REHABILITATION TECHNOLOGY:
MORE THAN ASSISTIVE TECHNOLOGY FOR MULTICULTURAL CONSUMERS

YOLANDA V. EDWARDS
DOTHEL W. EDWARDS, JR.
DION F. PORTER

Chapter Highlights

➡ Assistive technology

➡ Technology used in career development and job placement

➡ Technology used in career assessment on multicultural consumers

➡ Computer competency among rehabilitation professionals

➡ Technology used in training rehabilitation professionals

➡ Summary

$\mathcal{R}$ehabilitation technology has lead to accessible environments for all people including paving the way for greater productivity and self-sufficiency among consumers with disabilities. Technology has had a profound impact on the knowledge, services, employment, and social exchange opportunities available for consumers with disabilities (Ritchie & Blanck, 2003; Bricout, 2004).

Rehabilitation professions now use rehabilitation technology in research, information dissemination, case management, job development, placement procedures, and even in education programs. In the past, rehabilitation technology has been synonymous with assistive technology. Technology in rehabilitation has also branched into areas including computer-assisted therapy. While there has been an enormous growth of technology in the field of rehabilitation, consumers with disabilities and minorities still have far less access to the Internet and assistive technology (Guo, Bricout & Huang, 2005). The "Digital Divide" has serious economic consequences for disadvantaged minority and disability groups, as demand for technical skills increases in the labor market.

This chapter will examine all areas of technology use in rehabilitation and some of the issues and emerging problems in each area for multicultural consumers and rehabilitation professionals. The areas that will be covered are assistive technology, technology in career and job placement and development, technology used in case management, computer competency among rehabilitation professionals, technology used in training rehabilitation professionals (e.g. distance education), and computer assisted therapy.

ASSISTIVE TECHNOLOGY

LEGISLATION, CATEGORIES, AND ATTITUDES PERTAINING TO ASSISTIVE TECHNOLOGY

Functional limitations are the limits to individual functioning that are experienced by consumers with disabilities, ultimately infringing on their independence or freedom (Riemer-Reiss, 2000; Rubin & Roessler, 2001). In order to minimize these functional limitations, assistive technology was developed for the purpose of greater productivity and self-sufficiency, thus allowing these consumers to better cope with social, vocational, and daily living demands (Rubin & Roessler, 2001; Scherer, 2000). Assistive technology was implemented to bridge the gap between a disability and its associated impairment, and promote further independence at home, work, and within society as a whole. Assistive technology, devices, and equipment have become very important for consumers who have experienced a loss, such as a limb or other major body part or organ (Falvo, 1999).

EARLY LEGISLATION

According to Rubin & Roessler (2001) and Cook & Hussey (2002), "the Technology-Related Assistance for Individuals with Disabilities Act of 1988 (Tech Act; P.L. 100-407) defines an assistive technology device as a piece of equipment, an item, or system which is used to increase, maintain, or improve the functional capability of a person with a disability, handicap, or impairment." These items or pieces of equipment were developed for consumers with disabilities in order to make their lives as independent as possible, both at home and at their place of employment. For the estimated 54 million Americans with disabilities, assistive technology has served, at times, as a medium between the individual with a disability and the world of work and independence (Rubin & Roessler, 2001; Scherer, 2000).

The Assistive Technology Act of 1998 was initially passed by Congress to provide grants to States in order to address the assistive technology needs of consumers with disabilities throughout this country (Scherer, 2000). When considering legislation such as Technology-Related Assistance for Persons with Disabilities Act, and Assistive Technology Act of 1998, we must remember that the focus of these important pieces of legislation was to assist not only consumers with disabilities, but also consumers with catastrophic and permanent disabilities (Galvin & Scherer, 1996).

CATEGORIES OF ASSISTIVE TECHNOLOGY

There are several different categories of assistive technology devices and equipment that are used by many of the estimated 54 million American consumers with disabilities. The following list provides just some of the categories of assistive technology devices that are commonly employed today:

- Aids for Daily Living
- Augmentative Communication Devices
- Computer Applications
- Environmental Control Systems
- Home/Worksite Modifications
- Prosthetics and Orthotics
- Seating and Positioning
- Aids for Vision/Hearing Impaired
- Wheelchairs/Mobility Aids
- Vehicle Modifications

(Rubin and Roessler, 2001, p. 402)

These various categories of assistive technology have enabled many consumers with disabilities to not only live a more independent and higher functioning life, but also to use these devices to improve their productivity at the worksite (Cohen, 2002). According to Cohen (2002), improvements in areas

226

such as voice recognition software, wireless technology, and other mainstream technology have had a tremendous impact on the vocational productivity of millions of consumers with disabilities, and their ability to readily complete job tasks and effectively do their jobs.

Scherer (2000) suggests that certain *design factors* contribute to the highest rate of use of assistive technology devices by consumers with disabilities. Some of these design factors include:

- Lightweight and portable
- Easy to use and set up
- Compatible with other devices
- Cost-effective to obtain and maintain
- Safe and reliable
- Attractive as well as durable
- The same or similar devices used by the non-disabled population

p. 133

Cohen (2002) suggests that consumers with certain disabilities, such as quadriplegia, paraplegia, and dexterity limitations as caused by cerebral palsy, can benefit from certain types of assistive technology products. One such type of assistive technology device is Keyboard Filters, which include typing aids like word prediction utilities and add-on spelling checkers. These products, which will suggest words based on the first one or two letters typed, assist in reducing the required keystrokes for an individual wanting to input large amounts of information (Cohen, 2000).

ASSISTIVE TECHNOLOGY IN HIGHER EDUCATION

It is estimated that 8 to 12 percent of students in the American higher education system have disabilities that may require special attention or some type of assistive technology device (Roach, 2002). According to Roach (2002), federal statutes dating back to the 1970's and the 1990 Americans with Disabilities Act (ADA) have played a very critical role in pushing schools to make their campuses physically assessable to consumers with disabilities. The National Center for Education Statistics at the U.S. Department of Education (2002) reports that 6% of all undergraduates enrolled in American institutions of higher education reported having a disability in 1995-1996, while 72% of all higher education institutions enrolled students with some type of disability in 1996-1998. Ninety-eight percent of community colleges enrolled students with disabilities in 1996-1998.

The explosion of the Internet and the World Wide Web has ushered in demands that institutions of higher education accommodate students with disabilities with what is known as assistive technology. Roach (2002) asserts that assistive technology, or technology that is information and media oriented, is just as important as the media technology that is provided to students, such as the Internet and the World Wide Web. The Center on Disabilities at the California State University at Northridge (CSUN) has developed a certificate program to train disabilities service professionals within higher education on various aspects of working with and providing services to students with disabilities. Roach (2002) contends that annually, some 4,000 people attend the "Technology and Persons with Disabilities" conference sponsored by CSUN, which has been rapidly expanding every year since its inception.

ATTITUDES TOWARD ASSISTIVE TECHNOLOGY DEVICES

Attitudes toward consumers with disabilities play an important role in how they view society and non-disabled persons. There are certain attitudes that are directed toward assistive technology devices, not only by the non-disabled person who has never used the device, but also by the individual who actually uses the equipment (Reimer-Reiss, 2000; Rubin & Roessler, 2001). Attitudes toward the device by the user generally are based on specific characteristics of the device, including cost. Cohen (2002) asserts that one of the greatest perceived barriers to implementing assistive technology in the workplace is cost. Other than cost and operating expenses, there are specific factors that may lead an individual who uses a specific device to develop a negative attitude toward that assistive item or equipment. There may be certain characteristics of the assistive technology which may make a user abandon the device altogether. Scherer (2000) lists such characteristics:

- The device did not improve independent living functioning
- Servicing and repair were difficult to obtain and/or were very expensive
- The device was too difficult to use, performed unreliably, or required too much assistance from an outside person

p. 132

Reimer-Reiss (2000) contend that there are many factors that lead to consumers developing negative attitudes toward their assistive technology devices, and ultimately discontinuing their use. Some of these factors include compatibility and the degree to which the user could experiment with the device prior to acquisition.

Not all users of assistive technology hold the same sentiments concerning their devices. Attitudes and overall satisfaction with their assistive devices may come down to what their individual needs and requirements are (Riemer-Reiss, 2000; Scherer, 2000). Even though all attitudes toward assistive technology are not negative ones, overall satisfaction will depend on whether or not the device

228

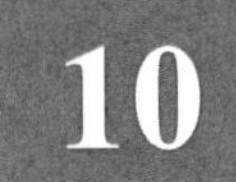

required by that individual will ultimately serve the individual's needs, and assist the person in becoming as independent and self reliant as possible.

MULTICULTURAL CONSUMERS USE OF AT DEVICES

While there have been several programs to increase the number of minorities who use assistive technology, large numbers of minorities with disabilities are still unable to access assistive technology because of their inability to secure low interest loans. Dalto (2003), working with an outreach program trying to increase the use of technology by minorities in the state of Maryland, found that 81% of the applicants surveyed had been turned down for assistive technology loans. One of the barriers for consumers with disabilities is limited income that prevents them from borrowing and/or making payments. Many consumers with disabilities do not qualify for low interest rate loans because of a poor credit history or having a debt to income ratio that is too high (Hammond, 2003). Success has been achieved, however, by employing targeted marketing strategies, partnerships with other agencies, and increasing consumers' incomes (Dalto, 2003; Hammond, 2003).

TECHNOLOGY USED IN CAREER DEVELOPMENT AND JOB PLACEMENT

The process of career development, as defined by Herr & Cramer (1996), involves the person's creation of a career pattern, a decision-making style, integration of life roles, values expression, and life roles self concepts. With this process, career counselors have been charged to provide the best possible career counseling to those that they serve. Prior to the mid 1960s, career counseling was practiced much as it was practiced in the early 20th century. Niles and Harris-Bowlsbey (2002) indicate that this form of career counseling involves the process of human-to-human interaction between the counselor and the consumer. The steps of career counseling include (a) self-assessment of one's interests, skills, values, goals, background, and resources; (b) study of all of the available options for school, additional training, employment, and occupations; and (c) a careful reasoning about which choice was best in light of information uncovered in the first two steps. The infusion of computer technology within these steps of career counseling became more prominent in the mid 1960s (Niles and Harris-Bowlsbey, 2002). Noted career counseling professionals, such as Joann Harris-Bowlsby, Donald E. Super, David Tiedemen, Martin Katz, and others, use the computer as a valuable tool in the career counseling profession (Niles and Harris-Bowlsbey, 2002). The field of career development has utilized a diverse cadre of technology such as test-scoring machines, telephone, and audio and video systems to provide career guidance and job placement. The advent of computers, however, has been of the most benefit to career counselors (Niles & Harris-Bowlsbey, 2002).

During the mid 1960s, through the 1980s, computer assisted career guidance systems were developed according to two methods (Issaacson & Brown, 2000). The first method utilized computers to present occupational and educational information. The second method utilized computers to provide self-information, decision-making strategies, and career development concepts (Issaacson & Brown, 2000). Prominent career theorists such as Donald E. Super, David Tiedeman, Martin Katz, and Anne Roe primarily developed and used computer assisted career guidance systems to foster their career development theories (Niles & Harris-Bowlsbey, 2002). These computer assisted career guidance systems also provided a means for the professional to record summaries of a person's use of the computerized system for the purpose of follow-through, and it allowed the user the take control of decision-making aspects of the process (Niles & Harris-Bowlsbey, 2002).

In the 1990s, computer assisted career guidance systems moved from large, mainframe systems that required the professional to spend large amounts of time and money to operate, to a more "dynamic" and "user friendly" tool (Issaacson & Brown, 2000). Currently, the nature of computer assisted career guidance systems infuse the procedures of storing and retrieving information about occupational data, educational settings, and training facilities with the career planning process (Issaacson & Brown, 2000). With this merger, the field of career counseling has evolved to include career planning and information systems as a stand-alone or a network system (Niles & Harris-Bowlsbey, 2002). As technology continues to improve, so will the capabilities of computer assisted career planning systems.

Niles and Harris-Bowlsbey (2002) indicated strengths of computer assisted systems include (1) test and inventory administration and interpretation; (2) database searches; (3) cross-walking that involves relating one database to another; (4) computers capable of delivering information and/or services in a consistent method; (5) computers with the ability to monitor a person's progress and be able to report the person's progress at any time to anyone who needs to know; and (6) computers that allow interactive instruction for a variety of career counseling related activities such as cyber counseling. With these capabilities, it would appear that computer assisted guidance systems would invariably signal the "end-all-be-all" solution for the profession. It is important to understand that despite the seemingly limitless potential of computer assisted career guidance systems, the use of technology such as the computer should always be considered a tool for the user. Caution should be taken to be aware of the potential limitations and ethical considerations when selecting technology, such as the computer, to assist with the career guidance process. Research indicates that consumers come to the career planning process with a plethora of personal and environmental backgrounds (Axelson, 1999). According to Tabor & Luzzo (1999), users of computer assisted career guidance systems should be given a combination of human-to-human interaction and computer assisted career guidance services. They further mention that counselors should first assess if the consumer is able to utilize the computer and apply the data retrieved from the system correctly and efficiently, and secondly, be able to explain the results of tests and inventories to consumers so that they will be able to make good career planning or placement decisions. Kilvinghan, Johnston, Hogan, and Mauer (1994) evaluated computerized career counseling and found that consumers who are highly motivated and goal directed benefited from computerized career counseling, and those consumers with less clear goals, who were less motivated for independence, did not benefit as much. They suggested that computer career counseling software be used as an adjunct to individual and group counseling.

Professional codes of ethics, such as the codes of the American Counseling Association (ACA) and the Commission on Rehabilitation Counselor Certification (CRCC), require the use of interventions such as computer assisted career planning and placement systems according to a consumer's needs and abilities. The operation and/or administration procedures should be explained, and follow-up by the career counselor should be conducted to determine if the consumer has difficulties or misunderstandings.

TECHNOLOGY USED IN CAREER ASSESSMENT ON MULTICULTURAL CONSUMERS

Shafer (2002) stated that there are no existing career development theories that have been developed specifically for one culture. Research has been done on the appropriateness of existing career development theories for specific cultural groups. For example, Shafer indicates that within the field of career development, more research has been conducted on African Americans than on other multicultural groups (Rojewski, 1994; Brown, 1997; Westbrook & Sanford, 1991; and Fouad & Kelly, 1992). There have been other studies that examined the career development of Hispanic Americans, Asian Americans, and Native Americans (Arbona, 1990; Leong & Serifica, 1995). However, there are no universal or culture specific career development theories. According to Niles & Harris-Bowlsbey (2002), this is due, in part, to the incompatible nature of the mainstream culture verses the specific culture of the person. The authors could find little research that has been done on multicultural consumers with disabilities as it relates to career development, and specifically, no research that has been done on multicultural consumers in regard to technology.

Axelson (1993) stated that much of computer interaction in technology career assessment is individually centered, which can lead to the possibility of "self-counseling." He believes that self-counseling will lead to a need for expertise in cross-cultural input, both for the content of programmed materials and for an appropriate and sequential format through which it is presented. While cross-cultural expertise for programming of authentic material might seem analogous to and suitable for culturally diverse consumers, the impact of technology on career guidance services still needs to emphasize the need for continuous planning to meet consumers' needs. Axelson suggested two basic questions we need to examine: (1) How will technology affect counselors' work environment and client interaction? and (2) What are the emerging trends? He envisioned future direct intervention of a human service professional to become more like a technician who provides consumers with the appropriate programmed materials. While this would standardize many of the career development opportunities, multicultural consumers have a variety of other factors that might affect career development technology, such as education, poverty, prejudice, and personal expectations.

Axelson (1993), for example, stated that access to education and employment opportunities is more difficult for consumers under poverty conditions. Developing a career can be expensive, and low-income people have fewer resources that might enable them to take advantage of available education, to commute to work, or to move to another geographical area where employment or occupational opportunities are more readily available. According to Axelson (1993), Hispanics and Blacks make up 47% of poor persons. Consumers with disabilities, particularly those with significant disabilities, remain the most marginalized group in America in terms of employment and economic opportunities, with employment rates of only 26% and earnings less than 50% of their non-disabled counterparts. For minority consumers with disabilities, the employment picture is even worse (U.S. Census Bureau, 2002).

Although standardized, the process of career development with technology will enhance the number of consumers served. Prejudice and discrimination against racial/ethnic/disability groups in employability in the workplace caused by preconceptions and stereotypes held by counselors tend to result in an underestimate of actual potentialities, and strengths are often overlooked. Axelson (1993) states that personal expectations of the counselors and consumers themselves generally reflect ingrained attitudes. Goals of the counselor must first revolve around altering states of mind or pessimistic expectations, rather than focusing on finding employment.

COMPUTER COMPETENCY AMONG
REHABILITATION PROFESSIONALS

In today's Information Age, rehabilitation professionals must operate with both an understanding of the profession and its place in the world (Warn, 1999). The major trend in rehabilitation services is new tools, and computerized approaches have expanded to case management. State vocational rehabilitation (VR) agencies and community based rehabilitation agencies have begun to move quickly toward incorporating computers into the day-to-day operation of their service delivery system. Andrew & Sabik (2001) surveyed 74 of the 80 state vocational rehabilitation directors. They reported word processing, email, and the ability to access the Internet as important computer skills. Although only 13 states required those computer skills, eighty-one percent (81%) expected new VR counselors to have those skills at employment.

Flynn (1997) examined computer access among VR professionals and found that all staff had computers on their desks. Participants indicated that the primary use of computers by VR agencies and community rehabilitation agency counselors is for case management, with 52 agencies use a counselor-accessible computerized case management system. Another important computer use is accessing the Internet. Thirty-five percent of counselors with computer access had total access to the Internet, while an additional 27% had partial (shared) access.

NEED FOR COMPUTER COMPETENT PERSONNEL

Andrew & Sabik (2001) identified a need for computer competent rehabilitation personnel. They indicated that VR agencies were requiring computer skills or expecting prospective counselors to have those computer skills. They recommended that rehabilitation education programs assume more responsibility for providing basic computer skills by offering instruction, peer tutoring, or any approach that would be cost-effective.

Edwards, Portman, & Bethea (2002) examined the computer competency of counselor education students and found that computer competency increased with an introductory course. Areas of weakness still existed, including assisting consumers with Internet searches, and using statistical packages, list serves, and CD-ROMs. Included in this same study was the measurement of students' motivation towards computers, which revealed that no group differences existed on motivational factors. Some researchers still believe that students' motivation is low toward computer use. Lee and Pulvino (1988) stated that counseling students were reluctant to use computers because they viewed the computers as having little relationship to the human qualities that are associated with their field. Although this may be a weakness in counselor education

233

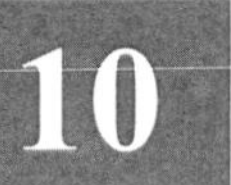

programs, it is something that can be remedied. Other studies have shown that inclusion of technology in courses can greatly improve students' attitudes. For example, Crimando and Baker (1984) compared the effects of regular lecture and computer assisted instruction (CAI) in teaching 30 students in a master's level rehabilitation education program. The CIA group achieved significantly better results on the post-test and responded more positively to the particular question on the attitude survey that stated, "I enjoyed this session." Crimando and Baker concluded that "If CAI and efficient formats like it are used for concept mastery, instructors and students will then have more time to critically examine the material, discuss its implications, and test its power in actual practice" (p. 54).

IMPLICATIONS FOR MULTICULTURAL PERSONNEL WHO ARE COMPETENT IN TECHNOLOGY

As the need for more competent personnel persists, there is going to be a need for multicultural personnel who are skilled in using technology. There still is disparity between racial and disability groups in their access to computers and the Internet. Caucasian American and Asian American households were twice as likely to have access to a computer and Internet in their homes as African Americans and Latina households. Some of the recent research shows an increase in computer and Internet usage for all racial groups, especially African Americans and Latina users, which are growing at a more rapid rate (NTIA, 2002). In addition to race, education and income are major variables that affect technology use. Education prepares people to learn new technology skills, and procedures required to enter the new technological world. NTIA (2000) reported that college educated consumers are six times more likely to have home computer or home Internet access than those with elementary school educations, regardless of race. Income was a major determinant to whether an individual can afford to buy a home or pay from Internet access. Consumers with fewer economic resources, including rural, female, minority, and disability households, do not access computers and Internet at home, because they are expensive.

Wilson, Wallin, and Reisser (2003) concluded that the gaps between race and disability would close as the cost of computers and access to the Internet decrease. They also concluded that disparities will close as difficulty of learning to use new and unfamiliar technology decreases and procedures become more user friendly and more commonplace. New technology will be perceived as being important to successful careers if parents and communities devote more resources toward it. One of the more significant findings is that African American and Caucasian Americans were equally willing to learn new job skills over the Internet, suggesting that the differences in material possessions should not be mistaken for differences in attitudes and beliefs.

TECHNOLOGY USED IN TRAINING REHABILITATION PROFESSIONALS

DISTANCE EDUCATION

The growing demand to serve a diverse population has increased the emphasis in higher education on training and retraining, coupled with trends toward multiple careers or changes in careers (Berge, 1996). Rehabilitation education programs have followed this trend by continuing to offer growing numbers of courses and programs of study through distance education technologies. There is a need in higher education to provide degree programs or certification that can be delivered to students without regard to place and time. There have also been problems accommodating the increasing number of adult learners in higher education. It is believed that these problems can be resolved by education or training through alternative classroom methods, such as distance education.

One of the potential problems in reaching diverse students is accommodating different cultures while paying attention to diverse learning styles associated with various ethnic groups and disability groups. Western views, for example, are individualistic, dualistic in thinking; their worldview is superior and task oriented. The non-western view is group cooperation, time is relative, worldview is other cultures and socially oriented. Sanchez & Gunawardena (1999) stated that educators must find a connection between culture and learning style to have effective education.

A second potential issue is reaching diverse students with disabilities. Little is known about diverse students with disabilities because the federal law prohibits requiring students to identify themselves on forms as disabled. Therefore, there are no statistics on this group. Paist (1995) estimated 3% of in-state students enrolled in the University of Wisconsin Extension Independent Study program have either visual, auditory, physical, or learning disabilities. Paist foresees that percentages will increase with greater availability of technology and accessibility for students with disabilities. More students are using university and college student disability services as the effects of the Americans with Disabilities Act spread. Many universities that make extensive use of distance education are putting an emphasis on services for students with disabilities. For example, Vincent (1995) stated that the Open University of the United Kingdom reported, of 5,000 undergraduate students, about 5% had a reported disability. Vincent further reported that the number of students with disabilities had grown approximately 10% per year; higher than the general enrollment rate. He ascribes this growth to convenience of home study, and the ability of information technology to overcome barriers to learning for students with disabilities.

COMPUTER ASSISTED THERAPY

Computer assisted counseling exists in a variety of forms. Some programs offer therapeutic consultation (Peterson 2003), clinical supervision (Peterson, 2003), computer based interpretation (Butcher, 1987; Fowler, 1985), and on-line therapy. As computer technology has become more affordable and desktop and laptop computers have grown in number, tasks such as written papers and face-to-face meetings have been transferred to computerized technologies. Meeting and interacting with each other online has become an everyday experience. One of the areas in which technology has improved is online therapy. Tyler and Sabella (2003) estimated that 275 practitioners offered direct counseling services via the Internet in 1996. More recently, Tyler and Guth (in press) performed an Internet search and found online counseling services, with 78% using email, 57% text chat (chat room), and 47% using the telephone as a mode for providing counseling services. It is clear that online counseling is a growing form of communication for consumers.

One of the problems for multicultural consumers is access to the technology itself. As the digital divide continues to grow, multicultural consumers show increasing disparity in their access to computers and Internet. A second problem is that computer assisted therapy is not well understood by the general public. Tyler and Sabella (2003) stated that traditional or face-to-face counseling, even with its long history, is still not well understood by the general public and multicultural groups. They believe that introducing online counseling will confuse the general public and multicultural groups even more.

SUMMARY

Technology shows tremendous potential for greater productivity and self-sufficiency among multicultural consumers with disabilities, especially within the areas of knowledge, services, employment, and social exchange (Ritchie & Blanck, 2003; Bricout, 2004). Rehabilitation professions and multicultural consumers are now using rehabilitation technology in research, information dissemination, case management, job development and placement procedures, distance education, and computer assisted therapy. While technology shows growth and promise for professionals and multicultural consumers, consumers still have far less access to the Internet and assistive technology (Guo, Bricout & Huang, 2005), which could have economic consequences and result in a lack of technical skills in the technological labor market. Multicultural consumers

236

and professionals must understand the potentials and opportunities technology affords to us, evaluate how technology is used, and consider the impact that technology has on our lives.

REFERENCES

Andrew, J. & Sabik, S. (1999). Computer skills expectations for rehabilitation counseling job applicants. *Rehabilitation Education, 13,* 349-356.

Arbona, C. (1990). *Career counseling research with Hispanics: A review of the literature.* The Counseling Psychologist, *18,* 300-323.

Axelson, J. A. (1993). *Counseling and development in a multicultural society* (2nd ed.) New York: Brooks/Cole.

Axelson, J. A. (1999). *Counseling and development in a multicultural society* (3rd ed.) New York: Brooks/Cole.

Bricout, J. C. (2004). Using telework to enhance return to work opportunities for consumers with spinal cord injuries, *NeuroRehabilitation, 19*(2), 147-159.

Brown, C. (1997). Sex differences in the career development of urban African American adolescents. *Journal of Career Development, 23,* 133-147.

Cohen, S. (2002). High-tech tools lower barriers for disabled: The latest generation of assistive technology. *Journal of Human Resources, 42,* 31-38.

Cook, A. M. & Hussey, S. M. (2002). *Assistive technologies: Principles and practices.* (2nd ed.). St. Loius, MO: Mosby.

Crimando, W. & Baker, R. (1984). Computer assisted instruction in rehabilitation education. *Rehabilitation Counseling Bulletin*, September, 50-54.

Dalto, M. (2003). Maryland' assistive technology loan program: Successful outreach and partnerships. *Journal of Disability Policy Studies, 14*(2), 91-94.

Edwards, Y., Portman, T. A. & Bethea, J. (2002). Counselor student computer competency skills: Effects of technology course in training. *Journal of Technology in Counseling, 2*(2). Retrieved from: http://jtc.colstate.edu.

Falvo, D. (1999). *Medical and psychosocial aspects of chronic illness and disability,* Pacific Grove CA: Aspen Publishers.

Flynn, C. (1997). Computer use in vocational rehabilitation agencies. *The Newsletter of the Rehabilitation Technology Associates, 15,* 2.

Fouad, N. A., & Kelly, T. J. (1992). The relation between attitudinal and behavior aspects of career maturity. *Career Development Quarterly, 40,* 257-271.

Galvin, J. C. & Scherer, M. J. (eds). (1996). *Evaluating, selecting and using appropriate. Assistive technology.* Gaithersburg, MD: Aspen Publishers.

Guo, B., Bricout, J. C., & Huang, J. (2005). A common open space or a digital divide?: A social model perspective on the online disability community in China. *Disability and Society, 20* (1), 49-66.

Hammond, M. (2003). The Utah assistive technology foundation: Program features and initiatives. *Journal of Disability Policy Studies, 14*(2), 95-97.

Herr, E., & Cramer, S. (1996). *Career guidance and counseling through the lifespan: Systematic approaches* (5th edition). New York: HarperCollins.

Issaacson, L. E., & Brown, D. (2000). *Career information, career counseling, and career development* (7th ed.) Needham Heights, MA: Allyn & Bacon.

Kivlighan Jr., D. M., Johnston, J. A., Hogan, R. S., Mauer, E. (1994). Who benefits from computerized career counseling? *Journal of Counseling & Development, 72* (3), 289-293.

Leong, F. T. L., & Serifica, F. C. (1995). Career development of Asian Americans: A research area in need of a good theory. In F.T.L. Leong (Ed.), *Career development and vocational behavior of racial and ethnic minorities* (pp. 76-102). Mahwah, NJ: Erlbaum.

National Telecommunications and Information Administration (2002). *A nation online: How Americans are expanding their use of the Internet.* Available Http://www.ntia.doc.gov/ntiahome/dn/index.html

National Telecommunications and Information Administration (2000). *Falling through the Net: Toward digital inclusion.* Available http://www.ntia.doc.gov/ntiahome/digitaldivide/

Niles, S. G., & Harris-Bowlsbey, J. (2002). *Career development in the 21sy century.* Upper Saddle River, NJ: Merrill Prentice Hall.

Peterson, D. (2003). Ethics and technology. In R. R. Cottone and V. Tarvydas (2nd Ed.), *Ethical and professional issues in counseling* (pp.169-202). Upper Saddle River, New Jersey: Merrill Prentice Hall.

Ritchie, H. & Blanck, P. (2003). The promise of the Internet for disability: a scenario of online services and web site accessibility at centers for independent living, *Behavioral Science and the Law, 21,* 5-26.

Riemer-Reiss, M. L. (2000). Factors associated with assistive technology discontinuance among individuals with disabilities. *Journal of Rehabilitation, 4,* 20-33.

Roach, R. (2002). Assistive technology comes into focus: With the push to from federal legislation, colleges and universities enhance learning for the disabled. *Black Issues in Higher Education, 4,* 56-61.

Rojewski, J.W. (1997). Career indecision types for rural adolescents from disadvantaged and non-disadvantaged backgrounds. *Journal of Career Assessment, 5,* 1-20.

Rubin, S.E., & Roessler, R.T. (2001). *Foundations of the vocational rehabilitation process* (5th ed.). Austin, TX: PRO-ED, Inc.

Scherer, M. J. (2000). *Living in a state of stuck* (3rd ed*).* CA: Brookline Books Inc.

Shafer, R. (2002). *Applying career development theory to counseling* (3rd ed). Pacific Grove: Brook/Cole.

Taber, B. J., & Luzzo, D. A. (1999). ACT research report 99-3: A comprehensive review of research evaluating the effectiveness of DISCOVER in promoting career development. Iowa City, IA: ACT, Inc.

Warner, M. (1999). Beyond the classroom: Instruction strategies and distance technologies that support lifelong learning. *Rehabilitation Education, 13*(1), 37-58.

Westbrook, B. W., & Sanford, E. E. (1991). The validity of career maturity attitude measures among Black and white high school students. *The Career Development Quarterly*, 40, 198-208.

Wilson, K., Wallin, J. S., & Reisser, C. (2003) Social stratification and the digital divide. *Social Science Computer Review, 21*(2), 133-143.

CHAPTER 11

REHABILITATION RESEARCH FROM A MULTICULTURAL PERSPECTIVE

PAUL LEUNG
CATHERINE MARSHALL
KEITH WILSON

Chapter Highlights

➡ Current status of rehabilitation research and ethnic populations

➡ The participatory action research model and inclusion of diverse populations

➡ Relevancy of rehabilitation research to diverse populations

➡ Evidence based research and diverse populations

➡ Assets and limitations of using existing databases

➡ Cultural mistrust and postcolonial traumatic stress

11

*T*he primary purpose of this chapter is to review the current status of rehabilitation research involving diverse ethnic/racial populations, explore the implications of quantitative and qualitative rehabilitation research from a multicultural perspective, and provide some thoughts about what may lie ahead in research related to multicultural rehabilitation. While much has occurred towards a more inclusive approach to rehabilitation research, much more remains to be done.

Over a decade ago, the National Council on Disability held a national conference in Jackson, Mississippi highlighting the "unique needs of minorities with disabilities." The Mississippi conference pointed to a lack of and a need for research related to underserved minority groups. Though that was 1992, that lack of attention to ethnicity and rehabilitation research remains just as relevant today. Any review of rehabilitation research, however cursory, can only lead to the conclusion that there is a long way to go before rehabilitation research can truly mirror the population of the United States. The need is as great today as it was a decade ago for research about diverse ethnic/racial persons who have disabilities.

The theme of this book is a multicultural approach to rehabilitation and highlights the need for an infusion of multiculturalism into all aspects of the rehabilitation process. This chapter will look at where we are in multicultural rehabilitation research and where we need to go. Strictly speaking, research in the multicultural arena is no different from any other rehabilitation research in considering both qualitative and quantitative approaches. We can assume that any rehabilitation research will involve good methodology and design along with appropriate analysis and interpretation to answer the questions asked. At the same time, this very assumption may be much of the problem. The bottom line is that we may need to rethink the assumption for it may very well be the key to understanding where we are, and what we need to do in multicultural rehabilitation research in order to find solutions that will improve the lives of persons with disabilities who are from diverse populations.

Lila Downs, [http://www.liladowns.com] who is of Mixtec-Indian and Scottish-American heritage, reminds us in her music that she, as are all of us, are creatures of our respective cultures. Though Downs has little to do with rehabilitation research, she directs us to think about who we are. Her message resonates as we think about rehabilitation research for she reminds us that we all are cultural beings. Our culture has an influence on us and on our behavior. This has often been taken for granted and too often ignored. Only recently have we begun the process of looking at culture's impact on research.

Rehabilitation research has drawn primarily on psychology to form our interventions and, as a result, we have tended to focus on the individual. However, given the push of the disability movement, rehabilitation practitioners now realize the importance of the environment and context in understanding disability. We now also accept context and environment as part of the definition of culture. Gergen, Gulerce, Lock, & Misra (1996), in groping with the influence of culture on psychology, asked, "To what degree and with what effects is psychological science itself a cultural manifestation? Starting from this perspective, it is immediately apparent that psychology and science are largely products of Western cultural tradition. "Suppositions about the nature of knowledge, the character of objectivity, the place of value in the knowledge generating process, and the nature of linguistic representation all carry the stamp of a unique cultural tradition" (p. 497).

In questioning the relevance of psychology for a changing international world, Mays, Rubin, Sabourin, and Walker (1996) shared a similar concern. They wrote that unless U.S. psychology is willing to learn from other nations, "the result will surely be an increasingly fragmented U.S. psychology that is at risk for failing to meet the psychological needs of its own U.S. population, with its rapidly growing multicultural, multinational, and multiracial population" (Mays et al, 1996, p. 486).

How science is defined and the extent to which science is a "cultural manifestation" depends on one's perspective. This notion mirrors arguments of feminist researchers (Du Bois, 1983; Gatens-Robinson & Tarvydas, 1992) who have long suggested the need to look at things differently. Du Bois (1983), for example, initiated her exploration of science and values by stating that "science is *not* 'value-free'; it cannot be. Science is made by scientists, and both we and our science-making are shaped by our culture" (p. 105). Dubois (1983) further observed that:

> In its conceptions of science and knowing, our society has embraced and reified the values of objective knowledge, expertise, neutrality, separateness, and *opposed* them to the values of subjective knowledge, understanding, art, communion, craft, and experience. Objectivity and subjectivity are modes of knowing, analysis, interpretation, and understanding. They are not independent of each other, and should not be.

p. 111

DuBois went on to write that it is the "*synthesis* of subjectivity and objectivity that is the source of intellectual power and responsibility—and truth" (p. 113). Harding (1986) argued that we must question the way science is

242

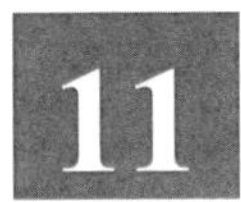

practiced so that there is not to be "an apparent immunity for the scientific enterprise from the kinds of critical and causal scrutiny that science recommends for all the other regularities of nature and social life. If we were to abandon these dogmas of empiricism, we could adopt the alternative view that science is a fully social activity—as social and as culturally specific as are religious, educational, economic, and family activities" (p. 56).

Given that rehabilitation research is a way for us to understand and describe multicultural people with disabilities along with what may assist in improving their lives, rehabilitation's research agenda must be committed to addressing cultural issues using culturally appropriate research design and instrumentation. There is general acceptance in psychometrics that an instrument developed and normed on one population should be used only with great caution with another population. Otherwise, interpretation and conclusions from that instrument have questionable validity and value (Marshall, Leung, Johnson, & Busby, 2003). However, equal caution is needed as we look beyond assessment and quantitative research "to the extent qualitative researchers carry their own cultural assumptions into the field, they risk imposing a foreign frame of reference in interpreting the experience and meanings of the people they study" (Tutty, Rothery, & Ginnell, 1996, p. 18).

Hughes, Seidman, and Williams (1993) noted "the selection of a research problem is constrained by Western mindscapes" and cautioned that "researchers need to develop culturally anchored methods that avoid ethnocentric biases in research and also take into consideration the role of cultural phenomenon in shaping the outcomes of the research process" (p. 689). Hughes et al (1993) found that "a culturally anchored perspective draws attention to an ongoing debate regarding the relative utility of qualitative versus quantitative research methodologies" (p. 696). They also drew attention to the fact that "qualitative researchers tend to assess behavior in naturalistic settings . . .. Preconceived rules and categories for classifying behavior are de-emphasized: The meaning . . . emerges through inductive analyses of the data themselves" (Hughes, Seidman, & Williams, 1993, pp. 696-697). While errors associated with inappropriate and culture-bound instrumentation used for measurement may not be the concerns of qualitative research, erroneous culture-bound interpretation of data, such as personal narratives, may be.

CURRENT STATUS OF REHABILITATION RESEARCH AND ETHNIC POPULATIONS

An understanding of multicultural rehabilitation research requires that we briefly look at the current status of social science research related to diverse ethnic and racial populations. Though Sue (1999) addressed research and ethnic minority populations from the perspective of psychology, much of what Sue discussed holds true for rehabilitation research. Sue (1999) indicated the lack of psychological research on ethnic minority populations is both subtle and systemic. Sue (1999) believed "the culprit is how science has been practiced— an effect caused by the selective enforcement of the principles of science." (p. 1070). Sue pointed out the overemphasis on internal validity verses external validity as a basic flaw in how psychological research has been used and interpreted to the detriment of multicultural populations.

Good methodology and design must take into account concepts of culture. Tucker and Herman (2002), in looking at academic needs of African American children, pointed out that theories and interventions are often based on research with mostly European American middle class samples, and that such theory and research do not advance knowledge about the specific needs of children from other cultural backgrounds. Tucker and Herman (2002) make the assertion that not only must research design meet the usual criteria of internal, external, and construct validity, but must also have the added dimension of cultural validity. Rogler (1989) argued for using a "continuing and open-ended series of substantive and methodological insertions and adaptations" to "mesh the process of inquiry with the cultural characteristics of the group being studied" (p. 296). Rogler also suggested using pre-testing and planning the collection of data that ensures adaptations to the cultural milieu of the target population and described culturally sensitive research as the "incessant and continuing finely calibrated interweaving of cultural components and cultural awareness into all phases of the research process" (P. 302). In other words, the infusion of culture into research design requires forethought and deliberate action on the part of the researcher.

THE PARTICIPATORY ACTION RESEARCH MODEL AND INCLUSION OF DIVERSE POPULATIONS

The recognition that persons who are the target for research must benefit from that research led the National Institute on Disability and Rehabilitation Research (NIDRR) to promote what NIDRR termed a "new" paradigm. A

central focus of this paradigm is Participatory Action Research (PAR) where persons with disabilities are considered an integral part of the research process from inception to completion. The PAR approach requires an active role for individuals with disabilities in defining, analyzing, and solving research issues and problems. PAR is considered a research process that includes both scientists and consumers. Acceptance of the PAR model also implies an acceptance of the role culture plays in behavior, and thus, rehabilitation research as well. PAR implicitly accepts the fact that the environment, including culture, has an influence in defining or describing disability, and that disability is a social construct. Nonetheless, much of current rehabilitation research has followed fairly traditional methodologies utilizing notions and constructs that researchers can readily define using existing instrumentation and accessible participants. As a result, consumers often do not believe that research responds to what they perceive to be important or relevant. Bellini & Rumrill (2002) concluded that in rehabilitation research "constructs that are the easiest to measure tend to be less relevant in terms of providing solid findings for practice, whereas constructs that are more complex tend to be those that are most closely related to the valued social outcomes that are important goals for rehabilitation consumers" (p.131). White (2002) further elaborated that "in researchers' zeal to create a more robust methodology, they must not neglect the value of their research to those to whom it is often directed—the participants and their peers" (p.438).

Issues of potential bias become even more important when they are intertwined with participants who not only have disabilities but who also are members of diverse ethnic/racial groups. There has been a revisiting in traditional medical research regarding inclusion of diverse populations and the need to be specific about the populations being studied. Under the assumption that researchers must better describe and define participants in their research, the U.S. Dept. of Heath and Human Services (2003) recently released "Guidance for Industry" regarding the collection of race and ethnicity data in clinical trials. These guidelines recognize race and ethnicity to be particularly important in the understanding of biological and physiological responses. Though clinical trials are seldom done in rehabilitation research, some of the same issues apply. Rehabilitation researchers need to be specific in their descriptions of the populations they research. There are obvious differences in response to different medical products by racially and ethnically distinct groups that are not only attributable to intrinsic factors, such as genetics, but also to external factors, such as socio-cultural issues or the interaction between the two.

In a discipline closer to rehabilitation, Tucker and Herman (2002) found that nearly 40% of published articles in clinical, counseling, and school psychology between 1993 and 1997 did not report the ethnicity of their participants. Perhaps in response to these findings, the American Psychological Association (APE 2002) adopted as policy "Guidelines on Multicultural Education, Training, Research, Practice, and Organizational Change for Psychologists." The Guidelines reflect recognition that research may have ignored culture in the past, with culture being seen as a nuisance variable. Culture has now become a "central contextual" variable that explains human behavior. The APA guidelines further indicate that failure to consider "within group" differences to be particularly egregious (p 39).

RELEVANCY OF REHABILITATION RESEARCH TO DIVERSE POPULATIONS

Even though there has been an increase in culturally diverse participants in rehabilitation research, many studies continue to use predominantly White and middle-class persons as primary participants. These samples, often selected out of convenience, undoubtedly affect external validity as well as the outcomes reported. Thus, rehabilitation research relevancy is affected not only in terms of consumer perception but also in terms of validity.

Other research areas that have application to rehabilitation research and that may assist in moving rehabilitation research toward new areas include other social sciences. Increased knowledge in social psychology and advances in method have facilitated the emergence of several areas in minority research, such as false consensus, perceived group variability, stereotype threat, collective action, the self, perceptions of justice, system justification mechanisms, and coping with stigma. Findings in these domains involve not only research with minority/diverse populations in natural settings, but also experimental research aimed at separating the relative effects of power, status, and group size.

Another issue that is important involves comparing ethnic/racial groups. Much of existing and traditional research with diverse populations portrays these populations in opposition to the majority population for comparison purposes. Ethnic and racial minorities are placed not only in a deficit perspective, but these results may reinforce negative stereotypic images. Results from these studies may not only be misleading but even counter to the rehabilitation philosophy of focusing on strengths.

246

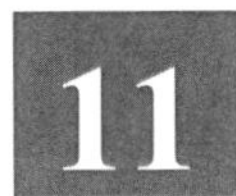

EVIDENCE BASED RESEARCH AND
DIVERSE POPULATIONS

Attention is currently being given to the use of interventions that are considered evidence or empirically based, i.e., having a "scientific" foundation in the research literature. A primary characteristic of evidence-based intervention involves identified and measured changes, along with evaluating the intervention against an alternate intervention (Coleman & Wampold, 2003). The problem with evidence-based intervention for diverse populations is that very little research data are available, along with the fact that some population groups are numerically quite small. Asian Americans, for example, have essentially been ignored in the literature. As Chwalisz (2003) noted, the definition of "evidence" is critical, as is the underlying assumption that "an objective reality exists that can be observed by researchers" (p.499). Chwalisz quoted Sturdee (2001) saying "scientific evidence cannot provide proof; it can only affirm our commitment to the conceptual structures and theoretical constructs provided by the paradigm within which what counts as evidence has already been defined" (p. 499). Chwalisz (2003) further characterizes psychological treatment evidence as hierarchical, triangulating, and dialectical, whose sources of evidence have been "too narrow to adequately capture the real-world activities of professional psychologists" (p.500). Chwalisz argues for an "expanded view of evidence" and a "philosophical shift in which all sources of evidence have the potential to contribute to the understanding of psychological phenomena" (p.500).

Wampold (2003), commenting on Chwalisz's methodological pluralism, raised a number of questions that provide a foundation for multicultural rehabilitation research. Wampold (2003) asked, What is the purpose of collecting evidence? Who evaluates the evidence? What are the theoretical, historical, political, and cultural contexts in which the evidence is embedded? What decisions are made based on the evidence (p.540)? Coleman and Wampold (2003) end by advocating processes for determining effectiveness of interventions "that are context driven; respect the interaction among the context, the disorder, and the individual; and systematically use evaluation methods that can capture that complexity" (p. 244).

Given the lack of inclusion of diverse populations in existing research, combined with the difficulty of identifying and locating participants from diverse groups, and especially persons who have disabilities, it is easy to come to a conclusion that it will be some time before enough evidence becomes available upon which to make truly evidence-based decisions. Second, adoption of current evidence-based research in rehabilitation may mean adoption of interventions that may not only be flawed but that may also present ethical dilemmas should they be adopted without further investigation. Sue (1999) cited his experience with a task force designated to determine which psychotherapeutic interventions met rigorous criteria to be designated as an empirically validated treatment. The task force found that no studies were ever conducted on the effectiveness of treatment for members of ethnic minority populations (Sue, 1999). Sue suggested that research is often used to assume generality of findings when it may not be warranted. The difficulty Sue indicated, is "our modus operandi is to assume that the work is universally applicable; the burden of proof is placed on researchers concerned about race, ethnicity, and bias to show that there are ethnic differences" (p.1073). Sue concludes by asking the question, "Whatever happened to the scientific notion of skepticism, where little is taken for granted, where conclusions are drawn from evidence and not from assumptions (p.1073)?"

Much of the currently available literature in rehabilitation on different ethnic/racial groups relates to access to rehabilitation services and, in particular, vocational rehabilitation. This area of research has been significant because it calls attention to inequities of access. In addition, research related to underutilization of rehabilitation services by different groups has brought about an emphasis to assure a more consumer oriented approach benefiting not only individuals from diverse populations but also all persons with disabilities. In part, changes to rehabilitation legislation, such as the Rehabilitation Act, were driven by recognition that diverse ethnic populations did not have equal access to the vocational rehabilitation system.

The majority of research into inequities or unequal treatment has used available databases as primary source documents. The next section will discuss the use of large databases and specifically their relationship to rehabilitation access questions.

ASSETS AND LIMITATIONS ASSOCIATED WITH USING EXISTING DATABASES

Databases are kept by government programs to document their activities and/or populations, and generally contain large amounts of information concerning persons served or those who benefit from activities of the program. Databases of interest to rehabilitation researchers include those kept by the United States Department of Education, Rehabilitation Services Administration (RSA) and the National Institute of Healths (NIH). Such databases contain national samples with similar data available for each state. For example, the national

RSA-911 will have similar variables as a state RSA-911 database. To ensure client confidentiality, most databases delete identifying information of individual clients. It is, therefore, not only difficult but also probably impossible to connect database demographics to a particular client or group within the database.

State/national databases are attractive for research for a number of reasons. First, databases generally provide access to large numbers of individuals. This is particularly important when there is need for power with a specific statistical analysis. Many statistics require a minimum number of participants to maintain critical statistical assumptions. Second, large databases can save time and money in identifying and locating participants. Using surveys to gain information on 300 participants, for example, will cost a lot more than using already collected data. The decision to survey participants may mean asking questions such as (1) What is the cost of a four-page survey? (2) Who will assist with distributing the survey to the participants? (3) Will participants receive a fee for successful completion of the survey? (4) Will the survey be done on the Internet? Finally, databases usually contain more variables than a survey instrument and, as a result, a researcher can investigate more research questions.

Database research can answer questions limited only by the creativity of the researchers. Using an RSA-911 state or national database, for example, answers can be found for the following types of questions: Are African Americans with disabilities accepted less for VR services than White Americans with disabilities? Is there a difference in successful closures (status 26) among African Americans and White American with disabilities?

At the same time, there are limitations to the use of databases or using recorded data from state and federal government programs. As with ex post facto research designs, independent variables cannot be manipulated or randomly assigned to a treatment group. Thus, cause-and-effect cannot be attributed to the results of studies using databases. For example, the conclusion that an individual who is a White American with a disability will cause that individual to be accepted into the public vocational rehabilitation program cannot be made. It is only possible to say that a correlation exists between the independent and dependent variables. Likewise, a conclusion that being an African American with a disability is the reason for not being accepted into vocational rehabilitation cannot be made. Basically, database results can only conclude there is a possible correlation between both the independent and dependent variables in the study.

Another challenge with using databases is that one can use only the variables that have been collected by the reporting program. The variance

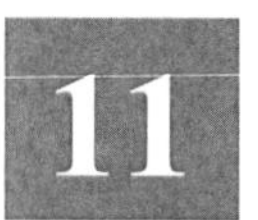

explained by the independent variable(s) is quite small for many of the studies exploring the acceptance into vocational rehabilitation at both the state and national levels. Wilson (2000) suggested that there are other possible variables that can be used to explain acceptance into vocational rehabilitation besides those variables that are already in the RSA-911 database. Because researchers cannot add to the database, researchers often must speculate about what may have brought about the results. This does not minimize the fact that speculation may provide additional perspectives often validating what is observed in everyday life. Speculation involves questioning and is a needed aspect of research.

ACCURACY OF DATABASE

Agencies and programs often "clean" databases of known errors and to make the database more accurate. The result is that databases presumed to be the same may actually be quite different. The total number of participants may vary, for example, depending on the specific database that is used. Researchers may be using quantitatively different databases for the same year. Using the same procedures (e.g., statistics and sampling) may produce different results. While having quantitatively different database may be unlikely, human error in entry, et cetera, does occur. In an effort to "clean-up" and continuously update the RSA 911 database for accuracy, variables within the database may quantitatively change during this "clean-up" procedure. Researchers need to examine the data closely for possible inconsistencies before using any database. Generally, it helps to ask the particular program about the details of the database and the proper protocol for reporting such inaccuracies. Using checks and balances will ensure results that are more accurate.

INTERPRETATION OF RESULTS

Though the cliché is that numbers do not lie, numbers have meaning that is based on an interpretation by the researcher. Because researchers who are members of the majority population may have a different worldview than African American researchers, we can perhaps not expect White American and African American researchers to be congruent in their interpretations of research findings. While there is nothing wrong with rehabilitation researchers interpreting findings differently, it is important to understand that similar results may produce different meanings depending on who is doing the interpretation.

Interpretations are also accepted or dismissed because of the perceptions and experiences of the persons reading a particular study. For example, results that indicate discrepancies in VR acceptance rates (accessibility) may have different meanings to African American and White American researchers. African American researchers/writers may pay more attention to discrimination in contrast with White Americans researchers who may attend to another possibility. One only has to examine the discussion sections of published research articles by White American and African American authors to see some of these differences. The different opinions expressed by researchers should not be the primary issue. Problems arise only when opinions are expressed that differ from the prevailing views. Perspectives expressed by researchers who are not considered part of the mainstream group tend to be devalued or discounted.

The discounting of positions and opinions based on whether the perspective is part of the mainstream thinking is the crux of the problem. An example of this was the conclusion by an Australian physician that the culprit for gastric ulcers was a bacterium. This was counter to prevailing opinion that gastric ulcers resulted from stress and dietary reasons (DuBois, 1995). Consequently, there was very slow acceptance of the bacterial theory and the use of antibiotics for the treatment of gastric ulcers. Well-designed empirically sound research may get the necessary attention needed to add diversity to vocational rehabilitation research, but as noted, there is no consensus about what is well-designed empirical research. This was particularly evident in some of the reactions to studies of the state/federal vocational rehabilitation program.

Given the importance of the VR program to persons with disabilities, including persons from minority racial backgrounds, eligibility and acceptance into the VR program by minority consumers were among the first multicultural rehabilitation research topics. Vocational Rehabilitation eligibility and race was first explored by Atkins and Wright in 1980. The Atkins and Wright (1980) study took a systematic look at vocational rehabilitation (VR) outcomes relative to race. Atkins and Wright reported that African Americans were accepted less for VR services than White Americans in the majority of Rehabilitation Services Administration (RSA) federal regions. As a result, Atkins and Wright generated a lot of controversy in the area of VR research regarding racial and ethnic minorities with disabilities (see the history chapter). Bolton and Cooper (1980) challenged the results of the Atkins and Wright study for what they considered to be small percentage differences that existed in VR acceptance between African Americans and White Americans with disabilities.

Since Atkins and Wright (1980), a number of studies on acceptance to Vocational Rehabilitation programs and race have appeared. Herbert and Martinez (1992) investigated whether race (Native American/Alaskan Native, Asian/Pacific Islander, African American, or White American) correlated with case service statuses 08 (closed not accepted for VR services), 26 (rehabilitated), 28 (closed other reason after the Individual Plan for

251

Employment [IPE]), and 30 (closed other reasons before the IPE. Herbert and Martinez came to a conclusion similar to Atkins and Wright that African Americans tended to be accepted less for VR services than White Americans.

A year after the Herbert and Martinez (1992) study, Dziekan and Okocha (1993) looked at the accessibility of VR services with regard to African Americans, Hispanics, Native Americans, Asian Americans, and White Americans. Dziekan's and Okocha's conclusions about African American experiences in VR coincided with those reported by Atkins and Wright and Herbert and Martinez. Two years later, Feist-Price (1995) found similar results in examining VR outcomes of another state. Results reported by four of five research teams exploring VR acceptance and ethnicity between 1980 and 1995 strongly suggested that race influences VR acceptance. Although the reasons for discrepancy in VR accessibility are somewhat unclear, many research teams (e.g., Atkins & Wright, 1980; Feist-Price, 1995) believed that prejudice and biased attitudes of White American VR counselors and administrators towards African Americans and people of color in the VR system may play an important role in disparate outcomes of the VR system.

Not long after the Feist-Price (1995) study, Wheaton (1995) published a study with a conclusion that a significant difference in the acceptance rates among African Americans and White Americans in the VR system did not exist. Likewise, Peterson (1996) and Wilson (1999) in separate studies came to the conclusion that there was no statistical difference between racial and ethnic minorities and White Americans in VR acceptance. Wilson (1999) revisited the notion of VR acceptance and race in response to the need for replication of studies related to VR acceptance and race. Wilson, Harley, and Alston (2001) replicated the Wilson (1999) study and found results similar to earlier research (e.g., Atkins & Wright, 1980; Feist-Price, 1995), namely that White Americans are more likely to be accepted for VR services than are African Americans with disabilities. These results challenged earlier findings that reported race and VR acceptance as independent of each other (Wheaton, 1995; Wilson, 1999). What is one to make of these different findings? An answer may lie in the nature of the data, the analysis of the data, the statistical techniques used, as well as in the interpretation of the data.

Addressing limitations of prior VR acceptance studies by using logistic regression, Wilson (2000) reported that the primary source of support at referral (entered first) and ethnicity (entered second) were the two variables that emerged as statistically significant in the regression model. Although the methodology in the Wilson (2000) study was different than some past studies (for example, Atkins & Wright, 1980), Wilson's results proved analogous with what the majority of studies reported regarding race and VR accessibility—

252

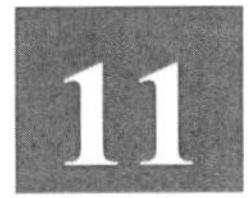

namely, African Americans and other racial and ethnic minorities are less likely to be accepted for VR services when compared to their White American counterparts.

More recently, Wilson (2002) found that African Americans with disabilities are more likely to be rejected for VR services when compared with White Americans with disabilities in the United States. In contrast to several other studies on VR accessibility and race, Wilson (2002) used a national sample, as did Atkins and Wright (1980) to investigate VR accessibility. Thus, the results of studies using large databases by Wilson and Atkins and Wright could be generalized to the entire population of individuals in the VR system rather than just one subset.

There have been other studies that focused on various ethnic/racial groups and the vocational rehabilitation program. For example, Wilson & Senices (in press) compared Hispanics to non-Hispanics (African American, White American, American Indian or Alaskan Native, and Asian or Pacific Islander) in the United States and their VR acceptance rates. Because people who self report as Hispanic are among the fastest growing ethnic group in the United States, attention to Hispanics is a necessary step in the progression of rehabilitation research with racial/ethnic groups. "Hispanics constitute an ethnic group rather than a racial category, and their members may classify themselves as White, Black, or some other race" (Rawlings & Saluter, 1994, p. xii) (also see RSA, 1995 & the United States Bureau of the Census, 2001, March). Wilson and Senice (in press) found a statistically significant difference between race/ethnicity and VR acceptance of Hispanics and non-Hispanics in the United States VR system. In particular, Hispanics were more likely to be accepted for VR services than non-Hispanics in the United States. Wilson and Senice (in press) were the first to compare people not only based on race and ethnicity, but also skin color or hue. Most people in the VR system who classify themselves as Hispanic tended to select the White race. Wilson and Senices suggest that people with disabilities who are of a darker hue may be discriminated against because of skin color. Several authors (e.g., Bennett, 1995; Devine & Elliott, 1995; Freud, 1938; Hacker, 1995; Schulman et al., 1999) support the assertion that discrimination may be based on skin color. Not only are people who classify themselves as racial and ethnic minorities discriminated against in the VR system, but a large part of the discrimination encountered by racial and ethnic minorities occurs as result of the color of their skin: Specifically, the darker ones' skin the more salient the projected discrimination (Wilson & Senice, in press).

As researchers continue to debate the reasons why racial and ethnic minority groups encounter more Vocational Rehabilitation (VR) ineligibility

than other groups (Atkins & Wright, 1980; Bolton & Cooper, 1980; Feist-Price, 1995; Wheaton, 1995; Wilson, 1997), it is clear that these underrepresented groups tend to have different experiences prior to their entry into human services than White Americans (Atkins & Wright, 1980; Baker & Taylor, 1995; Hacker, 1995; Thomas and Sillen, 1972). Relative to access to VR services, it is also becoming increasingly apparent that racial minorities also have problems once they enter into the VR system as well.

Once racial minorities are accepted into VR, they may face additional infrastructure barriers that hinder successful rehabilitation outcomes. As part of their study, Atkins and Wright (1980) looked at VR case closure patterns among both African Americans and White Americans. Although Atkins and Wright reported that race and reason for closure was statistically significant, it was not clear as to the specific reason for unsuccessful closures after the initiation of the Individual Plan for Employment (IPE) among the participants in their study.

Ross and Biggi (1986) looked at access to rehabilitation services at referral while observing outcomes including status 28 (closed after the initiation of the IPE). Ross and Biggi (1986) reported that refusal of services emerged as the most cited reason among White American customers for closure when found eligible for VR services, while African Americans were more likely to be closed for failure to cooperate. However, Ross and Biggi (1986) did find that unsuccessful outcomes between African Americans and White Americans were not found to be statistically significant.

Herbert and Martinez (1992) sought to determine whether race influenced case service outcomes for Statuses 08, 26, 28, and 30. In contrast to the results reported by Atkins and Wright (1980) and Ross and Biggi (1986), Herbert and Martinez did not find differences between African Americans and White Americans for Status 28 closure. African Americans and White Americans appeared to differ only slightly in reasons for closures once Individual Plans for Employment (IPE) were initiated. Peterson (1996) in a similar study also found no differences in unsuccessful closures after the IPE was initiated.

In an attempt to identify what may account for these differences, Wilson (2003) found that African Americans with disabilities were more likely to be categorized "failure to cooperate" while White Americans with disabilities were more likely to appear in the "other" category. Although there is no consensus on reasons for closure after the initiation of the IPE, the fact that more racial minorities are closed "failure to cooperate" may be particularly significant.

REASONS GIVEN FOR VR DISCREPANCIES

Prejudice and bias affect people with disabilities who are racial and ethnic minorities in extraordinarily similar ways; notably, the devaluation of the race or ethnicity of the minority group by White Americans (Olkin, 1999). Considering the extent of diversity and the disproportionate number of unsuccessful racial minorities with disabilities in the VR system, a continued examination of issues related to racial minorities in VR is essential. While much work is needed related to diversity in the VR system, there is room for some optimism regarding outcomes for racial minorities with disabilities.

Wilson, Harley, McCormick et al (2001) explored not only the reasons why these particular discrepancies exist but also described the consensus that exists in vocational rehabilitation and human services literature. Wilson, Harley, McCormick et al (2001) put it this way:

> Acceptance into vocational rehabilitation services is a complex issue in which multiple variables are to be considered. While we recognize that types of services received, severity of disability, and type of disability, for example, are important variables to consider when examining possible reasons for VR acceptance, literature examining VR acceptance in relation to these and other variables was scarce.

p. 27

Wilson, Harley, McCormick et al. (2001) described multiple reasons for VR discrepancies. These reasons included (1) the differences in worldviews between racial and ethnic minorities and White American counselors, (2) bias discrimination against racial and ethnic minority clients, and (3) cultural mistrust by racial and ethnic minority customers towards White American VR counselors, to name a few. Undoubtedly, discrimination may be unintended but nevertheless real. Not withstanding the intention of discrimination, Wilson, Harley, McCormick et al (2001) concluded, "it is apparent that conscious or unconscious discrimination can hamper customers who seek services" (p. 28).

Rehabilitation research has identified issues that interfere with implementation of the basic intent of the Rehabilitation Act. There is need to resolve not only accessibility concerns of racial and ethnic minorities in the VR system but facilitate a more customer friendly milieu for all people with disabilities. There is no doubt of the need for more research that includes a racially and ethnically diverse perspective that will advance a welcoming VR program.

DATA MINING

Another approach to the use of large data sets that has potential in multicultural rehabilitation research has been the adoption of tools long utilized by business and market researchers (Chan, Wong, Rosenthal, Kundu & Dutta, 2004). Traditionally known as pattern recognition, this approach involves data mining or the "extraction of hidden predictive information from large databases." (Chan et al, p.4). Chan et al used a data mining approach to reexamine effects of demographic variables and acceptance rates of the RSA 911 data sets along with other factors that influence employment rates of vocational rehabilitation consumers who have orthopedic disabilities.

OTHER METHODS OF KNOWING

Qualitative research has been recognized in a number of social science disciplines as having particular value in gathering information from diverse groups that have not had the benefit of research. Lykes (1989) wrote about her desire to better understand Guatamalan culture. "It was the concrete problems I confronted in undertaking research with Guatemalan women that enabled me to depart more significantly from the quantitative methods of my training towards a more qualitative participatory model of research that would enable me both to better address the questions I was asking and to engage in research that is consistent with my social goals and commitments" (p. 172). Lykes used oral history interviews "as the appropriate method for this study because they are both sensitive to the single individual's experiences, enabling us to look at a woman's understanding of herself and her elaboration of the social meaning of her life, and to the Guatemalan community's long tradition of oral communication" (p.172).

Feminists have for some time brought attention to a set of conceptual dichotomies that provide further insight for the need to use different perspectives. Science and epistemology are constructed in dichotomous ways: reason vs. emotion and social value; mind vs. body; culture vs. others; objectivity vs. subjectivity; and knowing vs. being. In each dichotomy, the former often controls the latter lest the latter threaten to overwhelm the former, and the threatening 'latter' in each case appears to be systematically associated with the 'feminine' perspective. Observers of social hierarchies other than that of masculine dominance have pointed to these very same dichotomies as the conceptual scheme that permits subjugation. Harding (1998) in *Is Science Multicultural? Postcolonialisms, Feminisms, and Epistemologies* (1998) refers to "the multiplicity of local resources, and their potential for generating knowledge" (p. 194). Indigenous communities, such as experienced by Lykes

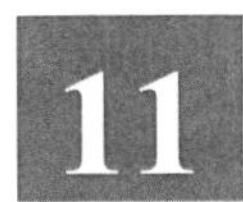

in Guatemala, offer rehabilitation researchers an alternative understanding of "ways of knowing."

In attempting to address disparities of access to health and human services, rehabilitation researchers may need to join others involved with groups where quantitative data are often labeled as "statistically unreliable" (Murray, 2003). To solve this problem, practitioners and researchers often recommend over-sampling (Murray, 2003; Schacht, et al, 2003), and pooling of data (Murray, 2003; Marshall & Largo, 1999), as well as other qualitative approaches (Marshall, Sanders, & Hill, 2001). Over-sampling is expensive and programs/agencies are often reluctant to do it. In support of qualitative methods, Murray (2003) reported that "more research is needed on many issues in occupational health and safety, and the health status of workers of color should be given a high priority. This research should use qualitative and ethnographic methods to examine risk [and] evaluate the effectiveness of interventions" (p. 224).

Researchers and practitioners across differing fields of work and intervention related to class, ethnically diverse populations, health disparities, access, and appropriate research and evaluation methods are asking similar and sometimes the same questions regarding moving beyond what can be perceived to be a "mafia-type hold" on what is considered rigorous research and ways of knowing. The processes and practices of researchers who work in indigenous communities are influenced by their own cultures as well as those they study. Awareness of this influence and adoption of appropriate research procedures are essential contributions to the validity of research. Yet funding sources and evaluators of "rigorous research" cannot seem to get away from the "gold-standard" of experimental research designs that call for the random assignment of individuals into control groups versus those who receive the intervention. The masses of people on the "lower decks" are telling researchers to consider research methods that are more appropriate to their cultural traditions.

We believe that how we go about knowing in indigenous communities, i.e. how we go about conducting research, is critical if disparities are going to be eliminated in health and human services. This issue is especially critical when a given research design may not be acceptable or appropriate to the community of interest (Davis & Keemer, 2002). For example, Linda Tuhiwai Smith (Ngati Awa and Ngati Porou), who works with indigenous people related to health and the author of *Decolonizing Methodologies: Research and Indigenous Peoples* (1999), writes that "story telling, oral histories, the perspectives of elders and of women have become an integral part of all indigenous research" (p. 144).

Tutty, Rothery, and Ginnell (1996) concluded that "good research is good research" and clarified their position by affirming that "fundamental to

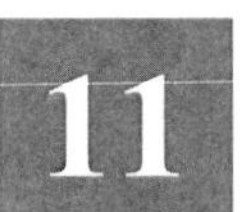

knowledge acquisition through quantitative and qualitative research studies is the idea that what we think should be *rooted in and tested against good evidence*, and that sound articulated methods—*systematic, disciplined inquiry*—are necessary to bring this about" (p. 15 [italics added]). However, what constitutes "good evidence?" Who determines the validity of the evidence? For Inuit whalers, hearing whales breathe constituted good evidence, while the International Whaling Commission's "scientific count" included only those whales that could be seen passing from the edge of the ice. Barreiro (1992) reported that while the count resulting from research methods that included hearing whales breathe was initially challenged, the Alaska Eskimo Whaling Commission's "population estimates were verified by successive aerial surveys" (pp. 27- 28).

Participatory action research calls for persons with disabilities and other community research partners to come together with academic researchers to determine appropriate research strategies (Bruyère, 1993). The lesson of the Inuit whalers is that we must learn to trust different views of what constitutes good evidence and how "disciplined inquiry" is to be structured. It may be that too frequently the options for research design rest squarely with academic researchers, and methods that fall below the "gold standard" of traditional experimental designs are suspect and of questionable value in the present political climate of evidence-based intervention.

We need to value the contributions and insights of community partners in research who suggest that research methods that mesh with their cultural traditions and "ways of knowing" may hold particular value in a given community. This was the case in a study involving the needs and resources of families with a relative who had a disability, and involving members of two southeastern American Indian Nations, i.e., the Eastern Band of Cherokee and the Mississippi Band of Choctaw (Marshall & Cerveny, 1994).

Research today tends to be so statistical and numbers-based that many not well versed in interpreting those numbers believe the human element to be missing. Qualitative researchers have to learn and understand that abstract factors not normally included in research design courses, such as communication style and non-verbal communication may be significant. In general, society perceives American Indians as stoic and nonverbal. Yet, qualitative data show the opposite (Marshall & Cerveny, 1994). Qualitative methodology can allow investigators to reach a personal level with research participants; however, for some, this may be too difficult, too draining, potentially lethal—a catharsis. On the one hand, telling one's story is difficult and painful, yet the irony here is that this is the way history, help, and medicine have been passed on for generations with Indian people. Some researchers may

consider qualitative research as too simple, yet such techniques transcend the past and can be a comfortable means of learning and explaining (Marshall, Sanders, & Hill, 2001). It is only through understanding history and culture, as well as appreciating different ways of knowing, that rehabilitation researchers enter into authentic partnerships in participatory research (Davis, Erickson, Johnson, Marshall, Running Wolf, & Santiago, 2002).

CULTURAL MISTRUST AND POSTCOLONIAL TRAUMATIC STRESS

Indigenous or native people often expect that rehabilitation researchers have an understanding of their culture, including history and environment, as part of the participatory research process. Stone (2002), a researcher and a member of the Blackfeet Nation, has written, "that in order to do ethical and moral research in the First Nations community, we must be aware of the postcolonial stress impact as an issue" (p. 114). Understanding the history and trauma of Native peoples is a responsibility of the researcher. The researcher must understand the impact of the dispossession, biological warfare, the boarding school era, termination, and federal government attempts at acculturation through urban relocation programs. Rehabilitation researchers must be concerned with how an indigenous, colonized, or low-income community might view the investigator as an oppressor "because it is the oppressor who defines the problem, the nature of the research, and, to some extent, the quality of interaction between him and his subjects" (Ladner, 1987, p. 77). Stone (2000) believes it both naïve and inappropriate for researchers to present themselves to a Native family that may be already carrying a psychological burden and say, "Hey, trust me. Throw yourself open for research. Let me interview you. Let me give you this questionnaire. Oh, don't worry. It won't hurt. It's for your own good. I'm here to help you" (p. 114). Similar examples can be found in African American rehabilitation research (Alston & Bell, 1996).

Rehabilitation researchers are in communities in order to help. While qualitative research and participatory strategies may give us an important opportunity for developing research procedures that are both culturally sensitive and result in valid conclusions, ultimately the goal is a "culturally grounded knowledge base" (Hughes, Seidman, & Williams, 1993, p. 699) that allows us to document needs, to intervene when appropriate, and to better serve people with disabilities. Our objective is to achieve culturally grounded knowledge, and that requires that we constantly check our research strategies and our data interpretations along with soliciting feedback from colleagues, from community research partners, and from research participants. This objective requires that we stay informed of both the history and the present social, cultural, and political circumstances of those we hope to help.

REFERENCES

Alston, R.J. & T. Bell (1996) Cultural mistrust and the rehabilitation enigma for African Americans. J. of Rehabilitation, 62(2) 11-15.

American Psychological Association (2002) Guidelines on Multicultural education, training, research, practice, and organizational change for psychologists. Washington, D.C.:

Angel, R. & Gronfein,W. (1988) The use of subjective information in statistical models, American Sociological Review 53, 464-473

Atkins, B. J., & Wright, G. N. (1980). Three views: vocational rehabilitation of Blacks: The statement. *Journal of Rehabilitation, 46,* 40, 42-46.

Barreiro, J. (1992). The search for lessons. *Akwe:kon Journal, 9,* 18-39.

Bellini, J. & Rumrill, P. (2002) Contemporary insights in the philosophy of science: implications for rehabilitation counseling research. *Rehabilitation Education 16*(2) 115-134.

Bennett, C. (1995). *Comprehensive multicultural education: Theory and practice* (3rd ed.). Needham Heights, MA: Allyn & Bacon.

Bolton, B., & Cooper, P. G. (1980). Three views: Vocational rehabilitation of Blacks: The comment. *Journal of Rehabilitation, 46*(2), 41, 41-49.

Bruyere, S. M. (1993). Participatory action research: Overview and implications for family members of persons with disabilities. *Journal of Vocational Rehabilitation, 3* (2), 62-68.

Chan, F., Wong, D., Rosenthal, D.A., Kundu, M., & Dutta, (2004) A. Eligibility rates of traditionally underserved individuals with disabilities revisited: a data mining approach. Journal of Applied Rehabilitation Counseling 36(3) 3-10.

Chan, F. Cheing, G., Chan, J. Y., Rosenthal, D., Chronister, J. (2005). Predicting Employment Outcomes of Rehabilitation Clients with Orthopedic Disabilities: A CHAID Analysis. Disability and Rehabilitation, 28(5) 257-270.

Chwalisz, K. (2003) Evidence-Based practice: a framework for twenty-first-century scientist-practitioner training. *The Counseling Psychologist 31*(5) 497-528.

Coleman, H. K. K. and B.E. Wampold (2003) Challenges to the development of culturally relevant, empirically supported treatment in Pope-Davis, D.B, Coleman, H.L.K., Liu, W.M.,& Toporek, R.L. (eds) Handbook of multicultural Competencies, Sage Publications: Thousand Oaks.

Davis, J. D., Erickson, J. S., Johnson, S. R., Marshall, C. A., Running Wolf, P., & Santiago, R. L. (Eds.). (2002). *Work Group on American Indian Research and Program Evaluation Methodology (AIRPEM), Symposium on Research and Evaluation Methodology: Lifespan Issues Related to American Indians/Alaska Natives with Disabilities*. Flagstaff: Northern Arizona University, Institute for Human Development, Arizona University Center on Disabilities, American Indian Rehabilitation Research and Training Center.

Davis, J. D., & Keemer, K. (2002). A brief history of and future considerations for research in American Indian and Alaska Native communities. In J. D. Davis, J. S. Erickson, S. R. Johnson, C. A. Marshall, P. Running Wolf, & R. L. Santiago, (Eds.), *Work Group on American Indian Research and Program Evaluation Methodology (AIRPEM), Symposium on Research and Evaluation Methodology: Lifespan Issues Related to American Indians/Alaska Natives with Disabilities* (pp. 9-18). Flagstaff: Northern Arizona University, Institute for Human Development, Arizona University Center on Disabilities, American Indian Rehabilitation Research and Training Center.

Devine, P. G., & Elliot, A. J. (1995). Are racial stereotypes really fading? The Princeton trilogy revisited. *Personality and Social Psychology Bulletin, 21*, 1139-1150.

DuBois, A (1995) Spiral Bacteria in the Human Stomach: The Gastric Helicobacters http://www.cdc.gov/ncidod/eid/vol1no3/dubois.htm April 26, 2004

Du Bois, B. (1983). Passionate scholarship: Notes on values, knowing and method in feminist social science. In G. Bowles and R. D. Klein, *Theories of women's studies* (pp. 105-116). Boston: Routledge and Kegan Paul.

Dziekan, K. I., & Okocha, A. G. (1993). Accessibility of rehabilitation services: Comparison by racial-ethnic status. *Rehabilitation Counseling Bulletin, 36, 183-189.*

Feist-Price, S. (1995). African Americans with disabilities and equity in vocational rehabilitation services: One state's review. *Rehabilitation Counseling Bulletin, 39,* 119-129.

Freud, S. (1938). *The Basic Writings of Sigmund Freud*. Trans. By A. Brill. New York: Modern Library.

Gatens-Robinson, E., & Tarvydas, V. (1992). Ethics of care, women's perspectives and the status of mainstream rehabilitation ethical analysis. *Journal of Applied Rehabilitation Counseling, 22*(4), 26-33.

Gergen, K. J., Gulerce, A., Lock, A., & Misra, G. (1996). Psychological science in cultural context. *American Psychologist, 51*(5), 496-503.

Graves, W. (1991, September). Participatory action research: A new paradigm for disability and rehabilitation research. *ARCA Newsletter*, pp. 8-11.

Hacker, A. (1995). *Two nations: Black and White, separate, hostile, unequal.* New York, NY: Macmillan.

Harding, S. (1986). *The science question in feminism.* Ithaca, NY: Cornell University Press.

Harding, S. (1998). *Is science multicultural?: Postcolonialisms, feminisms, and epistemologies.* Bloomington: Indiana University Press.

Herbert, J. T., & Martinez, M., Y. (1992). Client ethnicity and vocational rehabilitation case service outcome. *Journal of Job Placement, 8*, 10-16.

Hughes, D., Seidman, E., & Williams, N. (1993). Cultural phenomena and the research enterprize: Toward a culturally anchored methodology. *American Journal of Community Psychology, 21(6)*, 687-703.

Ladner, J. A. (1987). Introduction to tomorrow's tomorrow. In Harding, S. (Ed.) (1987). *Feminism and methodology.* Bloomington: Indiana University Press and Milton Keynes: Open University Press.

Lykes, M. B. (1989). Dialogue with Guatemalan Indian women: Critical perspectives on constructing collaborative research. In R. Unger (Eds.), *Representations: Social constructions of gender*, pp. 167-184. Amityville, NY: Baywood Publishing Co.

Marshall, C. A. & Largo, H. R., Jr. (1999). Disability and rehabilitation: A context for understanding the American Indian experience. *The Lancet, 354*, 758-60.

Marshall, C. A., Leung, P., Johnson, S.R., & Busby, H. (2003). Ethical practice and cultural factors in rehabilitation. *Rehabilitation Education, 17*(1), 55-65.

Marshall, C.A., Sanders, J. E., & Hill, C.R. (2001). Family voices in rehabilitation research. In C. A. Marshall (Ed.), *Rehabilitation and American Indians with disabilities: A handbook for administrators, practitioners, and researchers* (pp. 219-234). Athens, GA: Elliott & Fitzpatrick, Inc.

Mays, V. M., Rubin, J., Sabourin, M., & Walker, L. (1996). Moving toward a global psychology: Changing theories and practice to meet the needs of a changing world. *American Psychologist, 51*, 485-487.

Murray, L. R. (2003). Sick and tired of being sick and tired: Scientific evidence, methods, and research implications for racial and ethnic dispariteis in occupational health. *American Journal of Public Health, 93*(2) 221-226.

NIH Policy on Reporting Race and Ethnicity Data: Subjects in clinical research Release Date: August 8, 2001 NOTICE: NOT-OD-01-053 National Institutes of Health.

Peterson, G. E. (1996). *An analysis of participation, progress, and outcomeof individuals from diverse racial and ethnic backgrounds in the public vocational rehabilitation program in Nevada.* Unpublished doctoral dissertation, University of Northern Colorado.

Rawlings, S. W., & Saluter, A, F. (1994). *Household and family characteristics: U. S. Bureau of the Census, Current Population Reports*, P20-483.

Rehabilitation Services Administration (RSA). (1995). *Reporting manual for the case service report (RSA-911)* (RSA-PD-95-04). Washington, DC: Rehabilitation Services Administration.

Rogler, L. H. (1989) The meaning of culturally sensitive research in mental health. *American Journal of Psychiatry 146*(3) 296-303.

Ross, M. G., & Biggi, I. M. (1986). Critical vocational rehabilitation service delivery issues at referral (02) and closure (08, 26, 28, 30) in serving select disabled persons. In S. Walker, F. Belgrave, A. M. Banner, & R. W. Nicholls (Eds*.), Equal to the challenge: Perspective, problems, and strategies in the rehabilitation of the nonwhite disabled: Proceedings of the National Conference* (pp. 39-50). Washington, DC: The Center for the Study of Handicapped Children and Youth, School of Education, Howard University. (ERIC Document Reproduction Service No. ED 276 198).

Schacht, R. M., White, M., Daugherty, R., LaPlante, M., & Menz, F. (2003). *An analysis of disability and employment outcome data for American Indians and Alaska Natives.* Flagstaff: Northern Arizona University, Institute for Human Development, Arizona University Center on Disabilities, American Indian Rehabilitation Research and Training Center. (Available from the American Indian Rehabilitation Research and Training Center, Institute for Human Development, Northern Arizona University, PO Box 5630, Flagstaff, AZ 86011) National Institute on Disability and Rehabilitation Research. (1998, October). NIDRR 1999-2004 Long-Range Plan. Washington, DC: Author.

Schulman, K. A., Berlin, J. A., Harless, W., & Kerner, J. F., Sistrunk, S. Gersh, B.,Dubé., R., Taleghani, C., Burke, J., Williams, S., Eisenberg. J. M., & Escarce,. E. (1999). The effect of race and sex on physicians' recommendations for cardiac catheterization. *The New England Journal of Medicine, 340*(8) 618-628.

Smith, L. T. (1999). *Decolonizing Methodologies: Research and Indigenous Peoples.* London: Zed Books, Ltd.

Steinbeck, J., and Ricketts, E. F. (1971) [originally published in 1941]. *Sea of Cortez: A leisurely journal of travel and research.* Mamaroneck, NY: Paul P. Appel, Publisher

Stone, J. (2002). Focus on cultural issues in research: Developing and implementing Native American postcolonial participatory action research. In J. D. Davis, J. S. Erickson, S. R. Johnson, C. A. Marshall, P. Running Wolf, & R. L. Santiago, (Eds.), *Work Group on American Indian Research and Program Evaluation Methodology (AIRPEM), Symposium on Research and Evaluation Methodology: Lifespan Issues Related to American Indians/Alaska Natives with Disabilities* (pp. 98-121). Flagstaff: Northern Arizona University, Institute for Human Development, Arizona University Center on Disabilities, American Indian Rehabilitation Research and Training Center. (Available at http://www.wili.org/docs/AIRPEM_Monograph.pdf)

Sue, S. (1999). Science, ethnicity, and bias. *American Psychologist, 54*(12), 1070-1077.

Szymanski, E. M. (1993). Research design and statistical design. *Rehabilitation Counseling Bulletin, 36*(4), 178-182.

Thomas, A., & Sillen, S. (1972). *Racism and psychiatry.* New York: Carol Publishing Group.

Tucker, C. M & Herman, K. C. (2002) Using culturally sensitive theories and research to meet the academic needs of low-income African American children *American Psychologist 57*(10) 762-773

Tutty, L. M., Rothery, M. A., & Grinnell, R. M., Jr., (1996). *Qualitative research for social workers: Phases, steps, & tasks.* Boston: Allyn and Bacon.

United States Census Bureau (2001). Residential segregation of Hispanics or Latinos: 1980 to 2000. Census 2000 news releases [On-line]. http://www.census.gov/hhes/www/housing/resseg/ch6.html [2002, November. 27].

Walker, M. L. (1993). Participatory action research [editorial]. *Rehabilitation Counseling Bulletin, 37*, 2-5.

Wampold, B. E. (2003) Bashing positivism and revering a medical model under the guise of evidence. *The Counseling Psychologist, 31*(5) 539-545.

Wheaton, J. E. (1995). Vocational rehabilitation acceptance rate for European Americans and African Americans: Another look. *Rehabilitation Counseling Bulletin, 38*, 224-231.

White, G. (2002) Consumer participation in disability research: the golden rule as a guide for ethical practice. *Rehabilitation Psychology 47*(4) 438-446.

Wilson, K. B. (2000). Predicting vocational rehabilitation eligibility based on race, education, work status, and source of support at application. *Rehabilitation Counseling Bulletin, 43*, 97-105.

Wilson, K. B. (1999). Vocational rehabilitation acceptance: A tale of two races in a large Midwestern state. *Journal of Applied Rehabilitation Counseling 30*, 25-31.

Wilson, K. B., Harley, D. A., & Alston, R. J. (2001). Race as a correlate of vocational rehabilitation acceptance: Revisited. *Journal of Rehabilitation, 67*(3), 35-41.

Wilson, K. B. (2002). The exploration of vocational rehabilitation acceptance and ethnicity: A national investigation. *Rehabilitation Counseling Bulletin, 45*, 168-176.

Wilson, K. B. (2003). Vocational rehabilitation eligibility and unsuccessful closures after the initiation of the individual plan for employment (IPE): Are there really differences? *Journal of the Pennsylvania Counseling Association, 5, 2, 13-23.*

Wilson, K. B., & Senices, J. (2005). Exploring the vocational rehabilitation acceptance rates of Hispanics and non-Hispanics in the United States. *Journal of Counseling and Development 83(1), 86-96.*

Wilson, K. B., Harley, D. A., McCormick, K., Jolivette, K. & Jackson. R. (2001). A literature review of vocational rehabilitation acceptance and explaining bias in the rehabilitation process. *Journal of Rehabilitation, 32*, 24-35.

CHAPTER 12

THE SPIRITUAL REALM OF REHABILITATION COUNSELING

JOSEPH KEFERL
MARTI RIEMER-REISS

Chapter Highlights

➡ Is it spirituality or religion?

➡ Spirituality and rehabilitation counseling

➡ Spirituality and overall well-being

➡ Ethical considerations

➡ Ethical issues

➡ Conclusion

$\mathcal{A}$ holistic, multicultural model of working with humans involves attending to their spirituality. The significance of including spirituality in the helping process has been noted in several professions including psychology, counseling and (most recently), medicine. However, there is limited literature addressing the inclusion of spirituality in the field of rehabilitation counseling. Although the role of spirituality has been largely neglected in the past, the rationale for its inclusion in the field is vast. Within this context, one should be aware of the ethical responsibilities related to investigating the spiritual realm of rehabilitation counseling. This chapter will address the historical context and contributing factors for counselor avoidance of spirituality in practice, and will discuss implications of including spirituality as a legitimate component of the rehabilitation process. Ethical considerations of embracing spirituality in the rehabilitation counseling profession will also be presented.

The field of rehabilitation counseling prides itself in utilizing a holistic, multicultural model of service delivery. This model recognizes people as unique individuals with diverse values and experiences. Arguably, one of the most significant factors related to human values and experiences is one's spiritual perspective, which influences how one assigns meaning to life (Gibson, 2000; Lukoff, Turker, & Lu, 1992). The significance of relating spirituality to one's psychological well-being is evident in light of the fact that psychological and spiritual developments are deemed synonymous in many cultures (Fukuyama, 1999, 2000; Kain, 1996). Despite the importance of attending to spirituality, counselors frequently overlook their client's spiritual dimensions, and thereby run the risk of neglecting key cultural issues. A truly multicultural model of counseling must involve attending to one's spirituality (Evans, 2003; Fukuyama, 1999, 2000; Worthington, Kurusu, McCollough, & Sandage, 1996; Sue & Sue, 2003).

For some time, the field of rehabilitation counseling has aspired to adopt a holistic and culturally diverse model of service delivery that includes acknowledgment of an individual's medical, psychological, social, and spiritual realms. Efforts were made to develop and implement new methods and instruments of evaluation, service planning, and delivery designed to be more sensitive to the diverse needs of the whole person. While new evaluation instruments and diagnostic procedures have been adopted, the emphasis on capturing quantitatively measurable aspects of the person, such as medical condition, psychological status, and social aspects, persisted. Efforts to understand the importance of spirituality among clients remained stagnant in the rehabilitation community, despite evidence supporting the importance of including this component as an integral part of helping the person.

12

IS IT SPIRITUALITY OR RELIGION?

There exists a great deal of confusion and debate in the literature about the definitions and distinctions between religion and spirituality. In many contexts, the terms are used interchangeably. For the purpose of this chapter, the term "religion" will refer to an allegiance to a set of institutionalized beliefs or doctrines, while the term "spirituality" will be construed as a continued search for meaning and purpose in life. Spirituality is a deeply personal, individualized phenomenon that taps into human experiences, beliefs, values, culture, and behaviors. It is a multidimensional concept that may include transcendence, self-actualization, purpose, wholeness, balance, sacredness, altruism, and universality (Standard, Sandhu, & Painter, 2000). Spirituality is more cross-culturally applicable, unstructured, and inclusive than the concept of religion (Schulte, Skinner, & Claiborn, 2002). As a result, spirituality can occur in or out of the context of the institution of organized religion and not all aspects of religion are inherently spiritual (Chandler, Holden, & Kolander, 1992).

THE IMPACT OF SPIRITUALITY AND RELIGION

Although the concepts of religion and spirituality take on different meanings, they have both become significant influences in contemporary American society. For instance, nine out of ten adult Americans pray, 97% believe their prayers are heard (Steere, 1997) and 96% believe in a God or universal Spirit (Gallup, 1995). This influence impacts a wide array of professions such as counseling, occupational therapy, psychiatry, medicine, and treatment of addictions (Green, Benshoff, & Harris-Forbes, 2001; Priester, 2000; Standard, Sandhu, & Painter, 2000). In particular, the Council for Accreditation of Counseling and Related Educational Programs (CACREP) recently included religious and spiritual values as an aspect of social and cultural diversity in which students are required to demonstrate competency (Green et al., 2001). Further, within the discipline of occupational therapy, spirituality has been recognized as a factor that significantly affects a person's occupational performance and overall rehabilitation outcome (Engquist, Short-Degraff, Gliner, & Oltjenbruns, 1997).

Recently, the discipline of psychiatry expressed support for the inclusion of spirituality and religion in therapy. This support is demonstrated in the requirement for psychiatric residents to complete training in religion and spirituality (Sperry, 2000), and the fact that the psychiatric diagnostic manual now includes spiritual and religious problems (American Psychiatric Association, 1994). The field of rehabilitation psychology mandated that its professionals discuss spirituality with interested consumers (Kilpatrick &

268

McCullough, 1999; Richmond, 2004). The medical field embraced the spiritual movement by developing departments of behavioral medicine and prescribing meditation and prayer to treat physical illnesses (Chirban, 1992). Finally, treatment for addictions holds spirituality as one of the primary therapeutic features in recovery (Piedmont, 2001). The spiritually based Twelve-Step recovery programs (which originated in Alcoholics Anonymous) are applied widely, and are recognized as effective supplements to formal counseling. Many helping professions recognize the increased influence of religion and spirituality within modern society, and have established the value and necessity of including spiritual perspectives in practice.

SPIRITUALITY AND REHABILITATION COUNSELING

In addition to the previously mentioned professions, researchers have recently begun to examine the concept of spirituality as it pertains to rehabilitation counseling (Green et al, 2001, Havranek, 2003; McCarthy, 1995; Trieschmann, 2001). Because of the holistic orientation of rehabilitation counseling, which focuses on the importance of working with one's mind, body, and spirit, it would seem natural to explore the role of spirituality within the context of this profession. Despite this apparently natural connection, the spiritual dimension of the rehabilitation counseling client has commonly been excluded in rehabilitation counseling practice (Green et al., 2001; Havranek, 2003; Hinterkopf, 1996; Kilpatrick & McCullough, 1999; McCarthy, 1995). Thus, rehabilitation counseling might be more accurately described as "consumer driven," but not truly holistic (York, Miller, & Cecil, 1997).

NEGLECT OF SPIRITUALITY IN REHABILITATION COUNSELING

There are several reasons for the lack of recognition of spirituality in rehabilitation counseling practice. First, spirituality is viewed as a very subjective abstract concept. It is typically believed that spirituality is something that is uniquely defined and personalized by each individual and that can be influenced by a number of factors including culture. Because of the inherently subjective nature of spirituality, creating measurable research variables and methods to reliably demonstrate the impact of spirituality remains a challenge within the research community. As a result, there continues to be a lack of empirical evidence supporting the benefits of including it in practice. Many helping professionals are educated with the idea that scientific/empirical epistemology is the only true foundation of reality (Patterson, Hayworth, Turner, & Raskin, 2000). Therefore, until a greater range of empirical evidence is generated, rehabilitation professionals (and rehabilitation counselor training programs) may be unwilling or unprepared to assess spiritual issues or provide spiritual solutions or treatments.

Another possible contributing factor for why the field of rehabilitation counseling has ignored the concept of spirituality relates to an overemphasis on the separation of church and state. Because rehabilitation counseling is mainly funded and controlled by public institutions and policies, the emphasis on the separation of church and state is reinforced (McCarthy, 1995). Although religion and spirituality should not automatically be construed as synonymous, this civic separation often results in an unspoken prohibition against assessing rehabilitation clients' spirituality. Many rehabilitation counselor training programs are based in state institutions; therefore, the neglect may begin with one's education which lacks a spiritual component. As demonstrated by Kelly (1994), state-affiliated counselor education programs offer little or no consideration of religious or spiritual issues.

A third factor may relate to confusion in the field over the role and function of the rehabilitation counselor. Is the rehabilitation counselor really a counselor, or is he/she a coordinator of services? Current literature describes rehabilitation counselors as mediators with multiple roles to help people with disabilities enhance the quality of their lives (Chubon, 1992 as cited in Rubin & Roessler, 2001). Hershenson (as cited in Rubin & Roessler, 2001) emphasized that the role of rehabilitation counselors is multifaceted in that they need to be counselors, coordinators, and consulters. As a result of the many roles and multiple tasks required of rehabilitation counselors, the counseling dimension often becomes obscured. The lack of priority given to attending to the spiritual needs of clients may also be a function of large caseloads and agency pressure for case closures. The pressures and expectations of doing "more with less" has resulted in many rehabilitation counselors not having enough time to focus on the "counseling" aspects of the job. Most rehabilitation counselors are rewarded for achieving concrete results as opposed to the more nebulous concept of counseling for spiritual well-being. In general, the profession of rehabilitation counseling continues to focus on the quantifiable outcome related to the number of successful case closures. Counseling and spiritual growth are difficult to quantify, and thus these activities have not become a priority in the rehabilitation counselor's job role and function (Green et al., 2001).

Rehabilitation counselors may also avoid exploring issues of spirituality due to their own discomfort, confusion, and/or ambivalence over the meaning and role of spirituality. Spirituality is a complex construct to define and understand. Professionals often mistakenly equate the concept of spirituality with religion, which they perceive to be incompatible with their professional practice responsibilities (Engquist et al., 1997). The typical cultural belief in

America is that religion and spirituality should be confined to specifically religious settings and activities, and separated from the day-to-day affairs of the secular world (Kelly, 1994). Professionals also view spirituality as a personal matter that is not to be discussed or shared among one's clientele (Engquist et al., 1997; Green et al., 2001; Kilpatrick & McCullough, 1999).

The final reason rehabilitation professionals avoid the topic of spirituality in practice may be that they do not feel qualified due to insufficient formal training in its use (Green et al., 2001). To date, research on the infusion of spirituality in rehabilitation counselor education curricula has been sparse. Sentiments of a recent focus group comprised of rehabilitation counselors reflected concerns pertaining to a lack of training and preparation regarding the role of spirituality in rehabilitation counseling practice (York, Miller, & Duncan, 1997). A national survey of counselor education programs demonstrated that the majority of programs lacked any substantive coverage of spirituality in their curriculum (Kelly, 1994). This lack of training preparedness may stem from the fact that spirituality is not clearly defined in CORE (Council on Rehabilitation Education) standards, and thus may not typically be included in an already full curriculum (Green et al., 2001; Kilpatrick & McCullough, 1999). Literature on incorporating spirituality into rehabilitation counseling is limited (Green et al., 2001). In order to help future rehabilitation counselors feel comfortable with issues of spirituality, rehabilitation educators need to expand current rehabilitation counselor training program curricula to include the spiritual aspects of disability and rehabilitation (Kilpatrick & McCullough, 1999).

SPIRITUALITY AND OVERALL WELL-BEING

In a study by Larson, Swyers, and McCullough (1997), correlations between overall health and spirituality were found. Positive relationships were reported between spirituality, religion, and health, inferring that individuals who possessed strong spiritual and religious beliefs tended to have more outcomes that are positive related to physical wellness and mental health. They also experienced fewer alcohol and drug problems. A negative relationship was reported between spirituality and religion and disorders. Persons who maintained a strong spiritual or religious base tended to have lower rates of both physical and psychological disorders. These findings have particular relevance for persons with disabilities, particularly as they relate to progression, prognosis, and potential for incurring additional disabilities in the future.

Although based on generalized conjecture, there also appears to be a relationship between peoples' spirituality and their general desire to thrive. This

271

notion is taken from research conducted by Simmons (2001) in which results of a two-year study of hospitalized elderly patients were reported. In the study, persons who reported having spiritual struggles, or being disconnected from their God, had a significantly higher risk of dying. For persons who incur a severe disability, the importance of spirituality may be of primary importance as the person initially attempts to understand and reevaluate their feelings of value, identity, and self-worth.

BENEFITS OF INTEGRATING SPIRITUALITY IN REHABILITATION COUNSELING

The justification for integrating spirituality in rehabilitation counseling is multidimensional. At a philosophical level, spirituality is immersed in some of the most basic of human needs. Spirituality provides many with the necessary comfort and strength required to successfully navigate through challenging periods in their lives. People with disabilities and their families are often faced with significant challenges. These challenges can manifest in the individual in the form of cognitive, psychological, or physical transformations and events. The role of spirituality in working through the challenges associated with life and disability is to enhance the persons' ability to rationalize, find acceptance, and move forward with their life situation (Kilpatrick & McCullough, 1999). Despite this evidence, rehabilitation professionals may not fully recognize or understand the powerful role spirituality plays in the lives of many people who have disabilities. A substantial number of individuals with disabilities acknowledge spirituality as an important part of their lives and they find it to be useful in coping with their disabilities.

Despite the potential benefits of acknowledging the spirituality needs of clients, evidence suggests that rehabilitation counselors who work with people with mental illnesses may avoid addressing spirituality in practice, because they mistakenly fear that discussion related to spirituality and/or religion may trigger pathological symptoms (Fallot, 1998). Religion has been associated with maladaptive defense mechanisms, irrational and distorted views of reality, and dogmatic patterns of thinking among some people with mental illness. Counselors working with this population may be cautious about discussing spirituality and/or religion, as they do not want to risk reinforcing a client who may be operating from such a maladaptive perspective. Although exploring spirituality and/or religion might be risky for some, most people with mental illnesses do not become disorganized by discussion related to religious and spiritual experiences. Spirituality has been found to be a helpful tool for many clients as they cope with day-to-day challenges associated with mental illness. For instance, clients with mental illness often find that spirituality provides strength for coping, social support, and the feeling of being a "whole person" (Fallot, 1998). In general, spirituality has the potential to become a vital component in the recovery process for many people with mental illnesses.

Benjamin and Looby (1998) stated that in order for counselors to be able to assist clients in achieving true self-actualization and optimal wellness, counselors must be trained and prepared to meet the spirituality needs of their clients. A number of studies demonstrating the beneficial impact of spirituality were conducted in the counseling genre. Propst (1980) suggested that retention of clients might be improved when counselors recognize the religious and spiritual needs of their clients. Lack of follow-through due to low client investment is a common thread in cases of client detachment from rehabilitation services; therefore, the benefits of addressing spirituality to bolster client commitment are apparent (Propst, 1980). This finding supports the notion that understanding the spiritual needs of clients ought to become common practice among rehabilitation counselors—beginning in the earliest stages of rehabilitation and continuing throughout the course of service delivery. It connotes that people who feel that their religious and spiritual needs are recognized and valued will often feel compelled to invest themselves more fully in the rehabilitation service delivery system.

ETHICAL CONSIDERATIONS

Although there is sound rationale for including spirituality in the rehabilitation counseling process, one should be aware of the ethical implications of doing so. The Code of Professional Ethics for Rehabilitation Counselors (CRCC, 2002) emphasizes the value of cultural diversity in the training and work of all counselors. Counselors are expected to gain knowledge, personal understanding, and sensitivity applicable to working with diverse cultures. This is particularly important in light of the fact that religion and spirituality are understood to be associated with ethnic identity and multicultural values (Coughlin, 1992; Evans, 2003; Fukuyama, 1999, 2000; Pate & Bondi, 1995). Therefore, ethical counselors recognize and accept the spiritual values of clients as they would other important characteristics that contribute to client individuality. This is not to imply that counselors are expected to be knowledgeable about every religious and spiritual expression in this culturally diverse society. Counselors are, however, expected to recognize that part of their clients' cultural development may involve religion and/or spirituality. It is also important that counselors are aware of cross-cultural differences in understanding religious and spiritual beliefs and practices. In order to be truly empathic, counselors must not judge a client's religious and spiritual experiences using cultural values that differ from the client's. Effective responses to clients' spiritual concerns must be communicated in a manner independent of the counselor's belief system.

Coughlin (1992) indicated that all helping professionals must take into account the role that religious and spiritual values play in clients' overall mental health. Personality, attitudes, and behavior are all shaped by these cultural values, and relate to the meaning an individual attributes to his/her life circumstances. This is particularly important to the field of rehabilitation counseling, as it has a holistic and multicultural orientation. As indicated by Byrd (1997), rehabilitation counselors utilize medicine and psychology in their practice, and are increasingly aware of the need to incorporate the spiritual component of the client as well. In order to respect their clients' individual rights and personal dignity, rehabilitation professionals must also value the importance of spirituality and religion in the lives of their clients.

APPLICATION OF SPIRITUALITY
IN REHABILITATION COUNSELING

In order to attend to clients' spiritual values, it is helpful for counselors to recognize and understand their own spiritual beliefs and values. By developing such an awareness of their own spiritual views, counselors become sufficiently prepared to help clients enhance their own lives by finding meaning in them (Sue & Sue, 2003). Rehabilitation counselors working with clients devoted to a specific spiritual or religious expression can augment the rehabilitation process in the following ways. First, it is necessary that rehabilitation counselors acknowledge the importance of spirituality in their clients' lives. Clients may volunteer information related to their spirituality in a variety of ways. Issues of spirituality may be overtly communicated by the client, or they may be more veiled or hidden. In many cases, the client's choice to share aspects of their spirituality may be rooted in their culture. Cultural influences may impact the degree to which a client feels comfortable discussing issues of spirituality. It is important for the rehabilitation counselor to understand the cultural nature of spirituality (Bishop, 1992; Sue & Sue, 2003).

Second, rehabilitation counselors need to be willing to accept and consult with other spiritual and/or religious leaders in their clients' lives. For instance, the rehabilitation counselor may need to ascertain if the leader is a source of support within the client's spiritual world. If this is the case, then collaboration with the leader is necessary. Key components of this collaboration involve obtaining a signed release from the client, and respectfully communicating with the leader (Miller, 2003). This collaboration may provide the rehabilitation counselor with valuable insight into the client's worldview.

Rehabilitation counselors need to parallel their clients' worldviews with congruent terminology and imagery in conceptualizing vocational strengths and limitations. This is particularly relevant in terms of recognizing the client's value systems. Carefully choosing to use language and images that match the client's values strengthens the working relationship between the counselor and client, and also serves to facilitate a sense of holistic congruency (Sue & Sue, 2003).

Finally, it is necessary that counselors address spiritual themes that are meaningful to their clients and encourage the presence of those themes in the rehabilitation counseling process. Creating opportunities for thematic inclusion of spirituality in the rehabilitation process can bolster clients' sense of investment in their plan. The rehabilitation counselor can facilitate this process by focusing on spiritual themes that have relevancy to the client's culture and personal value systems.

ETHICAL ISSUES

Although there are some compelling reasons to involve spirituality in the counseling process, there are also some ethical considerations worthy of considering. Per The Code of Professional Ethics for Certified Rehabilitation Counselors (2002), professionals are required to know the limits of their expertise, and not risk potential harm to clients by engaging in areas in which they lack basic training and experience. Many rehabilitation counselors may not have the expertise to address specific questions about religious doctrine. Therefore, attempting to address such issues would constitute an overstepping of the counselor's limits of competence. It is important for counselors to make appropriate referrals when they cannot ethically handle a client's spiritual or religious needs.

There is an ethical tenet to respect individual dignity, uniqueness, and freedom of choice (CRCC, 2002). Ethical counselors avoid forcing their spiritual values on clients, as it would conflict with this ethical tenet. Similarly, it is unethical for rehabilitation counselors to direct clients toward any particular spiritual or religious orientation, as this could constitute an imposition of values, and represent a violation of the code of ethics.

Within ethical guidelines, there still remains an opportunity for appropriate and beneficial spiritual exploration. Spiritual values are certainly related to basic questions about oneself, and the meaning of life. Bound by the same ethical limits of not overstepping competence or imposing values, counselors can help clients understand the relationship between themselves, their disabilities, and the spiritual questions that arise. It is appropriate and ethical to encourage client exploration of spiritual issues related to the concerns being addressed in the context of rehabilitation counseling.

The following case demonstrates an ethical use of spirituality in rehabilitation counseling.

CASE EXAMPLE

Carrie, a 40-year-old female was severely injured while riding her motorcycle. She was referred to a vocational rehabilitation counselor, as she can no longer do her previous job of nursing. While discussing possible jobs for vocational exploration, Carrie revealed to her counselor that she felt her calling was to be a nurse. The counselor explored Carrie's use of the word "calling" to find that she is a very spiritual person who believes that her identity with nursing is what makes her life meaningful. The counselor brainstormed with Carrie to come up with a list of other things in her life that gave her a sense of connection and meaning. Carrie revealed that she was very connected to her dog and felt a sense of spirituality on long walks in the forest. The counselor gave Carrie a homework assignment to keep a journal and record anything that felt spiritually meaningful to her in the next week. Carrie and her counselor discussed how her sense of spirituality and purpose might be helpful in choosing a new vocational path. As a result of this discussion, Carrie, despite initially feeling depressed about the possibility of leaving the nursing field, now reports that she feels hopeful that she will find an equally meaningful calling in a new employment setting that is better suited to her new self. Carrie's counselor reinforced this positive outlook by scheduling time to discuss the results of her homework and possible transition into vocational exploration when Carrie feels she is ready.

CONCLUSION

As demonstrated in the aforementioned case example, the key to integrating spirituality into rehabilitation practice is that it does not require a novel process—only receptivity to exploring new issues. Using basic elements of empathic counseling, rehabilitation counselors can effectively examine clients' spiritual issues as they arise. The basic underpinnings of counselor training provide the rehabilitation counselor with a foundation from which spirituality can be explored. Rehabilitation counselors are encouraged to become sensitive to the significance of clients' spiritual values, and the implications for the rehabilitation counseling process. It is expected that rehabilitation counselors understand their ethical responsibilities in this regard by respecting the client's spiritual world, and by not inadvertently influencing a client in the realm of his/her spiritual beliefs. Spirituality may be viewed as a component of multicultural counseling, which should be approached directly throughout the rehabilitation counseling process.

This chapter represents one opportunity to educate current and future rehabilitation counseling professionals about the essence of spirituality in practice. The related strengths, limitations, and ethics involved are offered to help counselors enhance their competence in working with clients' spirituality, and avoid the pitfalls associated with it. Additional empirical research is necessary in order to determine the best techniques for integrating spirituality into the rehabilitation process.

REFERENCES

American Psychiatric Association (1994). *Diagnostic and statistical manual of mental disorders, Forth Edition*. Washington, DC: Author.

Bishop, D. R. (1992). Religious values as cross-cultural issues in counseling. *Counseling and Values, 36*, 179-191.

Benjamin, P. & Looby, J. (1998). Defining the nature of spirituality in the context of Maslow's and Roger's theories. *Counseling and Values, 42*(2), 92-100.

Byrd, K. E. (1997). Concepts related to inclusion of the spiritual component in services to   persons with disability and chronic illness. *Journal of Applied Rehabilitation Counseling, 28*(4), 26-29.

Commission on Rehabilitation Counselor Certification. (2002). *Code of Professional Ethics for Rehabilitation Counselors*. Retrieved April 10th, 2003, from http://www.crccertification.com/pdf/code_ethics_2002.pdf.

Chandler, C. K., Holden, J. M., & Kolander, C. A. (1992). Counseling for spiritual wellness: Theory and practice. *Journal of Counseling & Development, 7*, 168-175.

Chirban, J. T. (1992). Healing and spirituality. *Pastoral Psychology, 40*(4), 235-244.

Coughlin, E. K. (1992, April 1). Social scientists again turn attention to religion's place in the world. *The Chronicle of Higher Education*, p. 6, A7, A8.

Engquist, D. E., Short-DeGraff, M., Gliner, J., & Oltjenbruns, K. (1997). Occupational therapists beliefs and practices with regard to spirituality and therapy. *The American Journal of Occupational Therapy, 51*(3), 173-180.

Evans, K. M. (2003). Including spirituality in multicultural counseling: Overcoming counselor resistance. *Multicultural competencies: A guidebook of practices* (pp. 161-171). Association for Multicultural Counseling & Development, Alexandria, VA, US.

Fallot, R. D. (1998). The place of spirituality and religion in mental health services. *Spirituality and Religion in Recovery from Mental Illness, 80*, 3-12.

Fukuyama, M. A. (2003). Integrating spirituality in multicultural counseling: "A worldview." *Culture and counseling: New approaches,* (pp. 186-195). Allyn & Bacon, Needham Heights, MA, US.

Fukuyama, M. A., & Sevig, T. D. (1999). *Integrating spirituality into multicultural counseling.* Sage Publications, Inc, Thousand Oaks, CA, US.

Gallup, G. (1995). *The Gallup Poll: Public Opinion in 1995.* Wilmington, DE: Scholarly Resources.

Gibson, T. L. (2000). Wholeness and transcendence in the practice of pastoral psychotherapy from a judeo-christian perspective. *The psychology of mature spirituality: Integrity, wisdom, transcendence,* (pp. 175-186). Brunner-Routledge, New York, NY, US.

Green, R. L., Benshoff, J. J., & Harris-Forbes, J. A. (2001). Spirituality in rehabilitation counselor education: A pilot survey. *Journal of Rehabilitation, 67*, 55-60.

Havranek, J. E. (2003). The spirituality exploration guide: A means to facilitate discussion of spiritual issues in the rehabilitation counseling process. *Journal of Applied Rehabilitation Counseling, 34*(1), 38-43.

Hinterkopf, E. (1996). *Integrating spirituality in counseling.* Alexandria, VA: American Counseling Association.

Kain, C. D. (1996). *Positive HIV affirmative counseling.* Alexandria, VA: American Counseling Association.

Kelly, E. W. (1994). The role of religion and spirituality in counselor education: A national survey. *Counselor Education And Supervision, 33*, 227-237.

Kilpatrick, S. D., McCullough, M. E. (1999). Religion and spirituality in rehabilitation psychology. *Rehabilitation Psychology, 44*(4), 388-402.

Larson, D. B., Swyers, J. P., & McCullough, M. E. (Eds.). (1997). *Scientific research on spirituality and health: A consensus report*. Rockville, MD: National Institute for Healthcare Research.

Lukoff, D., Turner, R., & Lu, F. (1992). Transpersonal psychology research review: Psychoreligious dimensions of healing. *The Journal of Transpersonal Psychology, 24*, 41-60.

McCarthy, H. (1995). Understanding and reversing rehabilitation counseling's neglect of spirituality. *Rehabilitation Education, 9*(2), 187-199.

Miller, G. A. (2003). *Incorporating spirituality in counseling and psychotherapy: theory and technique*. Hoboken, NJ: Wiley.

Pate, R. H., & Bondi, A. M. (1995). Religious beliefs and practice: An integral aspect of multicultural awareness. M. T. Burke and J. G. Miranti (Eds.), *Counseling: The spiritual dimension,* (pp. 169-176). Alexandria, VA: American Counseling Association.

Patterson, J., Hayworth, M., Turner, C., & Raskin, M. (2000). Spiritual issues in family therapy: A graduate-level course. *Journal of Marital and Family Therapy, 26*(2), 199-210.

Piedmont, R. L. (2001). Spiritual transcendence and the scientific study of spirituality. *Journal of Rehabilitation, 67*(1), 4-14.

Priester, P. E. (2000). Varieties of spiritual experience in support of recovery from cocaine dependence. *Counseling & Values, 44*(2), 107-112.

Propst, L. R. (1980). The comparative efficacy of religious and nonreligious imagery for the treatment of mild depression in religious individuals. *Cognitive Therapy and Research, 4*, 167-178.

Richmond, L. J. (2004). Religion, spirituality, and health: A topic not so new. *American Psychologist, 59*(1), 52.

Rubin, S. E., & Roessler, R. T. (2001). The role and function of the rehabilitation counselor. In S. E. Rubin & R. T. Roessler (Eds.), *Foundations of the Vocational Rehabilitation Process* (5th ed). (pp. 251-266). Austin, TX: ProEd.

Schulte, D. L., Skinner, T. A., & Claiborn, C. D. (2002). Religious and spiritual issues in counseling psychology training. *The Counseling Psychologist, 30*(1), 118-134.

Simmons, J. (2001). Headlines: Study: Lack of spirit may shorten life. *Counseling Today, 44*, 3.

Sperry, L. (2000). Spirituality and psychiatry: Incorporating the spiritual dimension into clinical practice. *Psychiatric Annals, 30*(8), 518-523.

Stanard, R. P., Sandhu, D. S., & Painter, L. C. (2000). Assessment of spirituality in counseling. *Journal of Counseling & Development, 78*, 204-210.

Steere, D. A. (1997). Spiritual presence in psychotherapy: A guide for caregivers. New York: Broner/Mazel.

Sue, D. W., & Sue, D. (2003). What is cultural competence? In D. W. Sue & D. Sue, *Counseling the culturally diverse: Theory and practice* (4th ed). (pp. 17-29). New York, NY: John Wiley & Sons.

Trieschmann, R. B. (2001). Spirituality and energy medicine. *Journal of Rehabilitation, 67*(1), 26-32.

Worthington, E. L., Kurusu, T. A., McCollough, M. E., & Sandage, S. J. (1996). Empirical research on religion and psychotherapeutic processes and outcomes: A 10-year review and research prospectus. *Psychological Bulletin, 119*, 448-487.

York, K. D., Miller, D. M., & Cecil, D. (1997). *Spirituality and rehabilitation: A focus group approach*. (ERIC Document Reproduction Service No. ED432705)

CHAPTER 13

PARTNERING WITH FAMILIES FOR SUCCESSFUL CAREER OUTCOMES

STACIE L. ROBERTSON
CARL R. FLOWERS

Chapter Highlights

➡ Family models

➡ Ethnic family development

➡ Family influence on career success

➡ Strategies for partnering with families

➡ Counselor competencies and characteristics

➡ Conclusion

13

$\mathcal{F}$amily is the foundation from which one learns about the world (Sue & Sue, 1990). Families influence many aspects of an individual's life choices, including education, political views, and in many cases, career choice, and outcomes. In exploring the role of family in successful career outcomes, the importance of family cannot be overstated. Given the important role and influences of family in successful vocational outcomes, it is understandable that programming and services must encompass the whole of an individual's lifestyle, including active involvement of nuclear or traditional family members, in addition to others such as extended family members and a wide variety of community support people. This chapter focuses on considerations and definitions of family explored from various ethnic groups; the role and importance of family in the vocational rehabilitation process; family influences on vocational outcomes; and partnering strategies with clients and families from diverse backgrounds (e.g., African American, Asian American, Hispanic American and Native American), based on counselor competencies and characteristics.

The notion that disability is a natural part of the human existence has been widely chronicled in the rehabilitation literature (Americans with Disabilities Act, 1990; Smart & Smart, 2006; U.S. Department of Education and Rehabilitation Services, 2000). So too has the idea that family, in various forms and models, is influential in the acceptance, adjustment, and life outcomes of individuals with a disabilities. Power (1988), for example, observed that disability is "a family affair" and that "client performance in vocational rehabilitation is a function of both the person and the family involvement" (p. 195). Parke (2004) further noted that family members are mothers, fathers, and siblings, who have both direct and indirect influence on one another. As noted above, the notion of family may invoke various images or various definitions, forms, and models. Landesman and Veitz's (1987) definition of family as a "social group with whom one resides" (p. 61) may be appropriate in some instances; while references to family as people one feels close to and or on whom one tends to depend or rely, may also fit. Another definition, Goldenberg and Goldenberg's (2004) observation of family as a system in which a set of rules are in place, where members are assigned ascribed roles and where intricate overt and covert forms of communication are in place, may seem more appropriate.

From a disability standpoint, 2000 census data indicated that more than 20 million (28.1%) families in the United States reported having at least one family member with a disability (U. S. Census, 2005). Of this group, more than 16% (12 million families) reported that at least one family member reported

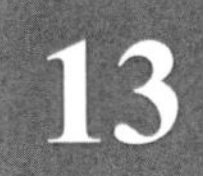

having a "condition that substantially limits one or more basic physical activities." These data suggest that disability is truly becoming "more common as a larger portion of the U. S. population (Smart and Smart, 2006, p. 29).

FAMILY MODELS

Hare and Gray (n. d.) observed that the traditional family model (e.g., married couple with their own children, where one parent works outside the home and all family members share a common dwelling) is less common than other familial structures. Data from the 2000 census suggests that this family model is now the *non-traditional* type in the United States, with less than 10% of all American families fitting the definition of a traditional or nuclear family. In its place, other family structure models, including extended, stepfamilies, single-parent families, and alternative families are emerging in the today's society (Benshoff & Janikowski, 2000).

Another increasingly common, frequently reported, familial model is the single-parent family. Recent statistics indicate that more than 90% of single-parent households are headed by females (Hare & Gay, n.d.). In this pattern, only one parent is responsible for establishing and maintaining family traditions and culture. Another quite common family model is the extended family, where the family unit includes informal kin (who may not be parents and or grandparents), as well as great grandparents, siblings, and other relatives who have maintained relationships with family members. Paniagua (1996) observed that the extended family often includes both "biologically related individuals as well as non-biologically related individuals" (p.128) where supports (e.g., instrumental and emotional) are provided. The non-biologically related extended family members often include friends, ministers, and healers.

Sue and Sue (1990) noted that the extended family plays important roles in decision-making among African Americans, Asians, Hispanics, as well as Native Americans. The influence of the extended family members in decision-making is often based, in part, on the instrumental supports (i.e., financial) and emotional (e.g., advice and counseling) provided (Paniagua, 1996). Other family forms include blended families, where families are created by divorce and/or remarriage; and grandparent-led families, in which children are reared by grandparents when the biological parents are no longer able to serve as family leaders, for one reason or another. According to the U.S. Census Bureau (2005), nearly 6 million grandparents were listed as head of households in 2002, and about 4 million youth lived in households headed by a grandparent. Grandparent-headed households have grown by 105 percent since 1970.

Regardless of the family structure, the family influences several aspects of an individual's life choices, including career choice, education, and political views.

ETHNIC FAMILY DEVELOPMENT

AFRICAN AMERICANS

Literature suggests that African American families reflect vast within-group differences, including organizational units, socio-economic status, cultural values, and country of origin (Staples, 1988). In support, Parke (2004) observed that recent literature has shifted toward the African American family being viewed as "resilient (p. 381), as opposed to previous literature tending to focus on the African American family as being disorganized. This resiliency, the author notes, is characterized by several important areas, including a strong sense of family and familial obligations, willingness to absorb relatives, frequent interaction with relatives, and a system of mutual aid. This strong sense of family or strong kinship bond is highly adaptive for the African-American family in providing support and in combining resources. Also highly adaptive is the African-American family's ability for role flexibility (Diller, 2004). This family strength indicates that family members are better able to take on different family roles. This strength, while adaptive in nature, allows for adjustment to the changes in family roles that often come with the onset of a disability. As an example, when compared to other groups, more African American families are headed by single women than any other ethnic group (Census, 2005). McCollum's (1997) observation that, in many ways, the African American family is defined by the manner in which its members perform "based on the needs within the family itself" (p. 220). This supports the view that the African-American family is highly resilient.

ASIAN AMERICANS

In the United States, Asian Americans include populations from nearly 30 countries in the Far East and South Pacific region, including China, Guam, Japan, Korea, the Philippines, and Vietnam. Given the broad variance, Asian American family models tend to be diverse, based on a number of factors, including languages, reasons for immigrating to the United States, and number of familial generations within the country. Ishi-Kuntz, cited in Demo, (Allen, and Fine, 2000), observes that, while within-group diversity is present, one constant is the fact most Asian families are generally viewed as patriarchal. In this population, length of residence in this country is a contributing factor, and impacts on how the family is defined.

HISPANIC AMERICANS

The term Hispanic refers to a number of groups of Spanish speaking descent, including individuals from Central America, South America, Cuba, and Mexico (Rubin & Roessler, 2001). Census data (2005) indicate that the Hispanic population experienced more than a 3% increase (14 million) in the United States, and continues at a rate (3.6 percent) well above that of other ethnic groups. Regardless of their original country of entry, the Hispanic family unit tends to be a close-knit, family oriented group, where the larger family (i.e., extended family) unit is common. Observing that Hispanic family members are likely to live in close proximity of one another, Parke (2004) explains "there is a high level of cross generational co-residence arrangements and assistance (p. 383).

NATIVE AMERICANS

Given that these populations represents nearly 400 distinct ethnicities and speak more than 200 languages, the literature suggests that it is almost impossible to define the typical family as a group. While different in many familial characteristics, Dykema, Nelson, and Appleton (1995) suggest that the extended family is one of the "greatest strengths common to American Indian cultures" (p. 150). Thomason (1991) suggests that at least four family types; Isolated, Traditional, Bicultural, and Acculturated, characterized by where the family lives and the family's participation in traditional within-group activities, are common among this population. The Isolated family usually lives in remote areas of their reservation and retains its preference for use of the native language. This is in contrast to the bicultural family, whose members also lives on the reservation, participates in tribal ceremonies, *and* who prefer speaking English (Thomason).

As can be seen, the term *family* has many different meanings across cultural populations. Who is considered a family member and how the family is involved in the counseling process, logically, also would differ based on cultural definitions of family. While this chapter offers examples of differences between cultural groups and family involvement in the counseling and career counseling process, multicultural competencies suggest that counselors increase their understanding of cultural differences through further research and involvement with different cultural groups.

FAMILY INFLUENCE ON CAREER SUCCESS

Providing career services to individuals with disabilities from various cultural backgrounds is multidimensional. Cultural differences, the individual's functional limitation, type, level, and onset of the disability, along with numerous other individual factors, may require that career services focus on assisting with independent or interdependent issues (i.e., housing, transportation, personal care assistance) and vocational issues (i.e., decision making skills, vocational development, vocational placement). As an example, an individual with severe mobility impairment, who is unable to drive, may need assistance with personal care and transportation issues before addressing general vocational issues. A holistic point of view is, therefore, necessary for successful career outcomes for individuals with disabilities and their families.

The onset of a disability is, in fact, a family affair (Power, & Dell Orto, 2004; Power, Dell Orto, & Gibbons, 1988; Power, Hershenson, & Fabian, 1991). Often, the family offers assistance with the individual's interdependent needs and influences the individual's vocational decisions. Family influence, therefore, is an important factor in human services and career counseling of individuals with disabilities, and is a strong factor in service treatment outcomes for individuals with disabilities. Family influence is especially important when working with those individuals who, based on their cultural beliefs, function in the collective. A collectivist view, inherent in many cultural groups (Skowron, 2004), indicates that disability is a reflection of the entire family as opposed to the individual (Hasnian, 2003; Sotnik, & Jezewski, 2005).

Independent living matters, such as transportation, self-care, housing, and money management skills often are matters of concern for both individuals from various racial/ethnic cultures and individuals with disabilities. Consequently, if the family's cultural values stress the importance of the family unit, an individual with a disability may remain living with the family, regardless of his or her abilities to live independently. Mexican families, for example, may expect a child to live in their home until they are ready to get married and start a family of their own. Within this type of family unit, the family often supports the individual with a disability financially as well as psychologically (Santana-Martin, & Santana, 2005). In addition to the family unit, the Mexican community is an important factor, and is often seen as family, providing assistance and support to the members of the community (Santana-Martin, & Santana, 2005). In this situation, the family and community members influence independent or interdependent matters. A Mexican-American with a disability may reside with his or her immediate family members, rely on a family member for personal assistance, and rely on a community member for transportation to and from work. Due to the interdependent nature of various cultural groups, working with the family to develop and implement an interdependent living plan for the person with a disability is vital.

Rehabilitation researchers have historically found that family involvement in the vocational process improves both the quality and quantity of placements (Drake, McHugo, Becker, Anthony, & Clarke, 1996; Newman, 1988). Factors such as family background, educational level, occupational attainment, and the family's location in the broader social context (i.e., socioeconomic status and cultural membership) affect vocational development (Kerka, 2000; Lankard, 1995; Schulenberg, Vondracek, & Crouter, 1984). The family's influence is apparent with regard to the opportunities provided by the family (i.e., educational, financial, role models, knowledge sources), the family's processes, which may include socialization practices, parent-child relations (Karka, 2000; Lankard, 1995; Schulenberg, et al., 1984), and the family's response to disability.

Family reactions to disabilities in general can significantly factor into the individual's counseling goals and outcomes, including vocational development and placement. This reaction may differ based on the family's cultural beliefs, with definitions of disability differing among cultures (Congress, 2004; Salas-Provance, Erickson, & Reed, 2002; Sotnik, & Jezewski, 2005). Causation, along with valued and devalued attributes of disabilities differ across cultures and dictate how disability is defined within the culture and/or the family (Groce, 2005). Sotnik and Jezewski provide an example

> … Southeast Asian beliefs related to disability and its causation range from those that focus on the behavior of the parents, particularly the mother, during pregnancy to sins committed by extended family memberships and reincarnation… A Southeast Asian individual with a disability may be segregated from the community because the disability represents a wrongdoing by the parents or ancestors and is considered a source of disgrace.

p.27

Taking Southeast Asian cultural beliefs into consideration, the counseling process may be hindered by the family, fearing that inclusion of the individual with a disability into the world of work may highlight the family's disgrace. While the cultural group may espouse a certain belief pertaining to work, beliefs regarding disability may supercede all other traditional beliefs. One individual of Asian decent indicates the following:

> There are many aspects of the way my parents have raised me that would have differed dramatically if I would have been able-bodied. In many ways the situation of me being disabled overshadowed many traditional Asian values they may have held. They did not exert the academic pressures that are

> common to Asian households, on me. … I know my parents
> would have pressured me a lot more to succeed academically if
> I did not have a disability.

Tsao, 2000

As noted by Tsao's personal experience, cultural beliefs regarding disability may override cultural beliefs regarding academic and, ultimately, career expectations. As cultural beliefs regarding disability may affect counseling outcomes, so too might cultural beliefs regarding meaningfulness of specific types of work (Hasnain, Sotnik, & Ghiloni, 2003). For some cultural groups, caregiver responsibilities, as they would be assigned to a person with or without a disability, may be considered a positive vocational outcome. With so many family factors influencing counseling and vocational outcomes, it becomes increasingly important to involve the family in the process.

STRATEGIES FOR PARTNERING WITH FAMILIES

Involving the family in vocational rehabilitation can be challenging for all counselors. Rehabilitation counselors, particularly, identify the following as challenges to family inclusion in the rehabilitation process: belief that there is an individual focus inherent in rehabilitation, lack of encouragement for family inclusion by rehabilitation agencies, limited funding, large caseloads, limited counselor time, and lack of training to provide services to families (Accordino, & Hunt, 2001; May & Hunt, 1994). Although this research is specific to rehabilitation, family inclusion is often neglected in other counseling and human service agencies, especially with regard to career counseling. While many road blocks and challenges to including families in the career counseling process may appear to be present for the counselor, the rewards for inclusion can be tremendous with regard to successful counseling outcomes. Given the various roadblocks to inclusion, it becomes up to the individual counselor to find creative ways in which to include the family.

Issues in working around time limits and caseload size are specific to the individual counselor and agency. There are, however, universal strategies that can assist in enhancing relationships with families who represent various cultural backgrounds. To enhance the relationship with the family, multicultural competencies and an ability to establish a working alliance with the family, is necessary. Conducting a family assessment to determine the family's ability to assist in the process or to determine if the family is a hindrance to the counseling process can help the counselor to determine strategies on how to involve the family. The remainder of the chapter will review several strategies for partnering with families, including basic competencies and characteristics needed to partner with the family, suggestions on establishing a working alliance with the family, and conducting a family assessment. This chapter concludes by using a rehabilitation model as an example of how families can contribute throughout the counseling process.

COUNSELOR COMPETENCIES AND CHARACTERISTICS

Partnering with multicultural families requires the counselor to possess basic competencies and characteristics. Multicultural competencies, essential when counseling at any level, include counselor knowledge of (a) their own cultural values and biases, (b) the client's cultural values and worldview (Sue & Sue, 1990), and (c) culturally appropriate intervention strategies (Arrendondo, et al., 1996). Multicultural competencies allow the counselor to understand the family's worldview, determine how the counselor's own biases may affect the counseling process, and determine treatment strategies and techniques that will aid in the counseling process.

Counselors with knowledge of their own cultural values and biases are better able to recognize the potential effects or the impact of their values on culturally diverse families (Middleton et al., 2000) and the impact these values may have on the counseling relationship. Knowledge of the family's cultural values and worldviews allows the counselor to determine if the counseling relationship style, techniques, and/or interventions fit with the family's cultural values, beliefs, and worldview. For example, Latino families often value distinct and highly structured family roles and duties. This authority structure of the family often influences how the family views authority in general, indicating that the family respects and may even be most comfortable in hierarchical structures. The counselor who attempts to lessen the power deferential, be less authoritative, more democratic, using indirect and subtle forms of communication may inadvertently alienate, disrespect, and/or confuse the Latino family that values authority structure (Diller, 2004). Values of importance to counselors that are often placed on the ethnic minority client are independence and achievement, along with self-disclosure and emotional expressiveness (Duncan, 2005; Sue, & Sue, 1990). Multicultural competency includes knowledge of how these values may come into conflict with a client who values collectivism, cooperation, and 'saving face' (Brown, & Landrum-Brown, 1995).

Inherent in multicultural competencies is the ability to recognize that variations exist within cultural groups, and the ability to avoid stereotyping individuals based on diversity group affiliation (Diller 2004; Groce, 2005). As Groce eloquently notes, "no ethnic background wholly explains the way any individual or family will think or act" (p. 2). Individuals and families differ in their affiliation with cultural values and beliefs. Individual diversity factors, such as socioeconomic status, may also impact a family's beliefs and values (Groce, 2005). Knowledge of the variations that are within ethnic/racial groups as they are often categorized within the United States, is necessary. Diller (2004) notes that it is common practice in the United States to divide the non-White population into four broad categories (Asian-American, African-American, Latino-American, and Native American). Although there are four broad categories, there is within each of these categories a great deal of variation. For example, the Asian-American category refers to "some twenty-nine distinct subgroups that differ in language, religion, and values" (Atkinson, Morten, & Sue, 1993, p. 195). Establishing a respectful relationship incorporates knowledge of the family's affiliation within their identified cultural group, knowledge of cultural values and beliefs that the family espouses, and knowledge of how these values and beliefs differ from other families or other cultural groups.

Along with multicultural competencies, specific characteristics are requisite to forming collaborative relationships with families. Sohlberg et al. (2001) note that role release, role replacement, interpersonal communication skills, self-confidence, and being well informed are all characteristics that families in the counseling process regarded favorably. Counselors, who acknowledge the expertise of the family and include the family in the counseling process while sharing their own expertise in counseling, successfully engage in role release and role replacement. Recognizing the expertise of the family along with acknowledging the individual's and the family's strengths and weaknesses (Sohlberg, et al., 2001) increases the likelihood that the family will participate in the counseling process.

As is true for any counseling process, interpersonal communication skills, along with basic counseling skills, are highly regarded in counseling that is inclusive of families. The success of the process is dependent on the counselor's ability to gather information from the family as well as convey information to the family. Equally important, the counselor works as a model to assist the family in developing positive communication within the family constellation (Bray, 1980). This includes becoming, to the extent possible, a part of the extended family referenced earlier in this chapter.

ESTABLISHING A WORKING ALLIANCE WITH THE FAMILY

The working alliance, or therapeutic relationship, has been found to be one of the most influential aspects of individual and family counseling. A working alliance has been established when the family perceives the counselor as trustworthy and helpful. A collaborative relationship forms when the family believes that they are working together as a team with the counselor (McMahon, et al., 2004). In establishing a working relationship with the family, establishing rapport in a culturally competent manner is vital. In working with culturally different individuals, it may be necessary to alter the standard "getting down to business" attitude customarily adopted in counseling procedures (Diller, 2004). Alvarez (1998), for example, observed that flexibility and acceptance of different views of time and punctuality are areas of importance when establishing early relationships with clients from differing backgrounds. In altering the standard "getting down to business" attitude, it may be necessary to spend additional time on mutual introductions, counselor self-disclosure, and providing information regarding the helping process (Diller, 2004).

While not intended as prescriptive, the following are additional considerations for human service professionals when working with families from diverse cultures in developing a working alliance that takes into consideration racial and ethnic diversity. Awareness can be important in achieving successful counseling outcomes. Hispanics, for example, share a common background and culture, and are considered a "family oriented people" (Alvarez, 1998, p74). While similar in many aspects, Alavrez (1998) observes that it is important to remember that this group also has "various ideas, values, and beliefs that may be different from those of other groups" (p. 73). As mentioned previously, recognizing the family's values and how they differ from that of the counselor increases the counselor's multicultural competencies and aids in developing a working alliance. Success with the family, and ultimately the client, is likely to be dependent on the acceptance of the service provider by the family.

Similar to the Hispanic family, knowledge of the values and beliefs of the African American family is also needed to develop a working alliance. Based on a history of discrimination and oppression within the United States, African American individuals and families may be distrustful of counselors and efforts to help (Alston, & Bell, 1996; Poston, Craine, & Atkinson, 1991). Mistrust may also be based on other family members' (i.e., grandparents, siblings, uncles) or community influences and perceptions, along with past racism and prejudice (Wilson & Stith, 1991). With African American families, the service provider's acknowledgement and understanding of the realities of racism and oppression can aid in developing a working alliance. Mitigating cultural distrust involves counselors developing their own multicultural competencies, recognizing and acknowledging differences, and understanding how conflicting values between counselors and families may affect the counseling process. Additional methods of mitigating distrust may include involving trusted members of the community, such as a family minister, into the counseling process (Diller, 2004).

Thomason (1991) observed that because the population is "extremely varied, it is impossible to make general recommendations regarding counseling that apply to all Native Americans" (p. 321). In working with the Native American population, Thomason recommends that counselor warmth, caring, and geniuses are important elements in successful outcomes. The counselor's ability to ascertain the client's family and tribal identification (e.g., linkage to tribal culture vs. mainstream culture) can also provide direction on if, how, and when the family might be involved in the client's rehabilitation program and success.

Sue and Sue (1990) observed that the admission of family problems or difficulties (e.g., family member seeking/receiving career counseling services) within Asian families is quite uncommon. As a result, gaining the confidence of inner-core family members will be critical to developing a working alliance as well as to the successful participation and outcome in the counseling process.

In many immigrant communities, the extended family is viewed as the norm and determines "where you live, with whom you live, where you work and at what occupation, whom you marry, and where and from whom you seek health care" (Groce, 2005, p. 9). In this situation, establishing a trusting relationship with the extended family, and possibly with the community in general, is necessary prior to establishing a relationship with an individual.

Multicultural counseling competencies are imperative during the initial relationship building stage, as well as throughout the counseling process. As mentioned, counselor self-awareness, awareness of the values and beliefs of others, along with an understanding of how values may conflict, assist the counselor in developing a working alliance. Recognizing how to build a relationship that is respectful of cultural values and beliefs allows for the development of a collaborative relationship involving the family.

FAMILY ASSESSMENT

A family assessment can generally aid in determining the family's functioning and to help ascertain the level of involvement the family may have with counseling, goal setting, and planning. Identifying the family's level of disability acceptance, determining the family's strengths and weaknesses, and assessing the family's beliefs about work and/or the family's work ethic all should be part of the family assessment. Bray (1980) also suggests assessing the family's power bases, communication patterns, and the effectiveness of the family's communication.

292

In working with a family from a diverse cultural background, an assessment of acceptance of disability status is warranted for both the family and the individual. The individual and the family may go through similar stages of acceptance, adaptation, or adjustment to the disability, including shock, anxiety, denial, depression, anger/hostility, and adjustment (Heiber Burns, 1980; Livneh, & Antonak, 2005; Livneh, Lott, & Anotack, 2004, Olney, & Kim, 2001; Vincent, 1990). The family's or the individual's stage of acceptance may affect acceptance of diagnosis, degree to which medical and/or psychological treatment is adhered to, and the extent to which the family or individual understands the individual's functional limitations and strengths (Vincent, 1990).

While the family and the individual may go through similar stages of disability acceptance, problematic adjustment behaviors may manifest themselves differently for the family and the individual. Specific to each stage of acceptance are issues that may need to be addressed in counseling. For example, in the denial stage, the individual and/or the family may exhibit a "blatant neglect of medical advice and therapeutic or rehabilitation recommendation" (Livneh, & Antonak, 2005). In this situation, a family member in denial may refuse to provide transportation to medical appointments or assistance in personal care needs. Talking with the family, providing medical information, and finding ways to assure that medical needs are taken care of becomes a vital part of the counseling process in this situation.

On the opposite end of the spectrum are those family members whose reaction to disability is to be overprotective of the individual with a disability. Croteau and Dorze (1999) define overprotection as the "underestimation of the recipient's capabilities that is manifested in unnecessary help, excessive praise for accomplishments, or attempts to restrict activities" (p. 432). This overprotection often has a negative affect on the motivation of the individual in regard to rehabilitation, counseling, and/or employment (Croteau, & Dorze, 1999). In working with families from diverse cultural backgrounds, assessing the family's acceptance of disability will also require knowledge of family roles and how the culture responds to disability. As an example, in many Puerto Rican families, it is the good and caring mother who continues to assist young or disabled children (Groce, 2005). The counselor who posses a multicultural awareness will recognize this ongoing assistance as an expected role of the mother, and not an attempt to overprotect or to intentionally discourage self-sufficiency.

Along with an assessment of the family's acceptance of disability and a general family assessment, when working with multicultural families it may prove helpful to assess cultural issues. These issues may include (a) the family's cultural identity, (b) the family's racial salience (Evans & Rotter, 2000), that is to say how important the family views race and/or cultural issues, and (c) the family's and the individual's level of acculturation, or the family's level of adhering to dominate cultural beliefs. In assessing the acculturation levels of the family and/or individual, the multicultural counselor will also look for any intergenerational conflicts with regard to acculturation and racial salience. Finally, in the family assessment the counselor may find it helpful to identify clients' worldviews and their experiences with prejudice and discrimination, along with how these factors affect the clients' vocational goals and outcomes (Evans and Rotter, 2000).

Family assessments can be gained through the use of interviews, observations, and techniques such as the genogram and/or the culturagram. The genogram, an instrument used to examine the internal family relationships, offers the client an opportunity to describe the importance of each family member and the family member's influence on counseling goals or career aspirations (Paniagua, 1996). The culturagram, similar to the genogram, is generally used in social work to explore the influence of culture on various aspects of the family's life (Congress, 2004). The ten areas of discussion addressed in the culturagram are identified in Table 1.

Table 1
TEN AREAS OF THE CULTURAGRAM

- Reasons for Relocation (if family is from a different country)
- Legal Status
- Time in Community
- Languages Spoken at Home and in the Community
- Health Beliefs
- Crises Events
- Holidays and Special Events
- Contact with Cultural and Religious Institutions
- Values about Education and Work
- Values About Family-Structure, Power, Myths and Rules

Congress, 2004

FAMILY CONTRIBUTIONS

Specific to vocational rehabilitation, Rubin and Roessler (2001) identify various areas in which the family can be included in the career counseling process. While this information is specific to vocational rehabilitation, other human service professionals can adapt the following information to fit within their work setting. Rubin and Roessler (2001) divide the vocational rehabilitation process into four phases: (a) the evaluation phase, (b) the planning phase, (c) the treatment phase, and (d) the termination phase. In moving through the vocational process, counselors must be mindful that individuals with disabilities may depend heavily on family for support, knowledge of job and social opportunities, residential and transportation services, and community awareness (Householder, & Jansen, 1999), to assist the individual through the phases of vocational rehabilitation, or career counseling.

The evaluation phase yields information regarding vocational choice options, functional limitations, interests, abilities, and aptitudes (Rubin & Roessler, 2001). In the evaluation phase, the family's values and beliefs will need to be assessed to determine appropriate vocational choice options and expectations. In this phase, and throughout the process, the family can be a valuable resource. Family members can add to the information gathering process by providing additional information and/or a different perspective with regard to the individual's functional limitations, strengths, interests, and abilities. During the evaluation phase, family members may also assist in a very practical manner through providing transportation, offering support, and assisting the individual in retaining information as it is received throughout this early stage of counseling.

The planning phase consists of consolidating information gained in the evaluation phase, determining appropriate counseling objectives, goal setting, and career exploration (Rubin & Roessler, 2001). Again, the family can provide basic assistance such as transportation to and from meetings, along with financial and residential support. Family input will be needed in determining family and culturally appropriate vocational objectives and goals. As mentioned previously, the family's ownership of the plan and objectives increases the probability of the individual's follow-through. Family members should, therefore, be included in the goal setting process as well as the placement process.

To acquire positive career outcomes, counselors secure and coordinate a variety of services to aid in rehabilitation. These rehabilitation services, as well as job placement itself, make up the treatment phase of vocational rehabilitation (Rubin, & Roessler, 2001). Rehabilitation services may include rehabilitation workshops consisting of transitional workshops and/or sheltered workshops, comprehensive rehabilitation centers, and/or work adjustment training. Throughout the treatment process, the individual may work with a variety of service providers, including, but not limited to, medical personnel, psychologist, speech-language pathologist, physical therapist, and occupational therapists. During this phase, the family may assist the counselor in locating culturally appropriate and/or culturally competent facilities and service providers. Similar to the other phases, families may assist in transportation to and from appointments, assure that treatment goals are adhered to, and in assisting the individual in retaining information obtained from service providers.

The treatment phase, by nature, involves a great deal of commitment from the individual with a disability. Family members can provide encouragement and general support, assisting individuals in increasing their belief in their ability to complete the career counseling process. Throughout the process, the family can also provide natural supports, and assist with job search tasks such job search organization, completion of applications, resume writing, and practicing interviewing skills. Family members can provide support through job search networking (Rogan, Banks, & Herbin, 2003), as well as socialization skill instructions.

Once an individual is successfully employed, the counselor begins to work toward the termination phases. Counselors, at this time, can provide education to the family in ways in which the family can support the individual in maintaining employment; provide emotional support; as well as residential, financial, and transportation support, if necessary. Family members can be trained by the counselor to provide follow-through support in assisting the individual with a disability in maintaining employment. Counselor commitment to inclusion of the family into the counseling process is an important first step. Counselors are encouraged to find ways to include the family that fit with the counseling goals, the family, and the individual's needs.

CONCLUSION

Successful career outcomes for individuals with disabilities from various cultural backgrounds is inclusive of the family and takes into account family influences on the individual, counseling goals, and outcomes. Partnering with the family involves careful assessment of the individual's definition of family, family influence, cultural factors, and cultural influences. The assessment takes into account the family's influence on the individual's beliefs about work and disability, in general, as well as the individual's career decisions. Through the use of multicultural counseling competencies, the successful counselor establishes a working alliance with the family, remaining flexible to the family's decision-making process. Incorporating the family throughout the various stages of the counseling process assures that the family supports the individual, the career counseling goals, and the process. Often it is this family support that makes for the most successful career outcomes for individuals with disabilities whose cultural heritage values family, the family's influence, and a collective sense of being. While this may be unusual for both the career counselor and the service-providing agency, it is often necessary to obtain successful career outcomes.

REFERENCES

Americans with Disabilities Act of 1990, 42 U.S.C. § 12101 et seq.

Alston, R. J., & Bell, T. J. (1996). Cultural mistrust and the rehabilitation enigma for African Americans. *Journal of Rehabilitation, 62,* 16- 20.

Alvarez, L. I. (1998). A short guide in cultural sensitivity training. *Teaching Exceptional Children, 31*(1), 73-77.

Accordino, M. P., & Hunt, B. (2001). Family counseling training in rehabilitation counseling programs revisited. *Rehabilitation Education, 15,* 255-264.

Arrendondo, P., Toporek, R., Brown, S.P., Jones, J., Locke, D.C, Sanchez, J., & Stadler, H. (1996). Operationalization of the multicultural counseling competencies. *Journal of Multicultural Counseling and Development, 24,* 42-78.

Atkinson, D. R., Morten, G., & Sue, D. W. (1993). *Counseling American minorities: A cross-cultural perspective,* (4th ed.): Dubuque, IA: William C. Brown.

Benshoff, J. J., & Janikowski, T. P. (2000). *The rehabilitation model of substance abuse counseling*. Belmont, CA: Brooks/Cole.

Bray, G. P. (1980). Team strategies for family involvement in rehabilitation. *Journal of Rehabilitation, 46,* 20-23.

Brown, M. T., & Landrum-Brown, J. (1995). Counseling supervision: Cross-cultural perspectives. In J. G. Ponterotto, J. M. Casas, L. A. Suzuki, & C. M. Alexander (Eds.) *Handbook of multicultural counseling* (pp. 263-286). Thousand Oaks, CA: Sage publications.

Congress, E. P. (2004). Cultural and ethical issues in working with culturally diverse patients and their families: The use of the Culturalgram to promote cultural competent practice in health care settings. *Social Work in Health Care, 39,* 249-262

Croteau, C., & Dorze, G. L. (1999). Overprotection in couples with aphasia. *Disability and Rehabilitation, 21*(9), 432- 437.

Demo, D. H., Allne, K. R., & Fine, M. A. (Eds.). (2000). *Handbook of family diversity*. New York: Oxford.

Diller, J. V. (2004). *Cultural diversity: A primer for the human services.* Belmont, CA: Wadsworth Publishing.

Drake, R. E., McHugo, G. J., Becker, D. R., Anthony, W. A., & Clarke, R. E. (1996). The New Hampshire study of supported employment for people with severe mental illness. *Journal of Consulting and Clinical Psychology, 64,* 391-399.

Duncan, L. E. (2005). Overcoming biases to effectively serve African American college students: A call to the profession. *College Student Journal, 39,* 702- 710.

Dykeman, C., Nelson, R. J., & Appleton, V. (1995). Building strong working alliances in American Indian families. *Social Work in Education. 17* (3), 148-158.

Evans, K. M, & Rotter, J. C. (2000). Multicultural family approaches to career counseling. *The Family Journal: Counseling and Therapy for Couples and Families, 8,* 67-71.

Goldenberg, I., & Goldenberg, H. (2004). *Family therapy: An overview* (6th Ed.). Belmont, CA: Wadsworth Publishing.

Groce, N. (2005). Immigrants, disability, and rehabilitation. In J.H. Stone (Ed.). *Culture and disability: Providing culturally competent services* (pp. 1- 14). Thousand Oaks, CA: Sage Publications.

Hare, J., & Gray, L. A. (n.d.). *Non-traditional families: A guide for parents.* Retrieved from http://www.cybernet.org/parent/nontradfam.html.

Hasnain, R., Sotnik, P., & Ghiloni, C. (2003). Person-centered planning: A gateway to improving vocational rehabilitation services for culturally diverse individuals with disabilities. *Journal of Rehabilitation, 69,* 10- 17.

Hayslip, B. & Goldberg-Glen, R., (Eds.) (2000). *Grandparents raising grandchildren: Theoretical, empirical, and clinical perspectives.* New York, NY: Springer Publishing.

Heiber Berns, J. (1980). Grandparents of handicapped children. *Social Work, 25,* 238-239.

Householder, D., & Jansen, D. (1999). Partnerships, families, employers, transition, disabled: Creating the best transition outcomes for moderate and multiply disabled individuals. *Journal of Vocational Rehabilitation, 13,* 51-55.

Kerka, S. (2000). *Parenting and career development* (Eric Digest No. 214). Columbus, OH: ERIC Clearinghouse on Adult Career and Vocational Education. (ERIC Document Reproduction Services No. ED440251).

Lankard, B. A. (1995). *Family role in career development* (Eric Digest No. 164). Columbus, OH: ERIC Clearinghouse on Adult Career and Vocational Education. (ERIC Document Reproduction Services No. ED389878).

Livneh, H., & Antonak, R. F. (2005). Psychological adaptation to chronic illness and disability: A primer for counselors. *Journal of Counseling and Development, 83,* 12- 20.

Livneh, H., Lott, S. M, & Antonak, R. F. (2004). Patterns of psychosocial adaptation to chronic illness and disability: A cluster analytic approach. *Psychology, Health, and Medicine, 9*(4), 411- 430.

May, K. M., & Hunt, B. (1994). Family counseling training in rehabilitation counseling programs. *Rehabilitation Education, 8,* 348-359.

McCollum, V. J. (1997). Evolution of the African American family: Considerations for family therapy. *Journal of Multicultural Counseling and Development, 25,* 219-229.

McMahon, B. T., Shaw, L. R., Chan, F., & Danczyk-Hawley, C. (2004). "Common factors" in rehabilitation counseling: Expectancies and the working alliance. *Journal of Vocational Rehabilitation, 20,* 101-105.

Middleton, R. A., Rollins, C. W., Sanderson, P. L., Leung, P., Harley, D. A., Ebener, D., & Leal-Idrogo, A. (2000). Endorsement of professional multicultural rehabilitation competencies and standards: A call to action. *Rehabilitation Counseling Bulletin, 43,* 219-240.

Newman, E. (1988). *Barriers to employment of persons with handicaps.* Temple University, 301 University Services Bldg., Philadelphia, PA 19122.

Olney, M. F., & Kim, A. (2001). Beyond adjustment: Integration of cognitive disability into identity. *Disability and Society, 16,* 563-583.

Paniagua, F. A. (1996). Cross-cultural guidelines in family therapy practice. *Family Journal, 4,* 127- 138.

Parke, R. D. (2004). Development in the family. *Annual Review of Psychology, 55*(2), 365-399.

Poston, W. S. C., Craine, M., & Atkinson, D. R. (1991). Counselor dissimilarity confrontation, client cultural mistrust, and willingness to self-disclose. *Journal of Multicultural Counseling and Development, 19,* 65-73.

Power, P. W., & Dell Orto, A. E. (2004). *Families living with chronic illness and disability: Interventions, challenges, and opportunities.* New York: Spring Publishing Company.

Power, P. W., Dell Orto, A. E., & Gibbons, M. B. (1988). *Family interventions throughout chronic illness and disability.* New York: Springer Publishing Company.

Power, P. W. (1988). Guide to vocational assessment. Austin, TX: Pro-ED.

Power, P. W., Hershenson, D. B., & Fabien, E. S. (1991). Meeting the documented needs of clients' families: An opportunity for rehabilitation counselors. *Journal of Rehabilitation, 57,* 11-16.

Rogan, P., Banks, & Herbein, M. H. (2003). Supported employment and workplace supports: A qualitative study. *Journal of Vocational Rehabilitation, 19,* 5-18.

Rubin, S. E., & Roessler, R. T. (2001). *Foundations of the vocational rehabilitation process.* Austin, TX: Pro-Ed.

Salas-Provance, M. B., Erickson, J. G., & Reed, J. (2002). Disabilities as viewed by four generations of one Hispanic family. *American Journal of Speech-Language Pathology, 11,* 151-162.

Santana-Martin, S., & Santana, F. O. (2005). An introduction to Mexican culture for service providers. In J. H. Stone (Ed.), *Culture and disability: Providing culturally competent services* (pp. 161-186). Thousand Oaks, CA: Sage Publications.

Schulenberg, J. E., Vonderacek, F. W., & Crouter, A. C. (1984). The influence of the family on vocational development. *Journal of Marriage and the Family, 46,* 129-143.

Skowron, E. A. (2004). Differentiation of self, personal adjustment, problem solving, and ethnic group belonging among persons of color. *Journal of Counseling and Development, 82,* 447-456.

Smart, J. F., & Smart, D. W. (2006). Models of disability: Implications for the counseling profession. *Journal of Multicultural Counseling and Development, 84,* 29-40.

Sohlberg, M. M., McLaughlin, K. A., Todis, B., Larsen, J., & Glang, A. (2001). What does it take to collaborate with families affected by brain injury? A preliminary model. *Journal of Head Trauma Rehabilitation, 16,* 498-511.

Sotnik, P., & Jezewski, M. A. (2005). Culture and the disability services. In J. H. Stone (Ed.) *Culture and disability: Providing culturally competent services* (pp. 15- 30) Thousand Oaks, CA: Sage Publications.

Staples, R. (1998). The emerging majority: Resources for non white families in the United States. *Family Relations, 37,* 348-354.

13

Sue, D. W., & Sue, D. (1990). *Counseling the culturally different: theory and practice* (2nd ed.). New York: Wiley.

Thomason, T. C. (1991). Counseling native Americans: An introduction for non-native-American counselors. *Journal of Counseling and Development, 69,* 321-327.

Tsao, G. (2000). Growing up Asian-American with a disability. Retrieved Aug. 27, 2005 from http://www.colorado.edu/journals/standards/V7N1/FIRSTPERSON/tsao.html.

U. S. Census Bureau (2005). Disabilities and American families 2000: Census 2000 special reports. Retrieved February 15, 200 from http://www.census.gov /prod/2005pubs/censr-23.pdf

U.S. Department of Education, Office of Special Education and Rehabilitation Services. (2000). *Long-range plan 1999-2003.* Washington DC: Author.

U. S. Census Bureau (2005). Hispanic population passes 40 million. Retrieved February 15, 200 from http://www.census.gov/prod/2005pubs/censr-23.pdf

Vincent, K. R. (1990). Coping with disability: The individual or a family member's. *Social Behavior and Personality, 18,* 1-6.

Wilson L., & Stith, S. (1991). Culturally sensitive therapy with Black clients. *Journal of Multicultural Counseling and Development, 19,* 32-42.

Index

A

Acculturation   76, 77, 138
Advocacy   190
African American   6, 7, 8, 10, 11, 51, 52, 53, 109, 132, 133, 134, 142, 161, 183, 185, 189, 234, 284, 285, 292
Alliance, Working   291
American Indian (Native American)   6, 12, 13, 48, 161, 164, 189
Americans with Disabilities Act (ADA)   29-33, 178, 189, 209, 282
Asian American   109, 132, 122, 142, 161, 189, 191, 234, 284
Assessment   49, 122, 129, 138, 139, 145, 231, 293
Assimilation   76
Assistive Technology   226, 227, 228
Attitudes   87
Assistive Technology   228

B

Beliefs   87, 160, 288, 290
Burnout   207

C

Capacity Building   12, 35, 36
Career Development   229-231
    Family influences   286
Case management   109, 114
CRUX Model   115-6
    Broker Model   117-8
    Rehabilitation Model   119-20
    Assertive Community Treatment   120-1

Strengths Model   121-2
Civil Rights   3, 156, 163, 164, 180
Civil Rights Act (1964)   4, 179, 180
Collectivism   120, 190
Comprehensive System of Personnel Development (CSPD)   208
Consortia of Administrators of Native American Rehabilitation
     (CANAR)   12, 13
Consumer   191
     Use of Assistive Technology   229
     Technology in career assessment   231
Consumerism   180
Counseling
     Peer   190
     Multicultural   75
Counseling
     Respectful Model   96
     Multicultural   3, 75, 111, 160, 289
     Addressing model   97
Cultural competence   48, 70, 84, 88, 290
Cultural Identity   74
Cultural Validity   244
Culturally aware counselors   98
Culturally competent counselors   85
Culture   71, 73, 100, 101, 210
     Work environment   210

D

Disability   131, 143, 156, 164,165, 167, 168, 169, 177, 179, 187,
     183, 188, 202, 212, 282, 286, 287
     Adjustment to   165
     Attribution of   164
     Energy model   159
     Medical model   157-8
     Social model   157-8
Distance Education   235
Diversity   2, 206, 212, 246

E

Ethics   131, 275
  Research   55
  Teaching/supervision   56
  Spirituality   273-5
  Codes   45, 214, 231, 275

F

Family   186, 192, 282, 283
  Decision making   283
  Development   284-5
  Reactions to disability   287

H

Hispanic American   7, 10, 54, 109, 133, 142, 143, 144, 146, 161, 183, 189, 191, 285
Human Resources   202, 203
  Recruitment   204, 211
  Retention   206
  Motivational theory   207

I

Illness
  Chronic   165
  Adjustment stages   165
Independent Living   29, 177, 184, 193, 195, 286
Individualism   83, 120, 186
Individuals with Disabilities Education Act (IDEA)   11, 26, 33

Language   47
Learning Styles   205

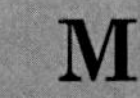

Mental Health   5-7
Minnesota Multiphasic Personality Inventory (MMPI)   135, 136
Mistrust   194, 259, 291

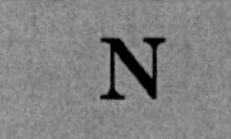

National Council on Disability (NCD)   11, 26, 28, 241
National Institute on Disability and Rehabilitation Research
     (NIDRR)   11, 26, 33, 216
National Rehabilitation Association (NRA)   4

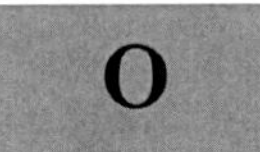

Oppression   78, 79, 81

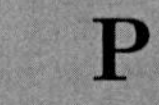

Privilege   80, 81

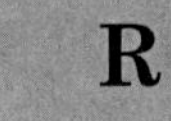

Race   5, 72
Randolph-Shepherd Act   19
Rehabilitation Act
     Amendments   21, 22

Section 21   11, 12
1973   23, 208
Section 501-504   23-4
Implementation   255
Rehabilitation Cultural Diversity Initiative (RCDI)   12, 208
Research
    Participatory Action   244
    Evidence Based   247
    Data Based   248-254, 256
    Indigenous   257-258

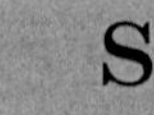

Segregation   20
Smith Fess Act   19
Spirituality   169, 170, 187, 267, 268, 269, 271
    Neglect in rehabilitation   269-271
    Overall well-being   271-2
    Application in rehabilitation   274-275
    Ethical considerations   275-6
Stereotype   82

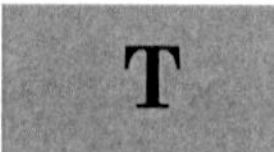

Technology and Related Assistance for Individuals with Disability   226
Tests
    Accommodations   144-5
    Bias   135,143
    Culture free   137
    Selection   139
    Translation   139
Ticket to Work   39

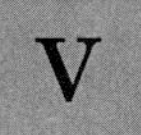

Vocational Rehabilitation
    Inequities   8, 9, 112, 255, 257

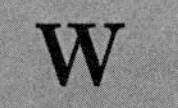

Wagner-O'Day   Act 19
White American (Caucasian)   110, 113, 132, 184, 210, 234
Workforce Investment Act   37
Worldview   83, 185, 255